# Statistics for Social and Behavioral Sciences

*Advisors:*
S.E. Fienberg
W.J. van der Linden

For further volumes:
http://www.springer.com/series/3463

John W. Graham

# Missing Data

Analysis and Design

Springer

John W. Graham
Department of Biobehavioral Health
Health & Human Development Bldg. East
The Pennsylvania State University
University Park, PA, USA

Please note that additional material for this book can be downloaded from
http://extras.springer.com

ISBN 978-1-4614-4017-8        ISBN 978-1-4614-4018-5 (eBook)
DOI 10.1007/978-1-4614-4018-5
Springer New York Heidelberg Dordrecht London

Library of Congress Control Number: 2012938715

© Springer Science+Business Media New York 2012

This work is subject to copyright. All rights are reserved by the Publisher, whether the whole or part of the material is concerned, specifically the rights of translation, reprinting, reuse of illustrations, recitation, broadcasting, reproduction on microfilms or in any other physical way, and transmission or information storage and retrieval, electronic adaptation, computer software, or by similar or dissimilar methodology now known or hereafter developed. Exempted from this legal reservation are brief excerpts in connection with reviews or scholarly analysis or material supplied specifically for the purpose of being entered and executed on a computer system, for exclusive use by the purchaser of the work. Duplication of this publication or parts thereof is permitted only under the provisions of the Copyright Law of the Publisher's location, in its current version, and permission for use must always be obtained from Springer. Permissions for use may be obtained through RightsLink at the Copyright Clearance Center. Violations are liable to prosecution under the respective Copyright Law.

The use of general descriptive names, registered names, trademarks, service marks, etc. in this publication does not imply, even in the absence of a specific statement, that such names are exempt from the relevant protective laws and regulations and therefore free for general use.

While the advice and information in this book are believed to be true and accurate at the date of publication, neither the authors nor the editors nor the publisher can accept any legal responsibility for any errors or omissions that may be made. The publisher makes no warranty, express or implied, with respect to the material contained herein.

Printed on acid-free paper

Springer is part of Springer Science+Business Media (www.springer.com)

*For Linda, Matthew, Joy, and Jazeya*

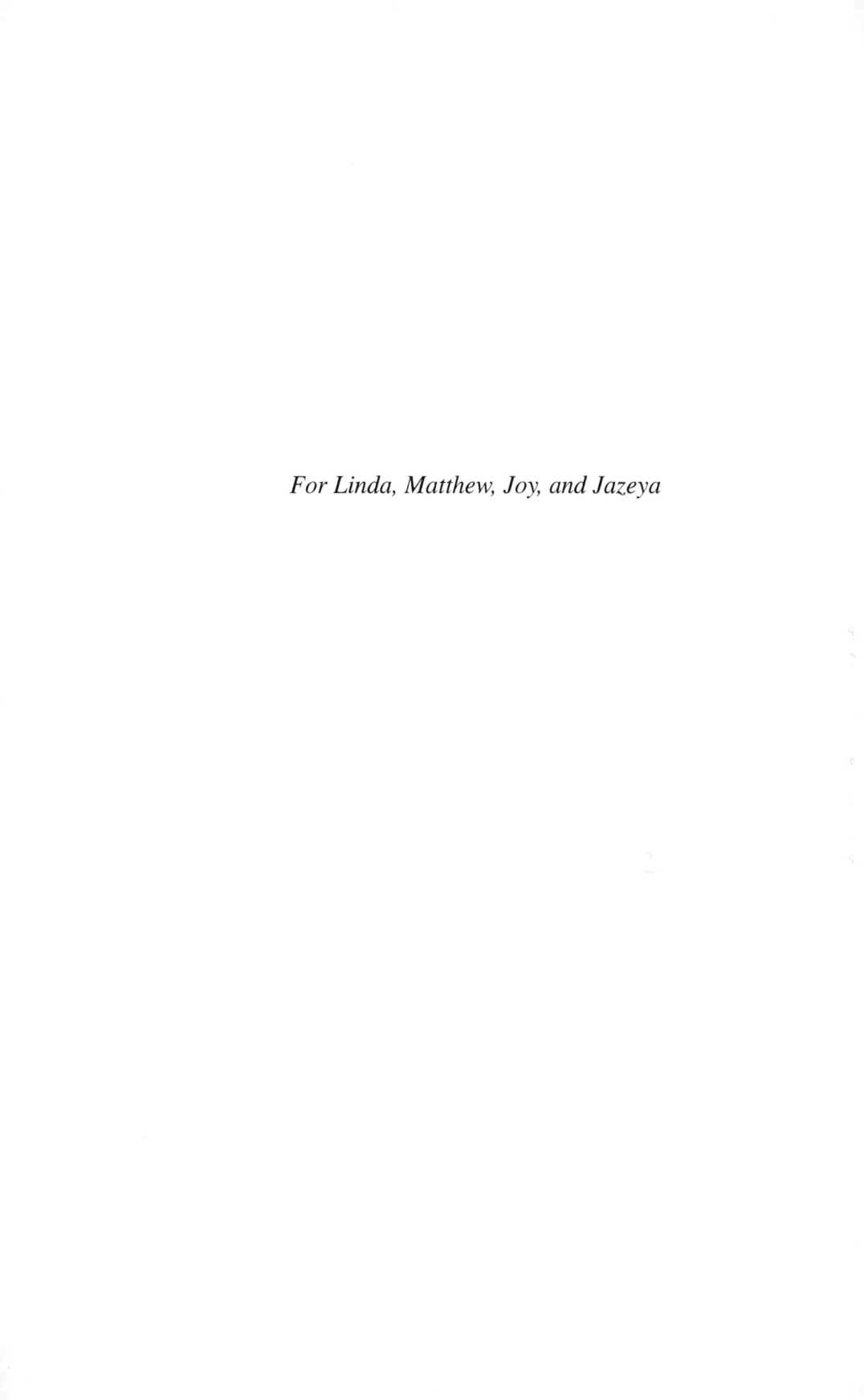

# Preface

My interest in missing data issues began in the early 1980s when I began working with the group that was to become the Institute for Health Promotion and Disease Prevention Research (better known as IPR) at the University of Southern California. This was my introduction to large-scale, longitudinal, field-experimental research. I had been trained in a traditional experimental social psychology program at the University of Southern California, and most of my colleagues at IPR (at least in the early days) happened also to have been trained as social psychologists. Given my training, much of my thinking in these early days stemmed from the idea that researchers had substantial control over the extraneous factors in their research. Thus, much of my early work was focused on gaining a degree of control in field experiment settings.

The challenges, of course, were numerous, but that is one of the things that made it all so interesting. One of the key challenges in those early days was missing data. The missing data challenge manifested itself as missing responses within a survey and as whole surveys being missing for some people at one or more waves of longitudinal measurement. Missingness within a survey often was due to problems with individual items (if students were confused by a question, a common reaction was to leave it blank) and problems with the length of the survey (slower readers would often leave one or more pages blank at the end of the survey). When whole surveys were missing from one or more waves of the longitudinal study, it was not uncommon that the student would return to complete a survey at a later wave. It was also common, however, that once a student was missing entirely from a measurement wave, that the student remained missing for the duration of the study.

In those days, there were no good analysis solutions for dealing with our missing data, at least none that one could expect to use with anything close to standard software. Our only real solution was to ignore (delete) cases with any missingness on the variables used for any statistical model. In fact, as I will discuss in Chap. 12, we even developed a planned missing data design (the first versions of the "3-form design") as a means of reducing the response load on our young student participants. Although this planned missing data design has proven to be an excellent tool for reducing response load, it further exacerbated our missing data analysis problems. My early thinking on this was that because the pairwise-deletion correlations produced in this context would be random samples of the overall correlations, this would somehow help with our analysis problems. Although that thinking turned out to be correct, it wasn't for another 10 years that our analysis solutions would catch up.

I started thinking in earnest about missing data issues in the late 1980s. The impetus for this new thinking was that statisticians and other researchers finally began making good missing data analysis tools available. In fact, what happened in the missing data literature in 1987 alone can be thought of as a missing data revolution. In that single year, two major missing data books were published (Little and Rubin 1987; Rubin 1987). These two books were the statistical basis for most of the important missing data software developments in the following decade and beyond. Also published in 1987 were two influential articles describing a strategy for performing missing data analysis making use of readily available structural equation modeling (SEM) software (Allison 1987; Muthen et al. 1987). These articles were important because they described the first missing data analysis procedure that was truly accessible to researchers not trained as statisticians. Also published in 1987 was the article by Tanner and Wong (1987) on data augmentation, which has become a fundamental part of some approaches to multiple imputation.

## Philosophy Underlying This Book

I feel it is important to give this brief history about the development of missing data theory and analysis solutions as well as the history of the development of my own skills in missing data analysis. It is important because my knowledge and experience in this area stemmed not from a background in statistics but from the need to solve the real problems we faced in the burgeoning discipline of prevention science on the 1980s and 1990s.

Because of my beginnings, my goals have always been to find practical solutions to real-world research problems. How can I do a better job of controlling the extraneous factors in a field experiment? How can I draw more valid conclusions about the success or failure of my intervention? Also, because I was trained as an experimental social psychologist and not as a statistician – not even as a quantitative psychologist – my understanding of the statistical underpinnings of various missing data techniques has often been couched in practical needs of the research, and my descriptions of these techniques and underpinnings have often relied more on plain English than on terms and language common in the statistical literature.

This practical basis for my understanding and descriptions of missing data techniques has caused some problems for me over the years. Occasionally, for example, my practical approach produces a kind of imprecision in how some of these important topics are discussed. To be honest, I have at times bumped heads a little with statisticians, and psychologists with more formal statistical training. Fortunately, these instances have been rare. Also, it has been my good fortune to have spent several years collaborating closely with Joe Schafer. This experience has been a huge benefit to my understanding of many of the important topics in this book.

On the other hand, my somewhat unusual, practical, approach to missing data techniques and underpinnings has gradually given me the ability to describe these things, in plain English, with a satisfying degree of precision. Further, my take on these issues, because it is so firmly rooted in practical applications, occasionally leads to discoveries that would not necessarily have been obvious to others who have taken a more formal, statistical, approach to these topics.

The long and short of this is that I can promise you, the reader, that the topics covered in this book will be (a) readable and accessible and (b) of practical value.

## Prerequisites

Most of the techniques described in this book rely on multiple regression analyses in one form or another. Therefore, I assume that the reader will, at the very least, already have had a course in multiple regression. Even better would be that the reader would have had at least some real-world experience in using multiple regression. As I will point out in later chapters, one of the most flexible of the missing data procedures, multiple imputation, requires that the output of one's statistical analysis be a parameter estimate and the corresponding standard error. Multiple regression fits nicely into this requirement in that one always has a regression coefficient (parameter estimate) and a standard error. Other common procedures such as analysis of variance (ANOVA) can be used with multiple imputation, but only when the ANOVA model is recast as the equivalent multiple regression model.

Knowledge of SEM is not a prerequisite for reading this book. However, having at least a rudimentary knowledge of one of the common SEM programs will be very useful. For example, some of the planned missing data designs described in Section 4 of this book rely on SEM analysis. In addition, my colleagues and I have found the multiple-group SEM (MGSEM) procedure (Allison 1987; Muthen et al. 1987) to be very useful in the missing data context. The material covered in Chaps. 10 and 11 relies heavily on these techniques. Finally, knowledge of one of the major SEM packages opens up some important options for data analysis using the full information maximum likelihood (FIML) approach to handling missing data.

Because my take on handling missing data is so firmly rooted in the need to solve practical problems, or perhaps because my understanding of missing data theory and practice is more conceptual than statistical, I have often relied on somewhat low-tech tools in my solutions. Thus, I make the assumption that readers of this book will have a good understanding of a variety of low-tech tools. I assume that readers are well versed in the Microsoft Windows operating system for PCs.[1] For example, it will be extremely helpful if readers know the difference between ASCII

---

[1] I know very little about the operating system for Apple computers, but with a few important exceptions (e.g., that NORM currently is not available for Apple computers), I'll bet that good knowledge of the Apple operating system (or other operating systems, such as Unix or Linux) will work very well in making use of the suggestions described in this book.

(text) files (e.g., as handled by the Notepad editor in Windows) and binary files (e.g., as produced by MS Word, SAS, SPSS, and most other programs). Although the Notepad editor for editing ascii/text files will be useful to an extent, it will be even more useful to have a more full-featured ascii editor, such as UltraEdit (http://www.ultraedit.com).

## Layout of this Book

In Section 1 of this book, Chaps. 1 and 2, I deal with what I often refer to as missing data theory. In Chap. 1, I lay out the heart of missing data theory, focusing mainly on dispelling some of the more common myths surrounding analysis with missing data and describing in some detail my take on the three "causes" of missingness, often referred to as missing data mechanisms. I also spend a good bit of space in Chap. 1 dealing with the more theoretical aspects of attrition. In Chap. 2, I describe various analysis techniques for dealing with missing data. I spend some time in this chapter describing older methods, but I stay mainly with procedures that, despite being "old," are still useful in some contexts. I spend most of the space in this chapter talking about the more theoretical aspects of the recommended methods (multiple imputation and maximum likelihood approaches) and the EM algorithm for covariance matrices.

In Section 2, I focus on the practice of multiple imputation and analysis with multiple imputed data sets. In Chap. 3, I describe in detail multiple imputation with Schafer's (1997) NORM 2.03 program. Chapter 4 covers analysis of NORM-imputed data sets with SPSS (versions 15, 16, and lower; and newer versions without the new MI module). In this chapter, I outline the use of my utility for automating the process of analysis with multiple imputed data sets, especially for multiple regression analysis. In Chap. 5, I describe multiple imputation with the recently released versions of SPSS (version 17–20) that include the MI module. In this chapter, I describe the process of performing multiple imputation with small data problems, staying within the SPSS environment, and performing automated analysis with regression and logistic regression. I also describe the limitations of this initial SPSS product (through version 20) and suggest the preferable alternative of doing MI with NORM 2.03 (along with my automation utility for reading NORM-imputed data into SPSS), but performing analysis and automation with the quite excellent automation features newly available in SPSS 17 and later versions. In Chap. 6, I cover the topic of imputation and analysis with cluster data (e.g., children within schools). I describe analysis of multilevel data with SPSS 17–20 Mixed module and also with HLM 6. I also describe a feature of my automation utility for analyzing NORM-imputed data with HLM 6–7. In Chap. 7, I discuss in detail multiple imputation with SAS PROC MI. In this chapter, I provide syntax for analysis with PROC REG, PROC LOGISTIC, and PROC MIXED and describe the combining of results with PROC MIANALYZE.

In Section 3, I focus on the practicalities of dealing with missing data, especially with multiple imputation, in the real world. In Chap. 8, I address the issue of spotting and troubleshooting problems with imputation. In Chap. 9 (with Lee Van Horn and Bonnie Taylor), I address the major practical concern of having too many variables in the imputation model. In Chap. 10, I cover the topic of doing simulation work with missing data. Given the popularity of simulations for answering many research questions, it is important to address issues that arise in the conduct of simulations relating to missing data. In addition to a brief description of the usual Monte Carlo approach to simulations, I also outline a more compact, non-Monte Carlo, approach that makes use of the multiple-group capabilities of SEM programs. In this section, I describe simulations based on MCAR missingness (this approach is at the heart of the material covered in Chap. 9), but I also extend this work in an important way to describe an approach to non-Monte Carlo simulations with MAR and MNAR missingness. In Chap. 11 (with Linda M. Collins), I cover the important area of including auxiliary variables in one's model. This chapter focuses mainly on addressing the problems associated with participant attrition. It touches on the value of auxiliary variables for bias reduction, but focuses on recovery of lost statistical power. The chapter covers practical strategies for including auxiliary variables in MI and FIML models. I outline an automation utility for determining the benefit of including auxiliary variables under a variety of circumstances.

Section 4 of the book describes the developing area of planned missing data designs. These designs allow researchers to make efficient use of limited resources, while allowing meaningful conclusions to be drawn. Chapter 12 describes the theory and practical issues relating to implementation of the 3-form design, a kind of matrix sampling design. Chapter 13 (with Allison Shevock; nee: Olchowski) describes a design we have called two method measurement. In this chapter, we present the theory and practical issues of implementing this SEM-based design.

# Acknowledgments

Writing this book has been a process. An important part of that process has been the development of my thinking over the years about issues relating to missing data analysis and design. The person who has had perhaps the biggest impact on my thinking about missing data issues has been Joe Schafer, with whom I have had the good fortune to collaborate for several years. The writings of Rod Little and Don Rubin formed the basis of my initial thinking about analysis with missing data, and Scott Hofer and Stewart Donaldson played important roles in the development of my early thinking. People with whom I have published over the past several years have also been important in the process, including Andrea Piccinin, Lori Palen, Elvira Elek, Dave MacKinnon, and Patricio Cumsille. People who have been especially supportive over the years, as consumers of my missing data skills, and particularly with this book, are Steve West, Wayne Velicer, David Hawkins, and Rico Catalano. Linda Collins, Sabrina Oesterle, Brittany Rhoades, Bob Laforge, and several blind reviewers provided me with critical feedback on one or more chapters of this book. Scott Hofer, Matthew Graham, and Liying Huang have helped in important ways with programming. Finally, I would like to thank Aaron Wagner and Stef Seaholtz for getting the book-related software and example data sets so well positioned on the Methodology Center web site.

# Contents

**Section 1  Missing Data Theory**

**1  Missing Data Theory** .................................................................. 3
   Overview ........................................................................................ 3
   Missing Data: What Is It? ............................................................. 4
   Missing Data: History, Objectives, and Challenges ..................... 5
   Terms ............................................................................................. 6
      Model ....................................................................................... 6
      Missingness ............................................................................. 7
      Distribution ............................................................................. 8
      Mechanisms of Missingness .................................................. 8
   Causes of Missingness .................................................................. 9
   Mapping Causes of Missingness onto the Three Missingness
   Mechanisms ................................................................................... 12
      Missing Completely at Random (MCAR) .............................. 12
      Missing at Random (MAR) ................................................... 13
      Not Missing at Random (NMAR; aka Missing Not
      at Random; MNAR) ............................................................... 15
   MAR Versus NMAR Revisited ..................................................... 17
      Can We Ever Know Whether MAR Holds? ........................... 17
      Maybe We Can Know if MAR Holds .................................... 18
      Measuring Estimation Bias .................................................... 19
      Factors Affecting Standardized Bias ...................................... 20
   Estimating Statistical and Practical Significance
   of Bias in Real Data ...................................................................... 21
      Percent Missing ....................................................................... 22
      Estimating $r_{XY}$ ....................................................................... 22
      Estimating $r_{ZY}$ ....................................................................... 22
      Estimating $r_{ZR}$ ....................................................................... 25

|   Sensitivity Analysis | 26 |
| --- | --- |
|     Plausibility of MAR Given in Tables 1.4 and 1.5 | 27 |
|     Limitations (Nuisance Factors) Relating to Figures in Tables 1.4 and 1.5 | 28 |
|     Call for New Measures of the Practical Significance of Bias | 29 |
|     Other Limitations of Figures Presented in Tables 1.4 and 1.5 | 32 |
|   Another Substantive Consideration: A Taxonomy of Attrition | 33 |
|     The Value of Missing Data Diagnostics | 34 |
|     Nonignorable Methods | 36 |
|     Sensitivity Analysis | 36 |
|   Design and Measurement Strategies for Assuring MAR | 38 |
|     Measure the Possible Causes of Missingness | 38 |
|     Measure and Include Relevant Auxiliary Variables in Missing Data Analysis Model | 43 |
|     Track and Collect Data on a Random Sample of Those Initially Missing | 43 |
|   References | 44 |
| **2  Analysis of Missing Data** | **47** |
|   Goals of Analysis | 47 |
|   Older Approaches to Handling Missing Data | 47 |
|     Complete Cases Analysis (aka Listwise Deletion) | 48 |
|     Pairwise Deletion | 51 |
|     Mean Substitution | 51 |
|     Averaging the Available Variables | 51 |
|     Regression-Based Single Imputation | 52 |
|   Basics of the Recommended Methods | 53 |
|     Full Information Maximum Likelihood (FIML) | 53 |
|     Basics of the EM Algorithm for Covariance Matrices | 54 |
|     Basics of Normal-Model Multiple Imputation | 56 |
|   What Analyses Work with MI? | 59 |
|     Normal-Model MI with Categorical Variables | 60 |
|     Normal-Model MI with Longitudinal Data | 60 |
|     Imputation for Statistical Interactions: The Imputation Model Must Be at Least as Complex as the Analysis Model | 62 |
|     Normal-Model MI with ANOVA | 63 |
|     Analyses for Which MI Is not Necessary | 63 |
|   Missing Data Theory and the Comparison Between MI/ML and Other Methods | 63 |
|     Estimation Bias with Multiple Regression Models | 64 |
|   Missing Data Theory and the Comparison Between MI and ML | 65 |
|     MI and ML and the Inclusion of Auxiliary Variables | 65 |
|     MI Versus ML, the Importance of Number of Imputations | 66 |
|   Computational Effort and Adjustments in Thinking About MI | 67 |
|   References | 68 |

## Section 2  Multiple Imputation and Basic Analysis

**3  Multiple Imputation with Norm 2.03** .................................... 73
   Step-by-Step Instructions for Multiple Imputation
   with NORM 2.03 ..................................................................... 73
      Running NORM (Step 1): Getting NORM ............................ 73
      Running NORM (Step 2): Preparing the Data Set ................ 74
      Writing Data Out of SPSS .................................................... 75
      Writing a Variable Names File from SPSS .......................... 76
      Empirical Example Used Throughout this Chapter ............. 76
      Running NORM (Step 3): Variables ..................................... 76
      Running NORM (Step 4): The "Summarize" Tab ................ 78
      Running NORM (Step 5): EM Algorithm ............................. 81
      Running NORM (Step 6): Impute from (EM) Parameters ... 86
      Running NORM (Step 7): Data Augmentation (and Imputation) ........ 88
      Running NORM (Step 8): Data Augmentation Diagnostics ............... 89
   References .............................................................................. 94

**4  Analysis with SPSS (Versions Without MI Module)
Following Multiple Imputation with Norm 2.03** .................... 95
   Analysis with the Single Data Imputed from
   EM Parameters ....................................................................... 95
      Before Running MIAutomate Utility .................................... 96
      What the MIAutomate Utility Does ...................................... 97
      Files Expected to Make Automation Utility Work ............... 97
      Installing the MIAutomate Utility ........................................ 98
      Running the Automation Utility ........................................... 98
      Products of the Automation Utility ...................................... 99
      Analysis with the Single Data Set Imputed
      from EM Parameters ............................................................. 99
   Analysis Following Multiple Imputation ............................... 100
   Automation of SPSS Regression Analysis with Multiple
   Imputed Data Sets .................................................................. 101
      Running the Automation Utility ........................................... 101
      Products of the Automation Utility ...................................... 102
      Rationale for Having Separate Input and Output
      Automation Utilities ............................................................. 103
      Multiple Linear Regression in SPSS with Multiple Imputed
      Data Sets, Step 1 ................................................................... 103
      Multiple Linear Regression in SPSS with Multiple Imputed
      Data Sets, Step 2 ................................................................... 104
      Variability of Results with Multiple Imputation ................... 106
      A Note About Ethics in Multiple Imputation ....................... 106
   Other SPSS Analyses with Multiple Imputed Data Sets ........ 107

## 5 Multiple Imputation and Analysis with SPSS 17-20 ... 111
Step-by-Step Instructions for Multiple Imputation
with SPSS 17-20 ... 111
- Running SPSS 17/20 MI (Step 1): Getting SPSS MI ... 112
- Running SPSS 17-20 MI (Step 2): Preparing the Data Set ... 112
- Empirical Example Used Throughout this Chapter ... 113
- Running SPSS 17-20 MI (Step 3): Variables ... 113
- Running SPSS 17-20 MI (Step 4): Missingness Summary ... 113
- Running SPSS 17-20 MI (Step 5): EM Algorithm ... 116
- Running SPSS 17-20 MI (Step 6): Impute from (EM) Parameters ... 118
- Running SPSS 17-20 MI (Step 7): MCMC (and Imputation) ... 118
- Running SPSS 17-20 MI (Step 8): MCMC Diagnostics ... 119

Analysis of Multiple Data Sets Imputed with SPSS 17-20 ... 120
- Split File ... 120
- Multiple Linear Regression in SPSS with Multiple Imputed Data Sets ... 120
- Binary Logistic Regression in SPSS with Multiple Imputed Data Sets ... 121

SPSS 17-20 Analysis of Norm-Imputed Data: Analysis
with the Single Data Imputed from EM Parameters ... 122
- Before Running MIAutomate Utility ... 123
- What the MIAutomate Utility Does ... 124
- Files Expected to Make the MIAutomate Utility Work ... 124
- Analysis with the Single Data Set Imputed from EM Parameters ... 126

SPSS 17-20 Analysis of Norm-Imputed Data: Analysis
of Multiple Data Sets Imputed with Norm 2.03 ... 126

Automation of SPSS Regression Analysis
with Multiple Imputed Data Sets ... 128
- Running the Automation Utility ... 128
- Products of the Automation Utility ... 129
- Setting Up Norm-Imputed Data for Analysis with SPSS 17-20 ... 130
- Multiple Linear Regression in SPSS with Norm-Imputed Data Sets ... 130
- Binary Logistic Regression in SPSS with Norm-Imputed Data Sets ... 130
- Other Analyses in SPSS with Norm-Imputed Data Sets ... 130

References ... 131

## 6 Multiple Imputation and Analysis with Multilevel (Cluster) Data ... 133
Imputation for Multilevel Data Analysis ... 134
- Taking Cluster Structure into Account (Random Intercepts Models) ... 135

Limitations of the Random Intercepts, Hybrid Dummy Coding,
Approach .................................................................................... 137
Normal Model MI for Random Intercepts and Random
Slopes Models ............................................................................ 138
Limitations with the Impute-Within-Individual-Clusters
Strategy....................................................................................... 138
Multilevel Analysis of Norm-Imputed Data with SPSS/Mixed................ 139
Preparation of Data Imputed with Another Program ........................... 141
Multilevel Analysis of Norm-Imputed Data
with SPSS 17-20/Mixed............................................................... 141
Setting Up Norm-Imputed Data for Analysis
with SPSS 17-20 ......................................................................... 142
Multiple Linear Mixed Regression in SPSS 17-20
with Norm-Imputed Data Sets ..................................................... 142
Multiple Linear Mixed Regression in SPSS 15/16
with Norm-Imputed Data Sets ..................................................... 143
Multilevel Analysis of Norm-Imputed Data with HLM 7 ........................ 145
Step 1: Imputation with Norm 2.03 ....................................................... 145
Step 2: Run MIAutomate Utility............................................................. 145
Step 3: Enter HLM Information Window: Executable
Information ................................................................................. 146
Step 4: Enter HLM Information Window: HLM Model
Information ................................................................................. 146
Step 5: MI Inference .............................................................................. 147
Limitations of the MIAutomate Utility for HLM ..................................... 148
Special Issues Relating to Missing Data Imputation
in Multilevel Data Situations ...................................................................... 149
Number of Level-2 Units ....................................................................... 149
Random Slopes Models ........................................................................ 149
3-Level Models ..................................................................................... 149
Other MI Models.................................................................................... 150
References........................................................................................................ 150

## 7 Multiple Imputation and Analysis with SAS ........................................ 151
Step-by-Step Instructions for Multiple Imputation
with PROC MI ............................................................................................ 152
Running PROC MI (Step 1): Getting SAS .............................................. 152
Empirical Example Used Throughout This Chapter.............................. 152
Running PROC MI (Step 2): Preparing the Data Set ........................... 153
Running PROC MI (Step 3): Variables.................................................. 155
Running PROC MI (Step 4): Summarizing the Missing Data............... 158
Running PROC MI (Step 5): EM Algorithm .......................................... 162
Running PROC MI (Step 6): Impute From (EM) Parameters ............... 168
Running PROC MI (Step 7): MCMC (and Imputation)......................... 169
Running PROC MI (Step 8): MCMC Diagnostics.................................. 170

Direct Analysis of EM (MLE) Covariance Matrix
with PROC FACTOR, PROC REG ............................................................. 174
    PROC FACTOR with an EM Covariance Matrix as Input ................... 174
    PROC REG with an EM Covariance Matrix as Input ......................... 175
Analysis of Single Data Set Imputed from EM Parameters
with PROC CORR ALPHA ...................................................................... 176
Analysis of Multiple-Imputed Data with PROC REG,
PROC LOGISTIC, PROC MIXED ............................................................ 177
    Analysis of Multiple-Imputed Data with PROC REG ......................... 177
    PROC MIANALYZE Output for PROC REG ..................................... 178
    Proc Reg with Multiple Dependent Variables ....................................... 181
    Analysis of Multiple-Imputed Data with PROC LOGISTIC .............. 183
    Analysis of Multiple-Imputed Data with PROC MIXED .................... 185
References .................................................................................................... 190

## Section 3   Practical Issues in Missing Data Analysis

## 8  Practical Issues Relating to Analysis with Missing Data: Avoiding and Troubleshooting Problems ............................................. 193
Strategies for Making It Work: Know Your Analysis ............................. 194
Strategies for Making It Work: Know Your Data .................................... 194
    Causes of Missingness ........................................................................... 194
    Auxiliary Variables ................................................................................ 196
    Bottom Line: Think FIML ..................................................................... 197
Troubleshooting Problems .......................................................................... 197
    Disclaimer ............................................................................................... 197
    Underlying Problem 1 ............................................................................ 198
    Solution 1 ................................................................................................ 198
    Underlying Problem 2 ............................................................................ 198
    Solution 2a .............................................................................................. 198
    Solution 2b .............................................................................................. 198
    Underlying Problem: Redundancies in Variable List
    (Matrix Not Positive Definite) ............................................................... 200
    Solution1 ................................................................................................. 203
    Solution1b ............................................................................................... 204
    Underlying Problem ............................................................................... 205
    First Conceptual Basis for This Missingness Pattern ........................... 208
    Solution ................................................................................................... 208
    Second Conceptual Basis for This Missingness Pattern ...................... 208
    Solutions ................................................................................................. 208
Summary of Troubleshooting Symptoms, Causes, and Solutions ............ 210
References .................................................................................................... 212

## 9 Dealing with the Problem of Having Too Many Variables in the Imputation Model .......... 213
Think FIML .......... 213
Imputing Whole Scales .......... 214
   Determining Whether a Scale Is Homogeneous or Heterogeneous .......... 215
   Decision Rules for These Scenarios .......... 219
   Decisions About Throwing Away Partial Data Versus Imputing at the Item Level .......... 220
   Issues Regarding Decision Rules .......... 222
Splitting Variable Set for Multiple-Pass Multiple Imputation .......... 223
   A Solution That Makes Sense .......... 224
   Comments .......... 228
References .......... 228

## 10 Simulations with Missing Data .......... 229
Who Should Read This Chapter? .......... 229
Background .......... 229
General Issues to Consider with Simulations .......... 230
   What Are the Goals of Your Simulation? .......... 230
   What Other Approaches Are Available to Achieve Your Goals? .......... 230
   What Should the Simulation Parameters Be? .......... 231
   What Should the Range of Parameter Values Be? .......... 231
Monte Carlo Simulations .......... 232
   Start with a Population and Generate Samples .......... 232
   Degrading the Sample .......... 233
   Automation Strategies .......... 237
   Technical Issues to Consider in Monte Carlo Simulations .......... 238
Non-Monte Carlo Simulation with the MGSEM Procedure .......... 239
   The Multiple Group SEM Procedure for MCAR Missingness: Overview .......... 240
   Examples of Good Uses of the MGSEM Procedure for MCAR Missingness .......... 241
   Overview of MGSEM Procedure for MAR/NMAR Missingness .......... 241
   Examples of Good Uses of the MGSEM Procedure for MAR/NMAR Missingness .......... 244
   What Simulations Cannot Be Addressed with the MGSEM Procedures? .......... 248
   Other Considerations with the MGSEM Procedures for MAR/NMAR Missingness .......... 250
References .......... 251

## 11 Using Modern Missing Data Methods with Auxiliary Variables to Mitigate the Effects of Attrition on Statistical Power ... 253
Effective Sample Size ... 254
An Artificial Data Demonstration of Improving Power Using a Missing Data Model with Auxiliary Variables ... 256
    Details of MGSEM Procedure ... 256
    Artificial Data Example for One Auxiliary Variable, 100 % of Eligible Subjects with Data ... 261
Artificial Data Demonstrations with More Realistic Attrition Patterns ... 262
    Less than 100 % of Eligible Subjects with Data for the One Auxiliary Variable ... 262
    Two Auxiliary Variables ... 264
    Two Auxiliary Variables with Different Values for $r_{YZ1}$, $r_{YZ2}$, $\%Z_1$, and $\%Z_2$ ... 264
Estimating $N_{EFF}$ with One or Two Auxiliary Variables: The General Case ... 267
    Automation Utility for Estimating $N_{EFF}$ in All One Auxiliary Variable Scenarios ... 267
    Automation Utility for Estimating $N_{EFF}$ in All Two Auxiliary Variable Scenarios ... 269
Implications of $N_{EFF}$ for Statistical Power Calculations ... 269
Loose Ends ... 271
    What Happens When Pretest Covariates Are Included in the Model? ... 271
    Multilevel Models ... 271
    "Highly Inclusive" Versus "Selectively Inclusive" Models ... 272
    What Other Factors May Affect the True $N_{EFF}$ Benefit? ... 275
References ... 275

## Section 4 Planned Missing Data Design

## 12 Planned Missing Data Designs I: The 3-Form Design ... 279
Who Should Read This Chapter? ... 279
    Reasons for Not Using the 3-Form Design ... 279
    Reasons for Using the 3-Form Design ... 280
The 3-Form Design: History, Layout, Design Advantages ... 280
    Matrix Sampling: Early Designs ... 281
    History of the 3-Form Design ... 281
    Basic Layout of the 3-Form Design ... 282
    Advantages of the 3-Form Design over Other Designs ... 282
    Disadvantages of the 3-Form Design Compared to the 1-Form Design ... 283

|     | The Disadvantage of the 3-Form Design Is Not Really a Disadvantage | 289 |
| --- | --- | --- |
|     | 3-Form Design: Other Design Elements and Issues | 290 |
|     | Item Order | 290 |
|     | The X Set | 290 |
|     | Variations of the 3-Form Design: A Family of Designs | 291 |
|     | Keeping Scale Items Within One Item Set Versus Splitting Them Across Item Sets | 293 |
|     | References | 294 |
| 13  | **Planned Missing Data Design 2: Two-Method Measurement** | **295** |
|     | Definition of Response Bias | 296 |
|     | The Bias-Correction Model | 297 |
|     | Benefits of the Bias-Correction Model | 298 |
|     | The Idea of the Benefit | 298 |
|     | How the Sample Size Benefit Works in Bias-Correction Model | 301 |
|     | Factors Affecting the $N_{EFF}$ Benefit | 302 |
|     | Real Effects on Statistical Power | 303 |
|     | Potential Applications of Two-Method Measurement | 307 |
|     | Cigarette Smoking Research | 307 |
|     | Alcohol Research | 308 |
|     | Blood-Vessel Health | 308 |
|     | Measurement of Hypertension | 308 |
|     | Nutrition Research | 309 |
|     | Measuring Body Composition/Adiposity | 309 |
|     | Assessment of Physical Conditioning and Physical Activity | 309 |
|     | Survey Research | 310 |
|     | Retrospective Reports | 310 |
|     | Cost Ratio Issues | 310 |
|     | Calculating Cost Ratio and Estimating Benefits in Studies with Narrow Focus | 311 |
|     | Calculating Cost Ratio and Estimating Benefits in Studies with Broad Focus | 312 |
|     | The Full Bias-Correction Model | 314 |
|     | A Note on Estimation Bias | 317 |
|     | Assumptions | 317 |
|     | Assumption 1: The Expensive Measure is More Valid than the Cheap Measure | 318 |
|     | Assumption 2: The Model Will "Work" Once You Have Collected the Data | 319 |
|     | Individual Versus Group Level Focus of the Research | 320 |
|     | Alternative Model: The Auxiliary Variable Model | 321 |
|     | References | 322 |

# Section 1
# Missing Data Theory

# Chapter 1
# Missing Data Theory

## Overview

In this first chapter, I accomplish several goals. First, building on my 20+ years of work on missing data analysis, I outline a nomenclature or system for talking about the theory underlying the modern analysis of missing data. I intend for this nomenclature to be in plain English, but nevertheless to be an accurate representation of statistical theory relating to missing data analysis. Second, I describe many of the main components of missing data theory, including the causes or mechanisms of missingness. Two general methods for handling missing data, in particular multiple imputation (MI) and maximum-likelihood (ML) methods, have developed out of the missing data theory I describe here. And as will be clear from reading this book, I fully endorse these methods. For the remainder of this chapter, I challenge some of the commonly held beliefs relating to missing data theory and missing data analysis, and make a case that the MI and ML procedures, which have started to become mainstream in statistical analysis with missing data, are applicable in a much larger range of contexts that typically believed.

Third, I revisit the thinking surrounding two of the central concepts in missing data theory: the Missing At Random (MAR), and Not Missing At Random (NMAR) concepts. Fourth, I describe estimation bias that is due to missingness that is NMAR, and outline several factors that influence the magnitude of this bias. In this section, I also make the case for thinking about the practical significance of the bias. Fifth, I pull together the information we have to date about the factors that influence missing data bias, and present a sensitivity analysis showing that missing data bias commonly described in studies may be much less severe than commonly feared.

Sixth, I extend the work on estimating missing data bias, introducing a taxonomy of attrition that suggests eight different attrition scenarios that must be explored in future research. Finally, I present design and measurement strategies for assuring that missingness is MAR. In this final section, I talk about measuring the plausible causes of missingness, about measuring "auxiliary" variables, and about the value of collecting additional data on a random sample of those initially missing from the main measure of one's study.

## Missing Data: What Is It?

Two kinds of missing data have been described in the literature. These are often referred to as ***item nonresponse*** and ***wave nonresponse***. In survey research, item nonresponse occurs when a respondent completes part of a survey, but leaves some individual questions blank, or fails to complete some parts of the survey. This type of missing value might occur because the person just did not see the question. It could occur because the person did not know how to respond to the question. It could be that the person intended to come back to the skipped question, but just forgot. It could be that the person leaves the question blank because of the fear that harm may come to him or her because of the response. It could be that the person leaves the questions blank because the topic is upsetting. Some people may not answer questions near the end of a long survey due to slow reading. Finally, it could be that the person fails to respond to the question because the question was never asked in the first place (e.g., in planned missing data designs; see Chaps. 12 and 13).

The concept of item nonresponse also applies to other types of research, where a research participant has some, but not all data from the measurement session. It could be that the data value was simply lost during the data collection or data storage process. It could be that the data value was lost because of equipment malfunction. It could be that the value was lost due some kind of contamination. It could be that the person responsible for data collection simply forgot to obtain that particular measure.

Wave nonresponse applies to longitudinal research, that is, research in which the same individuals are measured at two or more times (waves). Wave nonresponse describes the situation in which a respondent fails to complete the entire survey (or other measure); that is, when the person is absent from an entire wave of the longitudinal study. In some cases, the individual is missing entirely from one wave of measurement, but comes back to complete the measurement at a later wave. In other cases, the person is missing entirely from one wave of measurement, and never returns. I refer to this latter, special case as ***attrition***.

For a variety of reasons, which will become clear as you read through this book, I typically do not worry too much about item nonresponse. One upshot of this is that I typically do not worry too much about missing data in cross-sectional measurement studies. Of course, situations may occasionally arise in which item nonresponse causes serious problems for statistical inference, but I usually view this type of missingness more as a nuisance – a nuisance that can be dealt with extremely well by the missing data analysis strategies described in this book.

Even wave nonresponse is typically not a particular problem when the respondent returns to provide data at a later wave. Dealing with missing data involves making guesses about what the missing values might plausibly be, based on what is known about the respondent. If the researcher has data at a prior wave and data at a later wave on the same respondent, then these guesses are typically very good, because this is a kind of interpolation. With attrition, the researcher has information about the respondent only at a prior wave. Thus, making the guesses about the respondent's missing values involves extrapolation. And one is typically much less confident about guesses based on extrapolation. Still, as I describe in this chapter, much can be known, even in the case of attrition. So even with attrition, researchers can typically have good confidence in the performance of the missing data analysis procedures I describe throughout this book, provided they pay careful attention to all sources of information available to them.

## Missing Data: History, Objectives, and Challenges

The problem of missing data has long been an issue for data analysis in the social and health sciences. An important reason for this is the fact that algorithms for data analysis were originally designed for data matrices with no missing values. This all began changing in rather dramatic fashion in 1987 when two important books (Little and Rubin 1987; Rubin 1987) were published that would lay the groundwork for most of the advances in missing data analysis for the next 20 years and beyond.

These two published works have produced two rather general strategies for solving the missing data problem, MI and ML. I provide a more detailed discussion of these topics in Chap. 2 (under the heading, "Basics of Recommended Methods"). With either of these solutions to the missing data problem, the main objectives, as with any analysis procedure, are to obtain unbiased estimates of the parameters of interest (i.e., estimates that are close to population values), and to provide an estimate of the uncertainty about those estimates (standard errors or confidence intervals).

A good bit of missing data theory has been counterintuitive when viewed from the perspective of researchers with standard training in the social and health sciences. It was not until the software solutions began to emerge in the mid-to-late 1990s that it became possible to convince these scientists of the virtues of the new approaches to handling missing data, namely MI and ML. Although the use of these new approaches was undeniably a huge step forward, the theoretical underpinnings of these approaches have in large part remained a mystery.

Part of that mystery stems from that fact that the language used to describe missing data theory is as easy to understand for social and health scientists as ancient Aramaic. Although the language of the formal equation in statistical writing is beyond the ken of most nonstatistics researchers with standard training, an even bigger impediment to comprehending the underpinnings of modern missing data procedures is that the statistics books and articles on missing data commonly contain plain English words that have meanings in this context that are rather different from plain English.

## Terms

There are several terms that are at the heart of modern missing data theory that have been widely misunderstood outside of the statistics realm. Among these are model, missingness, distributions, and mechanisms of missingness. I would argue that to understand these terms fully, one must speak the language of statistics. Barring that, one must translate these fundamental concepts into plain English in a way that preserves their overall meaning with a satisfying degree of precision. The next sections tackle this latter task.

## *Model*

The word "model" appears in at least three ways in any discussion of missing data analysis. In order to avoid confusion, and to distinguish among the three different types of model, I define them here.

First, I will frequently mention the analysis model of substantive interest. I will refer to this model as the ***analysis model***. This is the model one tests (e.g., regression model; SEM model) to address the substantive research question.

The second type of model is the model that creates the missing data. I will refer to this type of model as the ***missing data creation model***. For example, in later sections of this chapter, I talk about a system of IF statements that can be used to generate MAR missingness. Such a set of statements might look like this:

$$\text{if } Z = 1, \text{ the probability that Y is missing } [p(Y\text{mis})] = .20$$
$$\text{if } Z = 2, \ p(Y\text{mis}) = .40$$
$$\text{if } Z = 3, \ p(Y\text{mis}) = .60$$
$$\text{if } Z = 4, \ p(Y\text{mis}) = .80$$

In this instance, the probability that Y is missing depends on the value of the variable Z, as shown in the IF statements.

It is important to realize that except for simulation work (and the kind of planned missing data measurement designs described in Chaps. 12 and 13), no one would want to create missing data. Also, although one typically does not know the details of this model, except in simulation work, it is often useful to have a sense of the kinds of models that create missing data. Later in the this chapter, for example, I will talk about sensitivity analyses in which one can make use of various missing data creation models to get a sense of the range of values that are plausible replacements for a missing value. Finally, a little later in this chapter I will mention that some missingness is often described as "ignorable." For that type of missingness, it is the details of the missing data creation model that are ignorable.

The third type of model is the model in which the missingness is handled. As I describe in this book, missingness will typically be handled with MI or ML procedures.

I will refer to the models that describe these procedures as the ***missing data analysis model***. For example, when I talk about whether a particular variable has been, or should be, included in the missing data analysis model, I am talking about whether the variable has been included in the MI (or ML) model. Finally, note that for the "model-based" (ML) missing data procedures (see Chap. 2, Basics of Recommended Methods), the ***Analysis Model*** and the ***Missing Data Analysis Model*** are the same.

## *Missingness*

Even this very fundamental term has been long misunderstood by nonstatisticians. Little and Rubin (2002) do not actually define this term, but their term ***missing data patterns*** seems closely related. Schafer and Graham (2002) talked about missingness by saying, "In modern missing-data procedures missingness is regarded as a probabilistic phenomenon (Rubin 1976)."

I believe that a definition that talks about probabilities is at the heart of the confusion about this concept. Being a probabilistic phenomenon may well make sense within the language of statistics. But it makes less sense in plain English. In my system, I begin by defining missingness using the standard rules of plain English:

***Missingness*** is the state of being missing.

There is nothing in this definition about probabilities. The phrase "state of being," which is a common descriptor for other English words ending in "ness," implies a static state, not a fluid or probabilistic one. The value is either missing or it is not. Please understand that what I am saying here does NOT deny the importance of probabilities in this context. It is just that I believe that the concept of probability, from the perspective of plain English, comes into the picture in a different way, and not in the definition of missingness itself.

In my system, my definition of missingness (the state of being missing) seems clear enough. However, in the next sections, I talk about the reasons for the missingness, and about variables that are related to, or explain missingness. That is, I will be talking about the causes of missingness. However, the first rule of causation is that the cause and effect must covary (e.g., Cook and Campbell 1979). And before the cause and effect can covary, each must first vary. That is, each must first be a variable (a quantity that takes on variable values). Thus, I will also need missingness to be a variable. A convenient operational definition of missingness is a binary variable, $R$, that takes on the value 1 if a variable (Y) is observed (i.e., not missing), and 0 if Y is missing.[1]

---

[1] Schafer and colleagues (Collins et al. 2001; Schafer and Graham 2002) have referred to this variable as $R$; Little and Rubin (2002; and Rubin 1976) refer to the same variable as $M$.

To be absolutely clear, at a conceptual level, I define missingness as the state of being missing. But as an operational definition:

$$\text{Missingness} = R$$

## *Distribution*

Schafer and Graham (2002) say, "[w]e treat $R$ as a set of random variables having a joint probability distribution." Note that they say that $R$ *has* a joint probability distribution, not that $R$ *is* a joint probability distribution. It is important in my system that the probability distribution is not $R$ itself. It is something outside $R$. That distribution is described in the next section.

## *Mechanisms of Missingness*

"In statistical literature, the distribution of $R$ is sometimes called the response mechanism or missingness mechanism, which may be confusing because mechanism suggests a real-world process by which some data are recorded and others are missed" (Schafer and Graham 2002; p. 150). Again, it is critical to see that these mechanisms are separate from $R$ itself. However, here there is an added layer of confusion having to do with the differences between the language of statistics and plain English. I am referring here to syntax. Note that Schafer and Graham referred to it as "… the process by which some data are recorded and others are missed." I believe that this statement is precise in plain English.

On the other hand, other writers refer to the idea of processes (or mechanisms) causing the missing data (i.e., $R$). It may seem that I am just being pedantic in making this point, but I believe statements such as this imply a model that is different from what researchers typically think of as addressing causal mechanisms. When researchers want to test whether it is reasonable to say "X causes Y," they would typically perform a regression (or comparable) analysis in which X (which can be a manipulated variable) predicts Y. That is,

$$X \Rightarrow Y.$$

In order to be consistent with this type of model, we should say that variables cause variables. In talking about missingness, we could say that some variable, Z, is the cause of missingness, that is,

$$Z \Rightarrow R.$$

Let me summarize my system on this point. First, we have mechanisms, which describe the process by which one or more variables causes missingness, that is the process by which some variable, Z, causes **R**. Second, we have the variables that represent the various causes of missingness.

## Causes of Missingness

What the statisticians refer to as the mechanisms of missingness generally fall into three categories: Missing Completely At Random (MCAR), Missing At Random (MAR), and Not Missing At Random (NMAR).[2] It makes sense that the various *causes of missingness* (i.e., variables that cause missingness) would fall into these three categories. Schafer and Graham (2002) suggest "[t]o describe accurately all potential causes or reasons for missingness is not realistic." However, and note that I am diverging somewhat from Schafer and Graham on this point, even if many causes are plausible, and I can think of only some of them, I believe that it is valuable to think in terms of causes of missingness.

In order to facilitate this discussion, Table 1.1 presents a list of all variables (by class) that are relevant to missingness (sometimes by not being related to it). It is customary in describing these concepts to refer just to MCAR, MAR, and NMAR missingness (although see Little 1995, who extends the list to include "covariate-dependent dropout"). However, in Table 1.1, I focus on the causes of missingness (the variables) rather than on the mechanisms. Also, I have attempted in Table 1.1 to provide an exhaustive list of all possible causes of missingness.

In discussing the various causes of missingness, some readers might be thinking that there is no way of knowing what the true cause of missingness is, so what is the point of this extensive list? Although it is true that we cannot know all the causes of missingness, I believe we can agree that all of the causes come from the categories on this list. And I believe that if we can at least conceive of a class of variables, then we should be able to think of at least some variables that would fall into that class. Further, I believe that this type of thinking can be useful in helping us make plausible guesses about the effects that these unknown variables have on our statistical estimation.

First in Table 1.1 is $R$, which I have already defined as a binary variable that is the operational definition of missingness, and that takes on the value 1 if Y is observed, and 0 if Y is missing.

---

[2] Little and Rubin (2002) refer to this as Not Missing At Random (NMAR). But Schafer and colleagues (Collins et al. 2001; Schafer and Graham 2002) refer to this same mechanism as Missing Not At Random (MNAR). I have decided to use NMAR here, because it makes sense that missingness should either be MAR or not (i.e., Not MAR). However, there are good arguments for using MNAR as well. I view the two terms to be interchangeable.

**Table 1.1** A taxonomy of all classes of variables and their relevance to missingness

| | |
|---|---|
| R | A binary variable that takes on the value 1 if Y is observed, and 0 if Y is missing. This variable is the operational definition of "missingness" – the state of being missing. |
| Y | A variable of substantive interest that is sometimes missing. I usually think of "Y" as the dependent variable (DV) in a regression model, but it can be any variable in the analysis model. |
| $Y_{Y1,R0}$ | It is related to Y (of course), but unrelated to R. |
| $Y_{Y1,R1}$ | It is related to Y, and also related to R. |
| X | Variables of substantive interest (will be included in the analysis model). |
| $X_{Y0,R0}$ | It is unrelated to Y and R. |
| $X_{Y1,R0}$ | It is related to Y, but not to R. |
| $X_{Y0,R1}$ | It is unrelated to Y, but it is related to R. |
| $X_{Y1,R1}$ | It is related to both Y and R. |
| V | Variables not of substantive interest; that is, not in the analysis model; but in the data set. (For now, these are never missing.) |
| $V_{Y0,R0}$ | It is unrelated to Y and R. |
| $V_{Y1,R0}$ | It is related to Y but not to R. |
| $V_{Y0,R1}$ | It is unrelated to Y, but it is related to R. |
| $V_{Y1,R1}$ | It is related to both Y and R. |
| W | Variables not in the data set (always missing) |
| $W_{Y0,R0}$ | It is unrelated to Y and R. |
| $W_{Y1,R0}$ | It is related to Y but not to R. |
| $W_{Y0,R1}$ | It is unrelated to Y but it is related to R. |
| $W_{Y1,R1}$ | It is related to both Y and R. |
| Q | A completely random process such as flipping a coin. Q is usually either always observed or always missing. Q is unrelated to all other variables, measured or unmeasured. |

In Table 1.1, I describe Y as a variable that is in the data set, but that is sometimes missing. I am describing the case where just one variable (Y) has missing data, but everything I say here can be applied to more complex missingness patterns (e.g., more than one variable with missing data and a variety of patterns of missing and observed variables). Also I am thinking here of this variable as the dependent variable (DV) in a regression analysis, but what I say also applies to other analysis models, and to models in which "Y" is some variable in the analysis model other than the DV (e.g., a mediation model with missing data for both the mediator and the outcome; or a growth model in which the variable being measured over time has missing data at more than one time).

The subscript $_{R0}$ means that Y is not related to its own missingness; $_{R1}$ means that Y is related its own missingness. For example, if Y was cigarette smoking, and if smokers were just as likely as nonsmokers to have missing data, then it would be $Y_{Y1,R0}$. However, if smokers were more likely than nonsmokers to have missing data, then it would be $Y_{Y1,R1}$.

Next, are variables labeled X. These variables are of substantive interest; they are in the data set, and are intended to be part of the analysis model. For example, if Y is smoking, I might be interested in several variables as predictors of smoking. I might be interested in personality variables like empathy and intellect (often referred to as agreeableness and openness), GPA, and rebelliousness. In this case, these variables would be in the X category.

I will talk here about the case where these variables are always observed, but what I say here can also be extended to the case in which these variables are also sometimes missing (e.g., see Chap. 11; also see Enders 2008). The four types of X variable shown in Table 1.1 vary in their relatedness (e.g., correlation) to Y and to $R$. In the table the $_{Y0,R0}$ subscripts denote that the variable is uncorrelated with both Y and $R$. For example, in one of my data sets, the personality variable empathy was found to be virtually uncorrelated with both smoking and missingness on smoking. The $_{Y1,R0}$ subscripts denote that the variable is correlated with Y, but not with $R$. For example, in my data set, the measure of rebelliousness was positively correlated with smoking, but was virtually uncorrelated with missingness on the smoking variable. The $_{Y0,R1}$ subscripts denote that the variable is uncorrelated with Y, but is correlated with $R$. For example, in my data set, the personality variable Intellect was virtually uncorrelated with cigarette smoking, but was negatively correlated with $R$ (higher intellect was associated with greater missingness on the smoking measure). Finally, the $_{Y1,R1}$ subscripts denote that the variable is correlated with both Y and $R$. For example, in my data set, the variable GPA was negatively correlated with cigarette smoking, and positively correlated with $R$ (higher GPA was associated with less missingness on the smoking measure). By the rules common in philosophy of science, no variable can be a cause of missingness unless it is correlated with $R$. That is, of the variables listed in Table 1.1, only those with $_{R1}$ as a subscript can be causes of missingness.

The next class of variables is V. Most data are collected with several purposes in mind. Thus, variables that are central to one set of analyses will be irrelevant to another set of analyses. It is these "irrelevant" variables that make up the V class. These variables are also in the data set, but they are not of substantive interest, and are thus not intended to be part of the analysis model. I am thinking of the case where these variables are always observed, but what I say can also be extended to the case in which these variables are sometimes missing (e.g., see Chap. 11; also see Enders 2008). With the V variables, the $_{Y0,}$ $_{Y1,}$ $_{R0,}$ and $_{R1}$ subscripts have the same meaning as with the X variables. The examples given above for the X class of variables could also apply here, except that as variables in the V class, the variables mentioned would not be part of the analysis model.

When they are causes of missingness, the two classes, X and V taken together, are the variables that relate to what Little (1995) referred to as "covariate-dependent dropout."

The next class of variables in Table 1.1 is W. These variables are not in the data set, and thus are always missing. These variables could have been omitted from the data set for a variety of reasons. They may have been deemed of less importance for the main goals of the research, or they may have been deemed important for the research, but omitted for cost reasons. Alternatively, they may not have been considered for measurement at all. With the W variables, the $_{Y0,}$ $_{Y1,}$ $_{R0,}$ and $_{R1}$ subscripts have the same meaning as with the X and V variables.

Finally, there is Q, a variable that represents a completely random process such as flipping a coin, or drawing a value from a valid random number generator. This variable can be entirely observed if the researcher happens to save it. However, it is often discarded after it has served its purpose, and therefore is entirely missing. An important property is that Q is unrelated (uncorrelated) to all other variables, measured or unmeasured.

I want to make use of another variable, Z, that is a different kind of variable than those appearing in Table 1.1. Z is a variable name I reserve as an "action" variable. Technically, Z can be any of the variables described in Table 1.1 (except *R*). Sometimes it will be the cause of missingness on Y, sometimes it will be related to Y, but not to *R*. Sometimes it will have been measured; sometimes it will not have been measured. Collins et al. (2001) made good use of this variable in their article.

## Mapping Causes of Missingness onto the Three Missingness Mechanisms

In this section, I will provide definitions of the three missingness mechanisms typically described in the missing data literature (MCAR, MAR, NMAR). I will begin each section with a classic example of that mechanism, and will show how the causes of missingness shown in Table 1.1 map onto that missingness mechanism. I will follow this with one or more definitions as they have appeared in the literature.

### *Missing Completely at Random (MCAR)*

#### Classic Example of MCAR

The classic example of MCAR missingness is that a researcher uses some completely random process to determine which respondent receives which of several planned missing data design options (e.g., which form of the 3-form design; see Chap. 12). The variable defined by this completely random process is in the Q class in Table 1.1. See Table 1.2 for a summary of how the variables from Table 1.1 map onto the three mechanisms of missingness.

**Table 1.2** Mapping causes of missingness onto the missingness mechanisms

MCAR: Any cause of missingness on Y is Q, $X_{Y0,R1}$, $V_{Y0,R1}$, or $W_{Y0,R1}$.

MAR: Any cause of missingness on Y is $X_{Y1,R1}$, or $V_{Y1,R1}$. After conditioning on X and V, the only residual relationships with *R* are $X_{Y0,R1}$, $V_{Y0,R1}$, $W_{Y0,R1}$, or Q.

NMAR: Some cause of missingness on Y is $Y_{Y1,R1}$, or $W_{Y1,R1}$. Even after conditioning on X and V, $Y_{Y1,R1}$ or $W_{Y1,R1}$ still have a residual relationship with *R*.

### Definitions of MCAR

The definitions for MCAR missingness vary in complexity. One of the more straightforward definitions for MCAR is " ... missingness does not depend on the values of the data Y, missing or observed ..." (Little and Rubin 2002). I often think of MCAR in this way: Cases with data for a variable, and cases with missing data for a variable, are each random samples of the total. This situation is achieved if the cause of missingness is a completely random process such as flipping a coin.

### Missingness That Is Essentially MCAR

Missingness can also be MCAR, or what I sometimes refer to as *essentially MCAR*, even when the cause is not a completely random process. This will be true if a particular variable causes missingness on Y, but happens not to be correlated with Y. One example is that parents, whose child was part of a drug prevention study, left an area to take a job in a new city. Their child will have dropped out of the measurement part of the study, so this variable (parents leaving) is a cause of missingness. However, as it turns out, this variable (parents leaving) is virtually uncorrelated with the DV, drug use. As shown in Table 1.2, the cause of missingness in this case could be a variable, $X_{Y0,R1}$, $V_{Y0,R1}$, or $W_{Y0,R1}$. In this instance, this variable behaves just like Q.

Table 1.2 summarizes the possible causes of missingness using the variables defined in Table 1.1.

## *Missing at Random (MAR)*

### Classic Example of MAR

A classic example here is reading speed. With a long, self-administered survey, for which there is a limited amount of time for completion (e.g., 50 min), fast readers will complete the survey, but slow readers will leave some questions blank at the end of the survey. However, reading speed is something that can be measured early in the questionnaire where virtually all of the respondents will provide data. Because of this, any biases associated with reading speed can be controlled by including the reading speed variable as in the missing data analysis model.

### Typical/Classical Definition(s) of MAR

Despite the occasional formality of its definition, the meaning of MCAR is what its label implies. And most researchers' intuition is reasonably accurate about its meaning. Unfortunately, this is not at all true of MAR. There is a sense in which the MAR missingness is random, but MAR does not mean that the missingness was caused by a completely random process (i.e., Q in Table 1.1).

A common definition of MAR missingness is that missingness ($R$) may depend on $Y_{OBS}$, but not on $Y_{MIS}$, where $Y_{OBS}$ represents data that are observed and $Y_{MIS}$ represents data that are missing. Using this definition, it is typically said that MCAR is a special case of MAR in which missingness also does not depend on $Y_{OBS}$.

## My Definition of MAR

As shown in Table 1.2, MAR means that once all of the known (and measured) causes of missingness (e.g., reading speed) are taken into account, that is, included in the analysis model or in the missing data analysis model, any residual missingness can be thought of as MCAR. What is important with MAR missingness is that one must take causes of missingness into account by including those variables in the analysis model or in the missing data analysis model. Otherwise, there will be estimation bias.[3]

## Define MAR by Creating MAR Missingness

I sometimes find it very useful for understanding MAR to see exactly how the MAR missingness is generated. For example, Collins et al. (2001) operationally defined three kinds of MAR missingness: MAR-linear, MAR-convex, and MAR-sinister. With MAR-linear, missingness on Y was a linear function of Z, and the values of Z represented the quartiles of Z:

if $Z = 1$, the probability that Y is missing $[p(Ymis)] = .20$
if $Z = 2$, $p(Ymis) = .40$
if $Z = 3$, $p(Ymis) = .60$
if $Z = 4$, $p(Ymis) = .80$

With MAR-convex, missingness on Y was a particular nonlinear function of Z:

if $Z = 1$, $p(Ymis) = .80$
if $Z = 2$, $p(Ymis) = .20$
if $Z = 3$, $p(Ymis) = .20$
if $Z = 4$, $p(Ymis) = .80$

With MAR-sinister, missingness on Y was a function of the correlation between X (another variable in the analysis model), and Z (the cause of missingness). With this type of missingness, Collins et al. (2001) divided the $N = 500$ into 50 clusters of

---

[3] Although as I demonstrate in a later section of this chapter, the amount of bias depends on many factors, and may often be tolerably low.

10 and calculated $r_{xz}$ within those 50 clusters. The groups were divided into the 25 with high correlations and the 25 with low correlations (median split). Then,

$$\text{if } r_{xz} = \text{high, } p(Y\text{mis}) = .80$$
$$\text{if } r_{xz} = \text{low, } p(Y\text{mis}) = .20$$

**MAR Does Not Refer to Missingness Alone**

One of most confusing aspects of MAR missingness is that MAR does not refer to missingness alone. Rather it refers also to the analysis model or the missing data analysis model. If the analysis model or the missing data analysis model does not take the causes of missingness into account, then missingness is NMAR (see next section), and not MAR.

This was so confusing, in fact, that Graham and Donaldson (1993) coined a new term to describe this kind of missingness. We referred to this kind of missingness as *accessible* missingness. We called it accessible, because the researcher had access to the cause of missingness. This captures the idea of MAR missingness that the cause of missingness is a variable that has been measured (e.g., X or V in Table 1.1). However, our new term applied to missingness itself and was independent of one's choice of whether or not to make use of the cause of missingness in one's analysis. That is, accessible missingness is a characteristic of the missingness (as defined here), whereas MAR is a joint characteristic of the missingness and the analysis used.

**MAR Missingness and Ignorability**

MAR missingness is sometimes referred to as *ignorable* missingness. But this is not ignorable in the way many researchers might think of ignorable. For example, MAR missingness is not ignorable in the sense that the cause of missingness (as I have defined it above) may be omitted from the missing data analysis model. What may be ignored here is the missing data creation model. For example, with MAR linear (e.g., as defined in the IF statements given above), it is sufficient to include the variable, Z (e.g., reading speed in my example), in the analysis model or in the missing data analysis model. It is not necessary to know precisely which IF statements generated the missing data.

## *Not Missing at Random (NMAR; aka Missing Not at Random; MNAR)*

**Classic Example of NMAR Missingness**

With this type of missingness, the cause of missingness, Z, is correlated with Y (the variable that is sometimes missingness), but Z has not been measured, so Z cannot be included in the missing data analysis model. The classic example of this kind of

**Table 1.3** Relationships between accessible/inaccessible and MAR/NMAR

| Missingness | Cause of missingness included in missing data analysis model | |
|---|---|---|
| | Yes | No |
| MCAR | MCAR | MCAR |
| Accessible | MAR | NMAR |
| Inaccessible | * | NMAR |

*Cause of missingness cannot be included in the missing data analysis model

missingness relates to the measure of income. It is common in survey research for people with higher incomes to leave the income question blank. But because income is missing for many respondents, including it in the missing data analysis model will not eliminate biases.

The classic definition of NMAR missingness is that missingness depends on $Y_{MIS}$. Using the logic presented in this book, NMAR missingness occurs when missingness on Y (i.e., $R$) is caused by Y itself, by some variant of Y,[4] or by some other variable that is related to Y, but which has not been measured (i.e., $W_{Y1R1}$, as shown in Tables 1.1 and 1.2). The important thing, however, is that even after taking all measured variables into account, residual missingness remains such that the cause of this residual missingness is $Y_{Y1R1}$ or $W_{Y1R1}$. The problem is that the data analyst would have no way of knowing whether the residual missingness was related to, or caused by some unmeasured variable ($Y_{Y1R1}$ or $W_{Y1R1}$) that was also related to Y.[5]

Graham and Donaldson (1993) defined this type of missingness as *inaccessible* missingness. It is inaccessible because the cause of missingness has not been measured and is therefore not available for analysis. The relationships between the Graham and Donaldson terms (accessible and inaccessible) and the classic terms (MAR and NMAR) are summarized in Table 1.3. For completeness, I also include a row for MCAR missingness.

An important point typically made about MAR and NMAR missingness is that the analyst cannot know which is working in a particular data set. Although I do agree to an extent with this point, I also believe that the analyst is not without relevant information in many data sets, especially in longitudinal data sets. I turn now to a detailed discussion of this issue.

---

[4] One common variant of Y, for example, could be Z, a 4-level, uniformly distributed variable where the four levels represent the quartiles of the original Y variable, which was continuous and normally distributed. In this example, the two variables are highly correlated ($r_{yz} = .925$), but they are not correlated $r = 1.0$.

[5] At the heart of all methods for analysis of NMAR missingness is a guess or assumption about the missing data creation model. Because all such methods must make these assumptions, methods for NMAR missingness are only as good as their assumptions. Please see the discussion in the next section.

## MAR Versus NMAR Revisited

Much of missing data theory revolves around the MAR and NMAR concepts. Part of the reason this distinction has been so important is that the recommended missing data analyses (MI and ML) assume that the missingness is MAR (or MCAR). So as long as the MAR assumption holds a good bit of the time, we are ok. But just as there has been confusion relating to the definitions of MAR and NMAR, there has also been a good deal of confusion about when the MAR assumption is plausible.

### *Can We Ever Know Whether MAR Holds?*

The conventional wisdom is that one cannot know whether the missingness is MAR or NMAR. For example, Schafer and Graham (2002) say "[w]hen missingness is beyond the researcher's control, its distribution is unknown and MAR is only an assumption. In general, there is no way to test whether MAR holds in a data set, except by obtaining followup data from nonrespondents ..." (p. 152).

Because of this apparent fact, writers simply assert that the conditions they want (i.e., MAR or NMAR) do, in fact, exist. Researchers who want MAR to hold often say nothing at all about it, and if they do say anything, it is simply to assert that it is reasonable to assume that MAR holds. In longitudinal studies, some researchers perform comparisons on pretest variables between those who drop out of the study and those who remain. Although such comparisons do little to address the issue of whether MAR holds, they are often used in this way (I talk in more detail about this practice later in this chapter under the heading, *The Value of Missing Data Diagnostics*).

Researchers who want to write about NMAR methods (e.g., pattern mixture models) simply assert that conditions exist in which the MAR assumption is untenable. We all know that such conditions can and most likely do exist, but researchers talking about NMAR methods generally do not make specific arguments about a particular data set. Some go no further than to say something such as, MAR methods are good, "... but also yield biased inferences under plausible models for the drop-out process" (Little 1995). In this vein, Demirtas and Schafer (2003) say, "[i]f we suspect that dropout is related to current response in some fundamental way, ignorability becomes dubious, prompting us to consider nonignorable alternatives." Similarly, Verbeke and Molenberghs (2000) say, "[i]n cases where dropout could be related to the unobserved responses, dropout is no longer ignorable, implying that treatment effects can no longer be tested or estimated without explicitly taking the dropout model ... into account" (p. 234).

Some researchers do go a bit further when discussing NMAR methods. Demirtas and Schafer (2003) offered the general possibility that people who do not seem to be responding well to treatment may drop out to seek alternative treatment. They also offered the possibility that people who seem to be responding exceptionally well to treatment may drop out because they think they are cured. The implication is that either scenario would be NMAR because the dropout is related to the dependent variable. Enders (2011) also takes the assertion a bit further, saying "[a]lthough the MAR mechanism is often reasonable, there are situations where this assumption is unlikely to hold. For example, in a longitudinal study of substance use, it is reasonable to expect participants with the highest frequency of use to have the highest likelihood of attrition, even after controlling for other correlates of missingness." But in cases like these, the authors make no attempt to tie their examples to real data, or to evaluate their assertions either on substantive or on statistical grounds.

## Maybe We Can Know if MAR Holds

Unfortunately, scenarios such as those described above do not really explain the missingness, and comments of this sort offer no guidance to data analysts for specific missing data scenarios. It is generally held that one cannot know whether missingness is MAR or NMAR in any particular case. However, I believe there is much that one can glean from one's data. And although it may be true that we cannot know the details regarding MAR versus NMAR, I argue that we often do not need the precise details to know that MAR holds, either in a statistical sense, or at least in a practical sense.

Schafer and colleagues have opened the door to this way of thinking (also see Little 1994; p. 482). Schafer and Graham (2002) to say,

> [i]n general, there is no way to test whether MAR holds in a data set, except by obtaining followup data from nonrespondents .... In most cases we should expect departures from MAR, *but whether these departures are serious enough to cause the performance of MAR-based methods to be seriously degraded is another issue entirely* .... Recently, Collins et al. (2001) demonstrated that in many realistic cases, an erroneous assumption of MAR (e.g., failing to take into account a cause or correlate of missingness) may often have only a minor impact on estimates and standard errors (p. 152; emphasis added).

And Collins et al. (2001) say,

> [i]t is highly doubtful that an analyst will have access to all of the relevant causes or correlates of missingness. One can safely bet on the presence of lurking variables that are correlated both with the variables of interest and with the missingness process; *the important question is whether these correlations are strong enough to produce substantial bias if no additional measures are taken* (p. 333; emphasis added).

This work, especially the simulations conducted by Collins et al. (2001), can be interpreted to suggest that it is sometimes possible to make judgments about whether MAR does or does not hold in a particular situation.

## *Measuring Estimation Bias*

### Bias That Is Statistically Significant

Let us suppose we have conducted a Monte Carlo simulation to test whether a regression coefficient deviates appreciably from the known population value for that parameter. Let us say we conduct 500 replications of the simulation. That means we have a sample of $N=500$ estimates of the regression coefficient. Let us say that the average b-weight was −0.46808, and that the population value was −0.481487. In this case the raw bias is 0.013407, that is, the estimates for the regression coefficient were a little too close to 0. Further, let us say the standard deviation of the sampling distribution for this parameter was 0.065973. So the mean bias for this parameter was .013407, and the standard deviation for this mean was .065973. We can calculate the standard error for this mean by dividing the standard deviation by the square root of $N$ (500 in this case). So,

$$SE = .065973 / \sqrt{500} = .00295$$

Thus, the bias, .013407, in this case was statistically significantly different from 0,

$$t(498) = .013407 / .00295 = 4.57, p < .0001$$

### Bias That Is Significant in a Practical Sense

As with many statistical analyses, an effect can be statistically significant, but lack practical significance. Collins et al. (2001) attempted to distinguish between bias that did and did not have important practical implications for the statistical decisions (i.e., distinguish between bias that would and would not materially affect the interpretation of the analysis model). They made good use of **Standardized Bias**, which can be thought of as the percent of a standard error the estimate is from the population value.

$$\text{Standardized Bias (SB)} = \frac{\text{Estimate} - \text{Population Value}}{SE} \times 100$$

where SE is the standard error of the estimate (standard deviation of the sampling distribution). Collins et al. suggested that the absolute value of SB greater than around 40 represents a potential problem for statistical inference; "... once the standardized bias exceeds 40–50 % in a positive or negative direction, the bias begins to have a noticeable adverse impact on efficiency, coverage, and error rates" (Collins et al. 2001; p. 340). This implies that |SB| < 40 could be thought of as bias that was not significant in a practical sense.

## Factors Affecting Standardized Bias

In this section, I address factors affecting SB that might be thought of as having substantive interest. In a later section I address other factors that affect standardized bias, but that might be thought of more as nuisance factors.

Collins et al. (2001) studied several factors that affect SB. They studied a simple regression model (X predicting Y), such that X was never missing, but Y was sometimes missing. In their simulations, 25 % or 50 % of the Y values were missing. With 50 % missing on Y, as shown previously, MAR-linear missingness was a function of Z based on the following IF statements.

if Z = 1, p(Ymis) = .20
if Z = 2, p(Ymis) = .40
if Z = 3, p(Ymis) = .60
if Z = 4, p(Ymis) = .80

With 25 % missing on Y, the statements used to generate MAR-linear were these:

if Z = 1, p(Ymis) = .10
if Z = 2, p(Ymis) = .20
if Z = 3, p(Ymis) = .30
if Z = 4, p(Ymis) = .40

Collins et al. also varied the degree to which the cause of missingness (Z) was correlated with Y. In their simulations, $r_{YZ} = .40$ or $r_{YZ} = .90$. The correlation $r_{YZ} = .40$ simulated the situation where Z was one of the best predictors of Y. This correlation ($r_{YZ} = .40$) was the highest substantive correlation observed in one of my data sets where Y was adolescent cigarette smoking, and Z was rebelliousness. The correlation $r_{YZ} = .90$ simulated the case in which a variant of Y itself was the cause of missingness on Y.

From their simulations, it was clear that percent missing was related to SB. For the regression coefficient of X predicting Y (for MAR-linear missingness when Z was omitted from the model), the average SB was −10.8 for 25 % missing and −66.4 for 50 % missing. The correlation $r_{YZ}$ was also clearly related to SB. In their MAR-linear simulations, SB averaged −15.3 for $r_{YZ} = .40$ and −61.9 for $r_{YZ} = .90$.

A factor not studied by Collins et al. (2001) was $r_{ZR}$, the correlation between Z (the cause of missingness) and R (missingness itself). The IF statements they employed for all 50 % missing conditions of their MAR-linear simulation were:

if Z = 1, p(Ymis) = .20
if Z = 2, p(Ymis) = .40
if Z = 3, p(Ymis) = .60
if Z = 4, p(Ymis) = .80

These statements produced $r_{ZR}=.447$. As it turns out, $r_{ZR}=.447$ represents a rather dramatic effect of the variable on its own missingness. In my experience with drug abuse prevention programs, I have never seen a correlation anywhere near $r=.447$. For example, I found estimates much closer to $r_{ZR}=.10$ (and below) with five different prevention data sets (Graham et al. 2008). IF statements producing $r_{ZR}=.10$ would be:

if Z = 1, p(Ymis) = .433
if Z = 2, p(Ymis) = .478      range = .567 − .433 = .134
if Z = 3, p(Ymis) = .522
if Z = 4, p(Ymis) = .567

where the quantity **range** (which will be employed extensively in this and other chapters of this book) is simply the difference between the highest and lowest probabilities in the MAR-linear IF statements.[6] To illustrate the dramatic effect of $r_{ZR}$ on SB, in a later simulation we (Graham et al. 2008) estimated SB for the situation very close to that examined by Collins et al. (2001), namely, 50 % missingness, $r_{XY}=.60$, $r_{XZ}=.555$, $r_{YZ}=.925$, all variances = 1, except that we also varied $r_{ZR}$. For the situation with $r_{ZR}=.104$ (range = .14), we found SB to be just −5.9 (Graham et al. 2008; also see Chap. 10). Compare this to SB = −114.5, where percent missingness, $r_{XY}$, $r_{XZ}$, and $r_{YZ}$ are the same values as in the above situation, but $r_{ZR}=.447$ (range = .60), as used in the Collins et al. simulation.

Finally, Collins et al. (2001) did not vary the substantive correlation, $r_{XY}$. In all of their simulations, $r_{XY}=.60$. However, standardized bias is also affected by $r_{XY}$. For example, with 50 % missingness, $r_{XY}=.60$, $r_{XZ}=.555$, $r_{YZ}=.925$, $r_{ZR}=.447$ (range = .60), and all variances = 1, SB = −114.5. However, for these same conditions, but with a much more modest $r_{XY}=.20$, SB = −45.7 (see Chap. 10 for a more complete description of these effects).

## Estimating Statistical and Practical Significance of Bias in Real Data

One conclusion to draw from the simulations presented by Collins et al. (2001) and the follow-up simulations by Graham et al. (2008; also see Chap. 10) is that estimation bias due to NMAR missingness is tolerably low in a wide range of

---

[6] I describe the range quantity in more detail in Chap. 10. One important point about this quantity is that for any given level of missingness, $r_{ZR}$ is a linear transformation of the range of probabilities in the MAR-linear IF statements. During our simulation work (Graham et al. 2008), Lori Palen discovered that $r_{ZR}$ was the product of a constant (0.7453559925 for 50 % missingness and Z as uniformly distributed variable with four levels) and the range between the highest and lowest probabilities for the IF statements. I refer to this constant as the Palen proportion.

circumstances. Still, it would be good if we researchers had means for examining the statistical and practical significance of bias based on data from existing empirical data sets. We can make reasonable judgments about the statistical and practical significance of bias if we can make reasonable judgments about the factors that affect this bias (percent missing, $r_{XY}$, $r_{ZY}$, $r_{ZR}$). I suggest some workable strategies in this section for estimating these quantities. The strategies I suggest, in a broad sense, are a little like performing a statistical power analysis after a study has been completed.

## *Percent Missing*

Estimating this value is never really an issue. It is easy to know if one's DV is missing. It is also easy to get precise estimates of missingness within the program and control groups in an intervention study.

## *Estimating $r_{XY}$*

This is the correlation between the IV (X) and DV (Y) in a study. The Y variable is assumed to be a measured variable. The X variable could be a treatment group membership variable (e.g., treatment = 1; control = 0), or it could also be a measured variable. The quantity one wants here is the unbiased value of $r_{XY}$. Because of the possibility for bias due to NMAR missingness, this value is unknowable, to an extent. However, knowing this value even approximately may be good enough in this context. With realistic values of the key factors affecting bias, for example $r_{ZR} = .22$ (range = .30), and 50 % missing on Y, differences as large as .10 for $r_{XY}$ caused differences of SB of only about 5 (see Chap. 10). Thus, it is very likely that the complete cases estimate for $r_{XY}$, or better still, the EM estimate for $r_{XY}$, with several other variables in the model, will provide a reasonable estimate for this quantity (details of the EM algorithm are given in Chap. 2).

## *Estimating $r_{ZY}$*

This is the correlation between Z, the cause of missingness on Y, and Y, the variable that is sometimes missing. If the cause of missingness, Z, is suspected to be some measured variable (category X or V from Table 1.1), then it will be an easy matter to estimate $r_{ZY}$ in the same manner as just described for $r_{XY}$. Even if Z is suspected to be in the W category from Table 1.1, it may be possible to approximate this correlation by comparing it to known correlations between measured variables and Y.

If the cause of missingness is suspected to be Y itself, the calculation is a bit more difficult, but not impossible. First, just because Y is the cause of its own missingness, it does not follow that $r_{ZY} = 1.0$. It is much more likely to be something at least a little lower. For example, if Z, the cause of missingness on Y, were the quartiled version of the normally distributed, continuous variable, Y (i.e., 4-level, uniformly distributed version of Y, where everyone in the first quartile of Y has "1" for Z; everyone in the second quartile of Y has "2" for Z, and so on), then $r_{ZY}=.925$, approximately. Of course, variants are possible. For this chapter, when the cause of missingness is assumed to be Y itself, I will assume that Z is actually the quartilized version of Y, and I will assume that $r_{ZY}=.925$.

$r_{ZY}=.925$ is a reasonable estimate of the zero-order correlation of Z with Y. However, in many studies, other variables will be available that will affect $r_{ZY}$ (These are *auxiliary variables*: variables that are not part of the analysis model, but that are correlated with the analysis model variables that are sometimes missing; see Chap. 11). In particular, in longitudinal studies, the main DV will have been measured multiple times. And the relevant version of $r_{ZY}$, that is, the *operative* $r_{ZY}$, will be the version of $r_{ZY}$ that controls for measures of Y from prior waves of measurement. In studies like these, the operative $r_{ZY}$ is the semi-partial correlation of Z with Y controlling for Y measured at prior waves.

## Example of Estimating $r_{ZY}$

I will use data from the Adolescent Alcohol Prevention Trial (AAPT; Hansen and Graham 1991) to illustrate one approach for estimating the operative $r_{ZY}$. The variables are lifetime cigarette smoking at seventh, eighth, ninth, and tenth grades ($Smoke_7$, $Smoke_8$, $Smoke_9$, and $Smoke_{10}$). Let us say that the quartilized version of $Smoke_{10}$ ($Z_{10}$) is the cause of missingness in $Smoke_{10}$. I can create the quartilized version in SAS using Proc Rank, as shown below.[7] I then use Proc MI to generate an EM covariance matrix for performing the various regression analyses (basics of the EM algorithm are given in Chap. 2; details about using SAS Proc MI in this manner are provided in Chap. 7).

The order and logic of the regression analyses is as follows.

Model (1): Predict $Smoke_{10}$ using the supposed cause of missingness, $Z_{10}$, the quartilized version of $Smoke_{10}$.
The $R^2$ from Model (1) indicates the zero-order relationship between $Z_{10}$ and $Smoke_{10}$. In these data, $R^2=.834$ for Model (1). The corresponding zero-order $r=.913$. This verifies that the zero-order version of $r_{ZY}$ is indeed large.

Model (2): Predict $Smoke_{10}$ using $Smoke_7$, $Smoke_8$, and $Smoke_9$ as predictors.
The $R^2=.688$ for Model (2). The three smoking variables prior to the tenth grade accounted for 69 % of the variance in the tenth grade measure.

---

[7] Note that the quartilized version of $Smoke_{10}$ ($Z_{10}$), had only three levels in the data used in this example (0, 2, 3). Despite this, however, the results shown in this section are representative of what will commonly be found with these analyses.

Model (3): add $Z_{10}$ to Model (2) as a fourth predictor.
Model (3) assesses the incremental benefit of $Z_{10}$ in predicting Smoke$_{10}$, over and above Smoke$_7$, Smoke$_8$, and Smoke$_9$. For Model (3), $R^2 = .884$. The $R^2$-improvement over Model (2) was .195. The corresponding semi-partial $r = .442$.

In sum, the operative $r_{ZY} = .442$ in this instance, not .913. This represents the value of $r_{ZY}$ that is over and above the effects of other variables in the model assessed in previous waves of measurement. And it is this value, $r_{ZY} = .442$, that should be used in estimating the impact of estimation bias. Let me illustrate the impact of the difference between $r_{ZY} = .925$ and $r_{ZY} = .442$. With 50 % missing on Y, $r_{XY} = .20$, $r_{ZR} = .373$ (range = .50), and all variances = 1.0, SB = −31 with $r_{ZY} = .925$, and SB = −6.8 with $r_{ZY} = .442$.

▶ **Sample Data.** The input data set for this example is ex1.dat. Sample SAS code for analyzing these data is given below.[8]

```
data a;infile 'ex1.dat';
   input smoke7 smoke8 smoke9 smoke10;
   array x smoke7 smoke8 smoke9 smoke10;
*** recode "-9" values to system missing (".");
     do over x;
        if x=-9 then x=.;
     end;
  *** generate "missingness" (R10) for smoke10;
  if smoke10=. then r10=0;else r10=1;
run;

*** produce a quartilized version of smoke10;
proc rank data=a out=b groups=4;var smoke10;ranks z10;
run;

*** Generate EM covariance matrix (see chapters 2 and 7
        for details;
proc mi data=b nimpute=0;
  em outem=c;
  var smoke7 smoke8 smoke9 smoke10 z10;
run;
*** Regression with EM covariance matrix as input (see
        Chapter 7 for details;
proc reg data=c(type=cov);
  model smoke10=z10;
  model smoke10=smoke7 smoke8 smoke9;
  model smoke10=smoke7 smoke8 smoke9 z10;
run;
quit;
```

---

[8] SPSS and other statistical packages can certainly be used for this assessment. The EM covariance matrix is used here mainly as a convenience. If you are making use of SPSS, please see Chaps. 3 and 5 for details of performing comparable analyses in SPSS.

## Estimating $r_{ZR}$

Estimating $r_{ZR}$ can be tricky, but it is possible with longitudinal data. Recall that missingness is operationally defined as a binary variable, $R$ ($R_{10}$ in this case), that takes on the value 1 if the data point is observed, and 0 if the data point is missing. Thus, it is an easy matter to create this variable for the same data I presented in the previous example. This variable is generated using the statement just before "run" in the first data step of the SAS code shown above.

The main problem in estimating $r_{ZR}$ is that it is not possible to perform a correlation or regression analysis with $R_{10}$ and $Smoke_{10}$ in the same model; $r_{ZR}$ is undefined because data for $Smoke_{10}$ are available only when $R_{10}=1$, and a correlation cannot be calculated when one of the variables is a constant. Therefore, there is no direct test of the relationship between $Smoke_{10}$ and $R_{10}$. However, it is often possible to examine other correlations and regressions that give one a sense of what the relationship might be between $Smoke_{10}$ and $R_{10}$. I recommend the sequence of models described below.

Model (1): A regression model with $Smoke_7$ predicting $R_{10}$.
For model (1), $R^2=.0141$. The corresponding $r=.119$. Clearly, $Smoke_7$, taken by itself, is not an important predictor of $R_{10}$, missingness at tenth grade.

Model (2): Add $Smoke_8$ to Model (1) as a second predictor.
For model (2), $R^2=.0174$; $R^2$-improvement$=.0033$. The corresponding semi-partial $r=.057$. It is clear that $Smoke_8$ did not add appreciably to the prediction of $R_{10}$.

Model (3): Add $Smoke_9$ to Model (2) as a third predictor.
For model (3), $R^2=.0175$. $R^2$-improvement$=.0001$. The corresponding semi-partial $r=.01$. It is clear (a) that $Smoke_9$ did not add appreciably to the prediction of $R_{10}$, and (b) that even taken together, the seventh, eighth, and ninth grade measures of smoking contributed very little to the prediction of $R_{10}$. I discuss the implications of these results in the next section.

▶ **Sample Data.** The input data set for this example is ex1.dat. The sample SAS statements would be added to the end of the code for the previous example.

```
proc mi data=b nimpute=0;
    *** details of proc mi are given in Chapter 7;
    *** basics of EM algorithm are given in Chapter 2;
    em outem=d;
    var smoke7 smoke8 smoke9 r10;
run;

*** regression analyses with EM covariance matrix as input;
proc reg data=d(type=cov);
    model r10=smoke7;
    model r10=smoke7 smoke8;
    model r10=smoke7 smoke8 smoke9;
run;
quit;
```

## Sensitivity Analysis

A sensitivity analysis (e.g., see Little 1993, 1994, 1995) in this context would examine the effect on estimation bias when a range of values is used, rather than a point estimate, for quantities (e.g., $r_{XY}$, $r_{ZY}$, and $r_{ZR}$) for which information is limited. If the results show that bias is small through the entire range of values examined, then one has greater confidence that the true level of bias is small.

The relevant quantities for doing a sensitivity analysis in this instance are percent missing, $r_{XY}$, $r_{ZY}$, and $r_{ZR}$. Estimates of the first three quantities are relatively straightforward, as described above. The first quantity, percent missing, is a given. The two correlations $r_{XY}$ and $r_{ZY}$, although not known precisely, are likely to be at least similar to the values estimated from EM analyses. The fourth quantity, $r_{ZR}$, is the biggest question mark.

In the analyses described above, I did not show anything that relates directly to the relationship between $Smoke_{10}$ and $R_{10}$. However, with longitudinal data, it is often reasonable to extrapolate that relationship by examining the trends for data that are available. In the three models just tested, for example, the $R^2$-improvements due to each smoking variable were .0141, .0033, and .0001, for smoke7, smoke8, and smoke9, respectively. The corresponding semi-partial correlations were .119, .057, and .01. With a trend like this, we are in a good position to posit plausible values for $r_{ZR}$ involving $Smoke_{10}$ and $R_{10}$. In this instance, would you be surprised to learn that the true $r_{ZR}=.01$? Would you be surprised to learn that the true $r_{ZR}=.10$? Would you be surprised to learn that the true $r_{ZR}=.30$? Although the first two correlations are clearly within the realm of plausibility, the third correlation, $r_{ZR}=.30$, seems high. I do not mean that $r_{ZR}=.30$ is not ever plausible; I just mean that in this scenario it seems too high. What possible psychological, social, or administrative process might produce such a jump in this correlation in this situation?

My point here is that we can make use of this information to develop values that can be used for a sensitivity analysis. Even setting $r_{ZR}=.30$, in the context of the other quantities that are more easily estimated, produces a level of bias that can be described as tolerably low, or even not statistically significant. For example, with 50 % missing on Y, $r_{ZR}=.30$ (which corresponds to range=.40 with 50 % missing), $r_{ZY}=.45$, $r_{XY}=.20$, and all variances set to 1.0, SB=−4.5. And with a simulation with 500 replications, this degree of bias would not be statistically significant (see below).

In a previous section, I noted that the statistical significance of estimation bias can be calculated using (a) the average bias, (b) the standard deviation of the bias, and (c) the number of replications of the simulation.

$$t(df) = (\bar{b} - \beta) / \left(S_b / \sqrt{Nreps}\right) \qquad (1.1)$$

where $\beta$ is the population parameter value, $\bar{b}$ is the average parameter estimate over the number of simulation replications (Nreps), $S_b$ is the standard deviation of b over the Nreps, and the df for the t is Nreps-2 ($df=498$ in this case). The *t*-value

# Sensitivity Analysis

**Table 1.4** Cutoffs for statistical nonsignificant estimation bias

| $r_{ZY}$ | Maximum $r_{ZR}$ for statistical non-signif. | Range | IF statement probabilities | | | |
|---|---|---|---|---|---|---|
| | | | Q1 | Q2 | Q3 | Q4 |
| .925 | .200 | .27 | .366 | .455 | .545 | .634 |
| .80 | .216 | .29 | .355 | .452 | .548 | .645 |
| .70 | .261 | .35 | .325 | .442 | .558 | .675 |
| .60 | .306 | .41 | .295 | .432 | .568 | .705 |
| .50 | .373 | .50 | .250 | .417 | .583 | .750 |
| .40 | .455 | .61 | .195 | .398 | .602 | .805 |
| .20 | .738 | .99 | .005 | .335 | .665 | .995 |

*Note*: In each row, $r_{ZR}$ less than or equal to the value shown yields nonsignificant estimation bias. These figures hold for N=500, Nreps=500, and $r_{XY}$ = .20. Q1, Q2, Q3, and Q4 represent the four quartiles of Z, the cause of missingness on Y. Range = Q4 − Q1

for testing the significance of the bias can also be calculated from the standardized bias (SB) as,

$$t(df) = SB \times \sqrt{Nreps} / 100. \quad (1.2)$$

So with a little rearranging, it is easy to see that when Nreps=500, |SB|≤8.7 represents statistically nonsignificant bias (i.e., $t \leq 1.95$).

The statistical significance of the bias is clearly dependent on Nreps. Simulations with large Nreps are much more likely to discover significant bias than are simulations with smaller Nreps, because as Nreps gets large, the denominator of (1.1) gets smaller, and t becomes larger. However, for comparison purposes, it is possible to fix Nreps at some reasonable value. Table 1.4, which is based on Nreps=500, can be used to help in sensitivity analyses. The left column of the table lists a range of values for $r_{ZY}$. The second column of the table shows the corresponding maximum values of $r_{ZR}$ for which estimation bias for the regression coefficient for X predicting Y remains nonsignificant. The values in the remaining columns show the range and IF statements for MAR-linear missingness that produce the value of $r_{ZR}$ shown.

Table 1.5 shows the maximum values for $r_{ZR}$ that correspond to estimation bias that is nonsignificant in a practical sense, using the criterion of SB<.40 used by Collins et al. (2001).

## *Plausibility of MAR Given in Tables 1.4 and 1.5*

The figures shown in Tables 1.4 and 1.5 paint a very optimistic picture about the plausibility of MAR. Let me focus for the moment on the figures shown in Table 1.4. Even when $r_{ZY}$=.925, estimation bias will not be statistically significant as long as $r_{ZR}$ is no larger than about $r_{ZR}$=.20. This will actually cover a rather wide range of circumstances, the example described above with AAPT data being one of them. But with the more realistic estimates of $r_{ZY}$ shown in Table 1.4 (e.g., .80, .70, .60,

**Table 1.5** Cutoffs for practical nonsignificant estimation bias

| $r_{ZY}$ | Maximum $r_{ZR}$ for practical non-signif. | Range | IF Statement Probabilities | | | |
|---|---|---|---|---|---|---|
| | | | Q1 | Q2 | Q3 | Q4 |
| .925 | .417 | .56 | .220 | .407 | .593 | .780 |
| .80 | .484 | .65 | .175 | .392 | .608 | .825 |
| .70 | .552 | .74 | .130 | .377 | .623 | .870 |
| .60 | .641 | .86 | .070 | .357 | .643 | .930 |
| .50 | .738 | .99 | .005 | .335 | .665 | .995 |
| .40 | .738 | .99 | .005 | .335 | .665 | .995 |
| .20 | .738 | .99 | .005 | .335 | .665 | .995 |

*Note*: In each row, $r_{ZR}$ less than or equal to the value shown yields nonsignificant estimation bias. These figures hold for $N=500$, and $r_{XY}=.20$. Q1, Q2, Q3, and Q4 represent the four quartiles of Z, the cause of missingness on Y. Range = Q4 − Q1

.50, or even lower), the probability is even higher that estimation bias will be nonsignificant in a statistical sense (with Nreps = 500).

If the figures shown in Table 1.4 are optimistic, those shown in Table 1.5 are striking. With $r_{ZY}=.60$, or .50, which will be realistic in many longitudinal studies, the chances are actually very slim that estimation bias will be significant in a practical sense.

## *Limitations (Nuisance Factors) Relating to Figures in Tables 1.4 and 1.5*

The new findings presented here are good news indeed. They suggest that MAR missingness will very often be a highly plausible assumption. However, there are issues that must be presented and dealt with. Some of these issues relate to the assessment of statistical significance of bias; other issues relate to the assessment of practical significance of bias.

### Nuisance Factors Affecting Statistical Significance of Bias

The main nuisance factor here is the fact that the same level of bias will be judged to be nonsignificant with a simulation involving Nreps = 500, but statistically significant with Nreps = 5,000. This is akin to the fact that an effect of a particular magnitude, say $r=.10$, is nonsignificant with $N=100$, $t(98)=0.99$, but is statistically significant with $N=500$, $t(498)=2.24$, $p<.05$. This would not be a huge problem if researchers could agree on some specific Nreps that would be used in this context, regardless of the number of actually used in the simulation. I believe that Nreps = 500 would be a reasonable starting place for this.

Table 1.6 Standardized bias with different study sample size

| $r_{XY}$ | $r_{XZ}$ | $r_{ZY}$ | Range ($r_{ZR}$) | Study $N$ | Standardized bias | Relative bias |
|---|---|---|---|---|---|---|
| .20 | .185 | .925 | .50 (.373) | 500 | −31.0 | −.1009 |
| .20 | .185 | .925 | .50 (.373) | 1000 | −43.8 | −.1009 |
| .20 | .185 | .925 | .50 (.373) | 2000 | −62.0 | −.1009 |
| .20 | .185 | .925 | .50 (.373) | 8000 | −124.1 | −.1009 |

**Nuisance Factors Affecting Practical Significance of Bias**

Similar nuisance factors affect the assessment of the practical significance of bias. In this instance, the study sample size is a big issue. The simulations conducted by Collins et al. (2001) and by Graham et al. (2008; also see Chap. 10) all used $N=500$. With larger sample sizes, however, SB would be larger. Table 1.6 shows a simple study that varies the sample size, keeping all other factors the same.

As shown in Table 1.6, SB doubles as the study N quadruples. As I suggested above, bias of 31 means that the $t$-value is (in this case) too small by .31. For example, a true $t=2.41$ would appear to be $t=2.10$. It makes sense that increased sample size would increase the $t$-value for differences between group (program and control). Thus it also makes sense that the amount by which the $t$-value would be off due to bias would also increase (as shown in Table 1.6).

A second nuisance issue in this context is the variance of the X, Y, and Z. As shown in Chap. 10, SB is substantially affected by these variances (higher variance is associated with higher SB).

The solution to these nuisance issues should be straightforward. The variance issue can easily be solved by standardizing all variables using variance = 1.0. For the study $N$, the solution might be the same as before. If researchers could agree, we could always estimate SB with study $N=500$.

## *Call for New Measures of the Practical Significance of Bias*

In Graham (2009), I encouraged researchers to begin using SB, but also to develop other indicators of the practical significance of bias. Statisticians have taken several approaches to assessing this kind of bias. Raw bias is the (average) difference between the parameter estimate and its population value. Although raw bias is not particularly valuable in and of itself, most other approaches to assessing bias start with this. One test, which I described above, is the statistical test of whether the raw bias is significantly different from 0 in a statistical sense. As I noted above, I believe this test can be quite useful, but it is limited because in simulation work the bias is more likely to be statistically significant as the number of simulation replications increases.

Another test compares the bias against the SE of the estimate. I also described this above (standardized bias; SB). I believe that this measure can also be very useful, but as I described above, SB is limited in the sense that its magnitude is positively related to the study sample size. Other quantities that have been used in this context include comparisons against the standard deviation (e.g., see Bose 2001), relative bias (comparison of the bias against the magnitude of the parameter), and root-mean-square error (square root of the average squared difference between the parameter estimate and its population value).

Other areas of statistics, most notably structural equation modeling (SEM), have made very good use of practical indices of related quantities. In SEM, goodness of fit was a critical issue. It is important that goodness of fit involves the comparison between some standard (the true covariance matrix) and something estimated (the covariance matrix implied by the SEM model). Thus, many of the concepts inherent in the assessment of measurement bias have been found in the SEM goodness of fit literature.

The SEM counterpart to raw bias is the residual covariance matrix, that is, the matrix showing the element-by-element comparison between the real and implied covariance matrices. The test of statistical significance is the chi-square test, which provides a statistical test for the element-by-element comparison between real and implied covariance matrices. Similar to what was said about the statistical test of bias, it has long been known that the chi-square significance test is seriously affected by sample size, such that with large sample sizes, even trivial deviations from good fit were statistically significant by this test.

In response to this problem, SEM researchers have developed several indices of practical fit that have enjoyed much popularity, for example, Rho (Tucker and Lewis 1973; also known as the non-normed fit index; NNFI; Bentler and Bonett 1980), the comparative fit index (CFI; Bentler 1990), and the root-mean-square error of approximation (RMSEA; Browne and Cudeck 1993; Steiger and Lind 1980).

I often think of the chi-square test as a comparison of one's model against the perfect model. That is, if the chi-square is significant, it means that one's model deviates significantly from the perfectly fitting model. Practical indices known as comparative fit indices (Rho/NNFI and CFI) seek to compare the fit of the model under study against a very bad-fitting model, often referred to as the "independence" model. The model most often used in this connection is one in which variances are estimated, but all covariances are fixed at 0. Conceptually, the indices of practical fit that make use of this independence model represent the percent of the way from the poor fitting model (0) to the perfect model (100). And it is generally considered good fit if the fit of one's model is 95 % of the way from poor fit to good fit (e.g., Hu and Bentler 1999).

One variant of the NNFI is the normed fit index (NFI; Bentler and Bonett 1980). Although seldom used in SEM because of its sensitivity to sample size, it is relevant in the estimation bias context because it is so similar to what has been referred to as *relative bias*, the comparison of the raw bias to the parameter value. The formula for the NFI is:

$$\text{NFI} = \frac{X^2_{\text{Indep.}} - X^2_{\text{Model}}}{X^2_{\text{Indep.}}}, \quad 1 - \text{NFI} = \frac{X^2_{\text{Model}}}{X^2_{\text{Indep.}}}$$

Sensitivity Analysis

where the independence model is one that estimates variances but not covariances. Although this index is scaled so that a large value (e.g., .95) represents good fit, it makes more sense in the estimation bias context to reverse scale it (1−NFI) so that small values reflect good fit. Of course, this rescaled version has the same form as what statisticians have referred to as relative bias:

$$\text{Relative Bias (RB)} = \frac{\text{Raw Bias}}{\theta_{Pop}} = \frac{\theta_{Est} - \theta_{Pop}}{\theta_{Pop}}$$

## Preliminary Evaluation of RB

RB has the advantage of not being sensitive to sample size. For example, given the scenarios shown in Table 1.6, RB=−.101 for all Ns shown in the table. However, RB *is* sensitive to the magnitude of the parameter. The relationship between SB and RB is a constant over all conditions within a single level of $r_{XY}$. However, that relationship varies over different levels of $r_{XY}$. For example, holding RB constant,

When $r_{XY}$ = .10, conditions that lead to SB =∼ 15 produce RB =∼ .10.
When $r_{XY}$ = .20, conditions that lead to SB =∼ 30 produce RB =∼ .10.
When $r_{XY}$ = .40, conditions that lead to SB =∼ 65 produce RB =∼ .10.
When $r_{XY}$ = .60, conditions that lead to SB =∼ 113 produce RB =∼ .10.

Alternatively, holding SB constant,

When $r_{XY}$ = .10, conditions that lead to SB =∼ 30 produce RB =∼ .21.
When $r_{XY}$ = .20, conditions that lead to SB =∼ 30 produce RB =∼ .10.
When $r_{XY}$ = .40, conditions that lead to SB =∼ 30 produce RB =∼ .045.
When $r_{XY}$ = .60, conditions that lead to SB =∼ 30 produce RB =∼ .026.

## Conclusions About Relative Bias

A strength of RB is that it is not sensitive to sample size. Another strength is that it is a percentage of the magnitude of the parameter. We could say, for example, that if the bias is no more than 10 % of the magnitude of the parameter value, then it is small enough to be tolerable. A weakness of RB is that 10 % of a large parameter can be associated with a very large *t*-value (in comparison to no bias), and even with a large SB.

One possibility is that RB and SB can be used together. For example, when SB < 40 and RB < 10, we can perhaps have greatest confidence that the level of bias is tolerably small. For example, the following conditions might produce bias that is judged to be tolerably small:

When $r_{XY} = .10$, conditions that lead to SB $=\sim 15.1$ produce RB $=\sim .10$.
When $r_{XY} = .20$, conditions that lead to SB $=\sim 30.7$ produce RB $=\sim .10$.
When $r_{XY} = .40$, conditions that lead to SB $=\sim 40$ produce RB $=\sim .060$.
When $r_{XY} = .60$, conditions that lead to SB $=\sim 40$ produce RB $=\sim .034$.

It could also be that bias should be judged tolerably small if either of these conditions is met (SB < 40 or RB < .10). With smaller effect sizes, SB would take precedence; with larger effect sizes, RB would take precedence.

One other index of bias that is commonly used in this context is the root-mean-square error (square root of the average squared difference between the parameter estimate and its population value). Other indices that have been used in SEM, and that may or may not find counterparts in this context, are the RMSEA (root-mean-square error of approximation), the AIC (Akaike information criterion), and the BIC (Bayesian information criterion). The concept for the RMSEA was to give up on the idea of statistically good fit, and settle for establishing whether or not one had "close" fit. The AIC and BIC have enjoyed some popularity, especially in the area of latent class model fit.

Time will tell whether any of the indices already in use will prove to be helpful in describing bias that is or is not of practical significance. Time will also tell whether some of the other indices (RMSEA, AIC, BIC) can find useful counterparts in the bias assessment domain. In the meantime, I continue to encourage researchers to develop new indices that can be used for this purpose. I also encourage researchers to adopt the approach taken by SEM researchers in developing, and gaining experience with, indices that can help us identify when bias is and is not of practical significance.

## *Other Limitations of Figures Presented in Tables 1.4 and 1.5*

In this chapter, I have painted a very optimistic picture regarding the appropriateness of using MAR methods for handling missing data problems. It would appear from my writing that MAR virtually always holds. Indeed I am very optimistic about the idea that MAR holds a great deal of the time. However, I also acknowledge that my research experience is based predominantly in the area of prevention research. An important characteristic of this research domain is that the research is conducted almost exclusively on nonclinical populations.

To be honest, the effect sizes of interventions on these populations are not substantial. It is not at all unusual in these populations, for example, to find program effect sizes that are considered "small" in Cohen's (1977) terms (i.e., $r = .10$ or $d = .20$). We would expect much more substantial effect sizes in clinical research. For example in the drug treatment study described by Hedeker and Gibbons (1997;

also see Enders 2011), the program effect size was much larger, between medium and large in Cohen's terms ($r=.40$). So it would appear that the variant of Ben Franklin's adage, "an ounce of prevention is worth a pound of cure" is also true in the sense that preventive (primary prevention, universal) interventions tend to have less impact on the individual participants' lives than do curative (including targeted and indicated) interventions.

My point here is that the MAR assumption may be very likely to hold (in a statistical or practical sense) in research studies that involve nonclinical populations because the interventions have relatively little impact on all factors relating to these study participants, including factors relating to study participation. That is, it will be rare for universal preventive interventions to have more than a small impact on participants' decisions about remaining in the program (this point also applies to longitudinal studies that do not involve an intervention).

For curative (or targeted/indicated) interventions, on the other hand, because they do have much more dramatic impact on all factors relating to the participants' lives, are much more likely to relate to the reasons why people remain in or drop out of a research study that involves a curative intervention.

I am NOT saying that MAR assumptions do not hold or are less likely to hold in such studies. Indeed, the figures presented in this chapter (e.g., the figures in Tables 1.4 and 1.5) are most certainly also relevant in studies involving curative interventions. All I am saying here is that I have very little personal experience with research on clinical populations.

## Another Substantive Consideration: A Taxonomy of Attrition

There is another important consideration in the study of missingness, especially as it applies to drop out or attrition in longitudinal studies. The simulations conducted by Collins et al. (2001) and the follow-up simulations conducted by Graham et al. (2008; Chap. 10) all dealt with a particular category of missingness. This prior work was all based on a relatively simple regression model in which X predicted Y. Missingness on Y was a function of a variable Z. In this chapter I have described the IF statements used to generate the missingness on Y. Virtually all of this prior work can all be thought of as dealing with the situation in which Y (or some variant of Y) was the cause of its own missingness (although see the MAR-sinister simulations by Collins et al. 2001). The variable X in the substantive model used in those simulations had nothing to do with missingness on Y.

Graham et al. (2008) suggested an expanded taxonomy of missingness that examined three possible causes of missingness in the context of attrition from a program: Program (P; or Treatment; same as X in everything presented up to now in this chapter), Y, and the interaction between them (PY).[9] We suggested eight

---

[9] Note that everything I describe in this section can also be applied to the situation in which the predictor variable is a measured variable and not a manipulated program intervention variable.

possible combinations of these three causes. I present a slight rearrangement of the eight cases here:

Case 1: none of these causes
Case 2: P only
Case 3: Y only
Case 4: P and Y (but no PY interaction)
Case 5: PY interaction only
Case 6: P and PY (but not Y)
Case 7: Y and PY (but not P)
Case 8: P, Y, and PY

Case 1 is essentially MCAR missingness and presents no problem due to attrition. Case 2 is MAR given that P will always be in program, or treatment effects models. Case 3 is the situation in which only Y is the cause of its own missingness. As I have noted above, based on the Collins et al. (2001) simulations, and on the follow-up simulations, despite being NMAR, Case 3 is also not a problem for program, or treatment effects analyses. The remaining cases (4–8), however, have not been studied systematically.

## *The Value of Missing Data Diagnostics*

Future research must focus on the other cases of attrition. The tools for studying these cases will come from, or be closely related to, the tools already described in this chapter for studying case 3. However, new tools must be brought to bear on the study of these other cases. Missing data diagnostics are one such tool.

**Pretest Comparisons**

I have often seen researchers compare pretest measures, where everyone has data, for those who drop out of a study and those who stay. This practice does have some value, to be sure, but its value is limited. It is commonly the case that those who drop out are different, so there is no real surprise there. Also, any variable for which there are differences may simply be included in missing data analysis model, and all biases related to that variable are removed. I often say that what you can see (i.e., what is measured) cannot hurt you. What can hurt you, in the sense of bias, are differences on variables for which you do not have data. It is important to note that pretest comparisons do not allow the researcher to determine whether the MAR assumption holds.

It is useful to conduct pretest comparisons in order to identify variables that are related to missingness, and that should be included in the missing data analysis. Occasionally, an important variable can be found in the process. However, unless the study is of very short duration (e.g., if the study has just two waves of measurement),

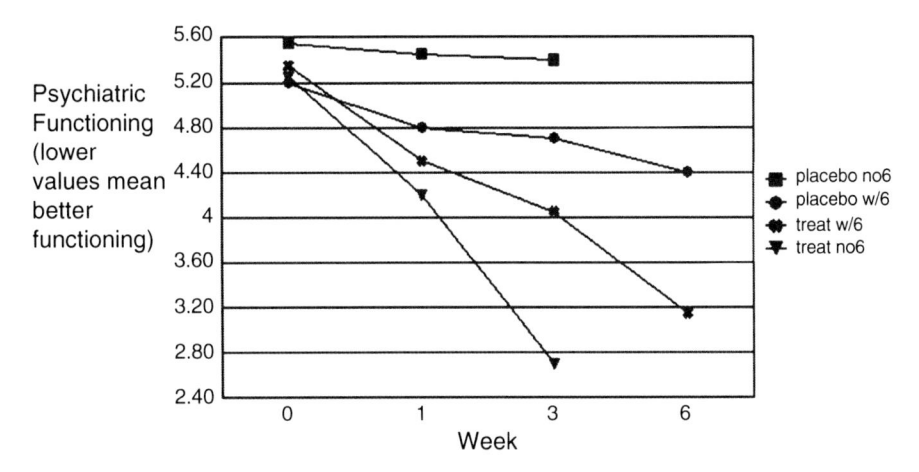

**Fig. 1.1** Psychiatric functioning at weeks 0, 1, 3, and 6. The four curves shown are based on approximate means for these four groups, from top to bottom: placebo control missing week 6 data; placebo control with week 6 data; drug treatment with week 6 data; drug treatment with week 6 data

the relationship between pretest variables and drop out is generally a weak one. And when the relationship is weak between pretest measures and missingness, the value of including such measures in the missing data analysis model is minimal.

It is certainly not a bad thing if no differences are found on pretest variables between stayers and leavers. But the lack of differences on pretest variables is inconclusive by itself; it amounts to arguing for the null hypothesis, which is a risky business. In any case, it is not the lack of difference on measured variables that matters; one really wants lack of difference on variables for which one does not have data.

**Longitudinal Diagnostics**

On the other hand, examining patterns of missingness over multiple waves of measurement can be extremely helpful. Hedeker and Gibbons (1997) presented data from a Psychiatric Clinical Trial on treatment for schizophrenia. Patients in the study were divided into the Drug Treatment and Placebo Control groups. The primary measurements were taken at weeks 0, 1, 3, and 6. In studying pattern mixture models, Hedeker and Gibbons plotted their data in four groups: Control with week 6 data missing; Control with data for week 6; Treatment with data for week 6; and Treatment with week 6 data missing. Figure 1.1 presents a representation of these plots, approximated from the 1997 paper, and combined into a single figure.

Imagine that the plots shown in Fig. 1.1 were such that the only data available were from weeks 0 and 6 (the two end points). Then one would have no clue where the missing values might be; they could plausibly be anywhere across the range of observed responses. In this situation, Little's (1994) "pessimist" would be correct in saying "… predictions of [the dependent variable] for nonrespondents could take any form, and thus nothing can honestly be said about [the mean of the dependent variable]" (p. 482).

But the plots shown in Fig. 1.1 are based on multiple time points, and thus they show clearly how each of the four groups is changing over time. As Little (1994) suggests, if information is available from other measured variables, then one is able to incorporate that information into the missing data analysis model, and the situation is not as dire as commonly supposed. The upshot here is that plots such as those in Fig. 1.1 can give one a degree of confidence in extrapolating to the missing data points.[10]

With the plots showing rather consistent changes over time within each of the four groups, it makes most sense that the missing point for the topmost plot is at least somewhere in the vicinity of the extension of that plot. Similarly, it makes most sense that the missing point for the bottom-most plot is at least somewhere in the vicinity of the extension of that plot. Although there may well be a plausible substantive theoretical explanation that would have the top curve bending downward, and the bottom curve bending upward, it makes little conceptual sense for the missing point for the top curve to be near the bottom of the range, or for the missing point for the bottom curve to be near the top of the range.

## *Nonignorable Methods*

Nonignorable methods, especially pattern mixture models (Demirtas and Schafer 2003; Hedeker and Gibbons 1997; Little 1993, 1994, 1995), may be useful when there is good reason to believe, and evidence to support the idea that the missingness goes beyond what can be handled by MAR methods (MI and ML). However, one must be careful about selecting the model that created the missingness. Using the wrong model with these methods can produce results that are more biased than are the MAR methods (Demirtas and Schafer 2003).

## *Sensitivity Analysis*

Little (e.g., 1994) has suggested the use of sensitivity analyses in conjunction with pattern mixture models. He talked about the idea that missingness on Y being a function of X (a measured covariate) and Y, and he posited a parameter $\lambda$, which indicated the degree to which Y, over and above X, was responsible for its own missingness. Rewriting his formula with my notation, it would be:

$$R_Y = X + \lambda Y$$

---

[10] Note that the plots shown in Table 1.1 could also be based on more than two levels of a measured independent variable.

Little suggested that one could examine the mean of Y and the 95 % confidence interval for several different values of $\lambda$. However, he also suggested that

> [a]nother way is to create draws from the posterior distribution, but with a different value of $\lambda$ for each draw sampled from a prior distribution of plausible values. The result would be a single wider interval for [the mean of Y]. Of course this interval is sensitive to the choice of prior, but a choice that provides for nonzero $\lambda$'s may be more plausible than the prior implied by the standard ignorable-model analysis, which puts all the probability at the value $\lambda = 0$ (pp. 480-481).

I really like this idea of taking random draws from a prior distribution of plausible values of $\lambda$ (also see Demirtas 2005 for a similar Bayesian strategy). But I would prefer to take a somewhat different approach. For starters, I would want to be very clear about who decides the plausibility of individual values of $\lambda$ (or comparable parameters). I would prefer that the substantive researcher, in close collaboration with the statistician, make these judgments. I would also prefer that the judgments about plausible values of the missing Y would come from substantive theory rather than from statistical theory. Then statistical theory would be matched with the substantive theory to help with the prediction.

It also makes sense, especially in longitudinal studies, that judgments be made about the missing values on a case-by-case basis. For example, look at the explanation given by Demirtas and Schafer (2003) as to why people in the Hedeker and Gibbons (1997) data were missing. Demirtas and Schafer suggested that dropouts from the placebo control group (the top curve in Fig. 1.1), who had the least favorable trajectory, may have dropped out because of the apparent failure of the treatment. They also suggested that dropouts from the drug treatment group (bottom curve in Fig. 1.1), who had the most favorable trajectory, may have dropped out because they judged that they were cured and no longer needed treatment. These possibilities do seem plausible given the trajectories shown in Fig. 1.1. However, these are average trajectories. Some individuals who showed this basic pattern may have dropped for the suggested reasons. However, some individuals with this basic pattern may still have dropped out for other reasons. Also, individuals who had different patterns are much more likely to have dropped out for other reasons.

My suggestion is that the substantive researchers should work hard to come up with several substantive theoretical models that would allow extrapolation from the known data. Each theoretical model would be matched as best as possible, with an appropriate statistical model to achieve the predictions about the missing values. Then the substantive researchers would make judgments about the relative plausibility of the various substantive theories. These judgments would generate a probability density function for the various theories, and random draws from that prior distribution would then produce the sensitivity analysis described by Little (1994).

I want to highlight two aspects of this approach. First, the models themselves should be derived from substantive theory, not statistical theory. Statistical theory would be applied as needed as a second step. Second, the relative plausibility of the various theoretical models would mean that the distribution of values would be based on substantive theoretical considerations and not on statistical ones.

## Design and Measurement Strategies for Assuring MAR

I have heard it said that the best way to deal with missingness, especially attrition, is not to have it. The same can be said for NMAR missingness, per se. It is best if one can convert NMAR to MAR. Three strategies have been described in the literature for helping to reduce or eliminate NMAR missingness, especially due to attrition. I present these below.

### *Measure the Possible Causes of Missingness*

Little (1995) talked about the importance of information about the missing data process. Schafer and Graham (2002; also see Demirtas and Schafer 2003) have argued for including measures about intention to drop out of later survey sessions. Leon et al. (2007) simulated the inclusion of intent to drop out, and showed that this approach can be useful for reducing bias associated with attrition.

Graham et al. (1994) suggested a broad list of the potential causes of a variety of types of missingness. They suggested measuring a wide variety of causes, including slow reading speed, lack of motivation (e.g., for completing a survey), rebelliousness, transiency, reasons for parents refusing to allow participation, and indirect measures of processes associated with the dependent variable being the cause of its own missingness.

Most of the potential sources of missingness they suggested continue to have value, but I want to focus here on attrition. For a variety of reasons, other kinds of missingness generally prove to have less impact on study conclusions. In Table 1.7, following Graham et al. (1994), I suggest several measures as proxies for processes that could account for the person dropping out of the study after one or more waves of measurement.

The questions shown in Table 1.7 come from a recent school-based adolescent drug prevention study (Drug Resistance Strategies-Rural; DRSR; Colby et al. in press). These questions are part of a survey given to all participants. I would normally include these measures early in the survey. When I am using the 3-form design (which is very often in my school-based studies), these questions would always be in the "X" set of questions (i.e., asked of everyone; see Chap. 12).

Measuring possible causes of attrition is a good strategy because it is likely to reduce estimation bias. An important point here is that variables such as these need not account for all of the cause of missingness. If they even reduce the uncertainty, it is very possible that the amount of estimation bias is reduced to tolerably low levels. Examine Tables 1.4 and 1.5, for example. It is easy to see from examining these tables that the correlation between the cause and missingness itself, under realistic conditions, does not need to be $r=0$ for bias to be nonsignificant in a statistical or practical sense.

Table 1.7 Measuring possible causes of attrition

| Construct | Process; relationship with attrition | Specific questionnaire items | Notes |
|---|---|---|---|
| Reading speed | This question relates mainly to missingness at the end of a long survey, and not attrition, per se. However, it is also applicable to attrition from a school-based study in the sense that it fits with a general orientation toward one's education | **How fast can you READ in the language used in this survey?**<br>Very fast<br>Fast<br>Moderately fast<br>A little slow<br>Slow | Data for one wave of the DRSR study showed that this item had a small but significant correlation ($r=-09$) with the number of variables completed on the last page of the survey (faster reading corresponded with more data). However, the magnitude of this correlation may have been affected by the fact that only about 4 % of the respondents failed to answer the questions on the last page of the survey |
| How far will you get in school? | This measures school orientation (or educational expectations). It is definitely relevant to attrition from a school-based study | **How far do you think you will get in school? Do you think you will: (please give just one answer)**<br>Finish 4 years of college<br>Finish 2 years of college<br>Finish a trade school or vocational school program<br>Finish high school<br>Finish eighth grade | In the DRSR study, 11 % of those measured at wave 2 (spring of seventh grade) were missing at wave 3 (spring of eighth grade). This variable was correlated $r=-.17$ with missingness at wave 3 (students expecting to complete more school were more likely to provide data at wave 3). This variable also had a small, but significant correlation ($r=-.05$) with completing the last page of the wave 3 survey (more school associated with more data) |

(continued)

Table 1.7 (continued)

| Construct | Process; relationship with attrition | Specific questionnaire items | Notes |
|---|---|---|---|
| Grades in school (GPA) | This measures school achievement. All things being equal, better students are more likely to respond better to school-based interventions; students with lower grades are more likely to drop out, or to miss school-based activities such as measurement sessions for school-based interventions | *What grades do you usually get in school?*<br>Mostly As<br>As and Bs<br>Mostly Bs<br>Bs and Cs<br>Mostly Cs<br>Cs and Ds<br>Mostly Ds<br>Ds and Fs<br>Mostly Fs | My colleagues and I have been using this question for years. It has proven to have value in predicting attrition. Based on EM algorithm correlations for AAPT data (Hansen and Graham 1991). Grades at ninth grade was correlated $r=-.25$ with missingness at tenth grade (students with higher grades were more likely to provide data at tenth grade)<br>In DRSR data, this variable in spring of seventh grade showed an EM correlation of $r=-.19$ with having data at spring of eighth grade (students with higher grades in seventh grade were more likely to provide data in eighth grade) |

Design and Measurement Strategies for Assuring MAR 41

| | | |
|---|---|---|
| General motivation; conscientious-ness; civic engagement | When I originally came up with this idea, it was focused on motivation to complete a long survey. However, in its more general form, conscientiousness can be predictive of many activities, including attrition from any kind of study | *How much are you like this: once I start something I want to do, I really want to finish it*<br>Exactly like me<br>Pretty much like me<br>Somewhat like me<br>A little like me<br>Not at all like me<br>*How much are you like this: if it is my duty to do something, I do it*<br>Exactly like me<br>Pretty much like me<br>Somewhat like me<br>A little like me<br>Not at all like me | DRSR data: these variables have proven to be related in important ways to other variables in our survey. However, thus far, we have seen only a modest correlation between these variables and drop out (multiple R = −.09 for the spring seventh grade version of these two variables predicting missingness at wave 3, spring eighth grade). These two variables (in spring of eighth grade) showed a disappointingly low correlation with missingness at the end of the survey |
| Civic engagement | This concept is related to conscientiousness, but I believe it applies more generally to taking part in society, however defined. It should also be related school engagement, and therefore should predict attrition | | I have not yet included measures of this construct in any of the studies in which I am involved |

(continued)

Table 1.7 (continued)

| Construct | Process; relationship with attrition | Specific questionnaire items | Notes |
|---|---|---|---|
| Mobility, transiency | These measures are clearly related to attrition; these are most consistent with what others have referred to as "intent to drop out" | *How likely is it that next year you will be in this school (or in the next higher school in this school system)?*<br>Extremely likely<br>Likely<br>Somewhat likely<br>A little likely<br>Not at all likely<br>*Since first grade, how many times have you changed schools because your family moved or because of some other family reason. Do NOT count times you changed schools just because you went to the next grade (like when you went from elementary to middle school or middle to high school)*<br>0 – I have not changed schools<br>1<br>2<br>3<br>4<br>5 or more | DRSR data: these two variables measured in spring of seventh grade were correlated with wave nonresponse at eighth grade, $r=-.27$ (those more likely to be in school were more likely to provide data in spring of eighth grade), and $r=-.20$ (those with more school changes were less like to provide data in spring of eighth grade). The multiple $R=.31$ for these two variables combined |

Another particularly good thing about this strategy is that it is easy and relatively inexpensive to implement. The specific measures that will help with attrition bias will vary across different research contexts, but the classes of variables described here will typically have counterparts in other research contexts. In addition, adding a few measures (along the lines of those described above) to one's measurement arsenal will typically be relatively easy and within one's budget.

## *Measure and Include Relevant Auxiliary Variables in Missing Data Analysis Model*

In Chap. 11, the chapter coauthor (Linda M. Collins) and I present a more detailed look at the use of auxiliary variables. Collins et al. (2001) showed that estimation bias could be reduced if an auxiliary variable (a variable highly correlated with Y, sometimes missing, but not part of the analysis model) were included in the missing data analysis model. Auxiliary variables are typically included as a matter of course in longitudinal studies. The same variable as the main DV, but measured at previous waves, is generally most highly correlated with the main DV. If such a variable is not already part of the analysis model, (e.g., as a covariate or part of a growth curve analysis), it can be added in a number of ways in the missing data analysis model. We describe this in more detail in Chap. 11, but for now, I will mention that the easiest way to take such variables into account is simply to add them to one's MI analysis (see Chaps. 3, 7, and 11).

## *Track and Collect Data on a Random Sample of Those Initially Missing*

Tracking and collecting data on those who are missing at the conclusion of the last wave of measurement represents perhaps the best approach to turning possible NMAR missingness into missingness that is clearly MAR. The logic here is that one identifies a random sample of those initially missing, and then tracks these individuals down, and measures them (see Glynn et al. 1993; Graham and Donaldson 1993). If the researcher is successful in measuring a large proportion (e.g., 80 %) of the targeted sample, then the data from the sample can be generalized to the remaining missing individuals, and the missingness becomes MAR.

Tracking and measuring respondents who were not available at the main measure can be expensive. However, one thing that makes this strategy feasible is that the costs of measuring the individuals in the targeted random sample can be focused on a relatively small number of individuals. That is, rather than having to spend, say, $200 per respondent on the full sample of 200 individuals initially missing (total costs: $40,000), one could expend, say, $500 per respondent, to track and measure 40 individuals from the targeted sample of 50 (total costs $25,000). Of course, these are hypothetical figures, but the point is that this strategy can be relatively cost-effective.

One problem, of course, is that tracking and measuring individuals who were initially missing from the main measurement wave can be a daunting task. When we attempted this kind of thing in the AAPT project, for example (see Graham et al. 1997), we were able to track and measure a percentage of the originally targeted sample that was much smaller than 80 %. However, even under these circumstances, one is still able to make good use of the new data collected (e.g., see Glynn et al. 1993). As I have said in this chapter, it is not necessary to remove all of the NMAR missingness in order to achieve bias that is tolerably small. Future research must bear this out, but I believe that even when one is able to track and measure only some of the targeted sample, and perhaps augment this with others tracked and measured from the group of those initially missing, one will generally convert enough of the NMAR missingness to MAR to make MAR methods reasonable.

**Follow-Up Measures as Auxiliary Variables**

When one speaks of tracking those initially missing and measuring them (or a random sample of them), one is often talking about collecting data, not on the missing DV, but on an excellent proxy for the missing DV. That is, it often happens that the procedures used to collect data from the sample of those initially missing will be different from the procedures used in the main study (e.g., follow-up phone survey versus a paper-and-pencil, in-class survey in the main study). Time will generally also be different. For example, the time frame for the main measurement might be, say, 2 months (e.g., all of April and May of a given year). The follow-up measures may take 2–3 months longer (taking place in June, July, or even August of that year).[11] When this is true, it makes more sense to think of these measures, not as direct replacements for the missing measures, but as excellent auxiliary variables. However, in order for these follow-up measures to work as auxiliary variables, one must also collect follow-up data on a random sample of respondents who did provide data at the main measure.

# References

Bentler, P. M. (1990). Comparative fit indexes in structural models. *Psychological Bulletin, 107*, 238–246.
Bentler, P. M., & Bonett, D. G. (1980). Significance tests and goodness of fit in the analysis of covariance structures. *Psychological Bulletin, 88*, 588–606.
Bose, J. (2001). Nonresponse bias analyses at the National Center for Education Statistics. Proceedings of the Statistics Canada Symposium, 2001, Achieving Data Quality in a Statistical Agency: A Methodological Perspective.

---

[11] Of course, the distinction between main measure and auxiliary variable becomes blurred when the methods used for collecting data on the follow-up sample are the same as, or very similar to, the methods used for the main measure of the DV, and when the follow-up measure occurs at a time not too far removed from the main measure.

# References

Browne, M. W., & Cudeck, R. (1993). Alternative ways of assessing model fit. In K. A. Bollen & J. S. Long (Eds.) *Testing structural equation models*. Newbury Park, CA: Sage, pp. 136–162.

Cohen, J. (1977). *Statistical power analysis for the behavioral sciences*. New York: Academic Press.

Colby, M., Hecht, M. L., Miller-Day, M., Krieger, J. R., Syvertsen, A. K., Graham, J. W., and Pettigrew, J. (in press). Adapting School-based Substance Use Prevention Curriculum through Cultural Grounding: A Review and Exemplar of Adaptation Processes for Rural Schools. *American Journal of Community Psychology*.

Collins, L. M., Schafer, J. L., & Kam, C. M. (2001). A comparison of inclusive and restrictive strategies in modern missing data procedures. *Psychological Methods*, 6, 330–351.

Cook, T. D., & Campbell, D. T. (1979). *Quasi-experimentation: Design & analysis issues for field settings*. Chicago: Rand McNally.

Demirtas, H. (2005). Multiple imputation under Bayesianly smoothed pattern-mixture models for non-ignorable drop-out. *Statistics in Medicine*, 24, 2345–2363.

Demirtas, H., & Schafer, J. L. (2003). On the performance of random-coefficient pattern-mixture models for nonignorable dropout. *Statistics in Medicine*, 21, 1–23.

Enders, C. K. (2008). A note on the use of missing auxiliary variables in full information maximum likelihood-based structural equation models. *Structural Equation Modeling*, 15, 434–448.

Enders, C. K. (2011). Missing not at random models for latent growth curve analysis. Psychological Methods, 16, 1–16.

Glynn, R. J., Laird, N. M., and Rubin, D. B. (1993). Multiple imputation in mixture models for nonignorable nonresponse with followups. *Journal of the American Statistical Association*, 88, 984–993.

Graham, J. W. (2009). Missing data analysis: making it work in the real world. *Annual Review of Psychology*, 60, 549–576.

Graham, J. W., & Donaldson, S. I. (1993). Evaluating interventions with differential attrition: The importance of nonresponse mechanisms and use of followup data. *Journal of Applied Psychology*, 78, 119–128.

Graham, J. W., Hofer, S. M., and Piccinin, A. M. (1994). Analysis with missing data in drug prevention research. In L. M. Collins and L. Seitz (eds.), *Advances in data analysis for prevention intervention research*. National Institute on Drug Abuse Research Monograph Series #142, pp. 13–63, Washington DC: National Institute on Drug Abuse.

Graham, J. W., Palen, L. A., Smith, E. A., and Caldwell, L. L. (2008). Attrition: MAR and MNAR Missingness, and Estimation Bias. Poster presented at the 16th Annual Meetings of the Society for Prevention Research, San Francisco, CA, May 2008.

Graham, J. W., Hofer, S. M., Donaldson, S. I., MacKinnon, D. P., and Schafer, J. L. (1997). Analysis with missing data in prevention research. In K. Bryant, M. Windle, & S. West (Eds.), *The science of prevention: methodological advances from alcohol and substance abuse research.* (pp. 325–366). Washington, D.C.: American Psychological Association.

Hansen, W. B., & Graham, J. W. (1991). Preventing alcohol, marijuana, and cigarette use among adolescents: Peer pressure resistance training versus establishing conservative norms. *Preventive Medicine*, 20, 414–430.

Hedeker, D., and Gibbons, R. D. (1997). Application of random-effects pattern-mixture models for missing data in longitudinal studies. *Psychological Methods*, 2, 64–78.

Hu, L. T., and Bentler, P. M. (1999). Cutoff criteria for fit indexes in covariance structure analysis: conventional criteria versus new alternatives. *Structural Equation Modeling*, 6, 1–55.

Leon, A. C., Demirtas, H., and Hedeker, D. (2007). Bias reduction with an adjustment for participants' intent to dropout of a randomized controlled clinical trial. *Clinical Trials*, 4, 540–547.

Little, R. J. A. (1993). Pattern-Mixture Models for Multivariate Incomplete Data. *Journal of the American Statistical Association*, 88, 125–134.

Little, R. J. A. (1994). A Class of Pattern-Mixture Models for Normal Incomplete Data. *Biometrika*, 81, 471–483.

Little, R. J. A. (1995). Modeling the drop-out mechanism in repeated-measures studies. *Journal of the American Statistical Association*, 90, 1112–1121.

Little, R. J. A., & Rubin, D. B. (1987). *Statistical analysis with missing data*. New York: Wiley.
Little, R. J. A., & Rubin, D. B. (2002). *Statistical analysis with missing data: Second Edition*. New York: Wiley.
Rubin, D. B. (1976). Inference and missing data. *Biometrika, 63*, 581–592.
Rubin, D.B. (1987). *Multiple imputation for nonresponse in surveys*. New York: Wiley.
Schafer, J. L., & Graham, J. W. (2002). Missing data: our view of the state of the art. *Psychological Methods, 7*, 147–177.
Steiger, J. H., and Lind, J. M. (1980). *Statistically based tests for the number of common factors*. Paper presented at the annual meeting of the Psychometric Society, Iowa City, IA.
Tucker, L. R., & Lewis, C. (1973). A reliability coefficient for maximum likelihood factor analysis. *Psychometrika, 38*, 1–10.
Verbeke, G., & Molenberghs, G. (2000). *Linear mixed models for longitudinal data*. New York: Springer.

# Chapter 2
# Analysis of Missing Data

In this chapter, I present older methods for handling missing data. I then turn to the major new approaches for handling missing data. In this chapter, I present methods that make the MAR assumption. Included in this introduction are the EM algorithm for covariance matrices, normal-model multiple imputation (MI), and what I will refer to as FIML (full information maximum likelihood) methods. Before getting to these methods, however, I talk about the goals of analysis.

## Goals of Analysis

The goal of any analysis is to obtain unbiased estimates of population parameters. For example, suppose the researcher wants to perform a multiple regression analysis to determine if the variable X has a significant, unique effect on the variable Y, after controlling for the covariate C. The first goal of this analysis is to obtain an estimate of the regression coefficient for X predicting Y that is unbiased, that is, near the population value. The second goal of analysis is to obtain some indication of the precision of the estimate; that is, the researcher wants to obtain standard errors or confidence intervals around the estimate. When these two goals have been achieved, the researcher also hopes to test hypotheses with the maximum statistical power possible. It is in this context that I will talk about the methods for handling missing data. In evaluating the various methods, I will talk about the degree of bias in parameter estimates, and whether or not there is a good way with the strategy for estimating standard errors. Where relevant, I will also evaluate the method with respect to statistical power.

## Older Approaches to Handling Missing Data

In this section, I will devote some space to each of these topics: (a) complete cases analysis, (b) pairwise deletion, (c) mean substitution, and (d) regression-based single imputation. With these older methods, the goal is not so much to present a historical overview of what was typically done prior to 1987. Rather, I want to mention the various approaches, say what is good and bad about them, and in particular, focus on what (if anything) is still useful about them. One thing is clear with these methods, however. None of them were really designed to **handle** missing data at all. The word "handle" connotes dealing effectively with something. And certainly none of these methods could be said to deal effectively with missing data. Rather, these methods, usually described as ad hoc, were designed to get past the missing data so that at least some analyses could be done.

## *Complete Cases Analysis (aka Listwise Deletion)*

Complete cases analysis begins with the variables that will be included in the analysis of substantive interest. The analyst then discards any case with missing values on any of the variables selected and proceeds with the analysis using standard methods. The first issue that arises with complete cases analysis relates to whether the subsample on which the analysis is done is a random sample of the sample as a whole. If the missingness is MCAR (see Chap. 1), then the complete cases are representative of the whole, and the results of the analyses will be unbiased. In addition, the standard errors from this analysis are meaningful in the sense that they reasonably reflect the variability around the parameter estimate (although if the estimates are biased, the meaningfulness of these standard errors is questionable).

However, because MCAR missingness is rather a rare occurrence in real-world data, it is almost always the case that cases with complete data for the variables included in the analysis are not representative of the whole sample. For example, in substance abuse prevention studies, it is virtually always true that drug users at the pretest are more likely than nonusers to drop out of the study at a later wave. This means that those with complete cases will be different from those who dropped out. And this difference will lead to estimation bias in several parameters. In particular, means at the posttest will be biased, and Pearson correlations between pretest and posttest variables will be biased.

On the other hand, when missingness is MAR, regression coefficients for pretest variables predicting posttest variables will often be tolerably unbiased. In fact, as noted in Chap. 1, when missingness on $Y_2$ (Y at time 2) is caused by $C_1$ (C at time 1; no missing data), then the regression coefficient for $X_1$ (X at time 1; no missing data) predicting $Y_2$ is unbiased when $C_1$ is included as a covariate. In this specific context, complete cases analysis yields b-weights that are identical to those obtained with ML methods (e.g., EM algorithm; Graham and Donaldson 1993).

With respect to bias, complete cases analysis tends to perform quite well, compared to MI and ML analyses, with ANCOVA or multiple regression analysis with several predictors from a pretest, and a single DV from a posttest. And because this type of model is so common, complete cases analysis can often be useful.

However, complete cases analysis fares less well when the proportion of cases lost to missingness is large. Thus, complete case analysis tends to fare much less well with more complex analyses, for example, with a mediation analysis with X, M, and Y coming from three different waves of measurement.

**Table 2.1** Hypothetical patterns of missing and observed values

| Variable | | | | | | Data |
|---|---|---|---|---|---|---|
| A | B | C | D | E | Percent | Points |
| 1 | 1 | 1 | 1 | 1 | 20 | 100 |
| 1 | 0 | 1 | 1 | 1 | 20 | 100 |
| 1 | 1 | 0 | 1 | 1 | 20 | 100 |
| 1 | 1 | 1 | 0 | 1 | 20 | 100 |
| 1 | 1 | 1 | 1 | 0 | 20 | 100 |

1 = observed; 0 = missing. 500 total data points

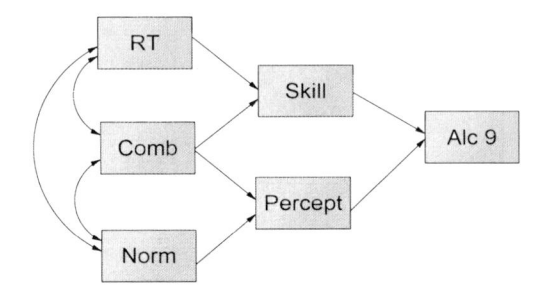

**Fig. 2.1** Theoretical mediation model for the adolescent alcohol prevention trial (Hansen and Graham 1991). RT = Resistance Training program vs. control; Norm = Normative Education program vs. control; Comb = Combined (RT + Norm) program vs. control; Skill = behavioral measure of skill in resisting drug use offers; Percept = measure of perceptions of peer drug use; Alc9 = measure of alcohol use at 9th grade

Also, because complete cases analysis involves discarding cases, it often happens that complete cases analysis will test hypotheses with less power. And this loss of power can be substantial if the missingness on different variables in the model comes from nonoverlapping cases. Table 2.1 shows the missingness patterns for such a data set. Although this pattern is somewhat extreme, it illustrates the problem. In this instance, 80 of 500 data points are missing. That is, just 16 % of the total number of data points are missing. However, in this instance, complete cases analysis would discard 80 % of the cases. Discarding 80 % of the cases because 16 % of the values are missing is unacceptable.

In situations such as the one illustrated in Table 2.1, MI or ML methods are clearly a better choice than using complete cases analysis. But even in much less extreme situations, I argue that MI/ML methods are the better choice. In fact, I argue that MI/ML methods are always at least as good as complete cases analysis, and usually MI/ML methods are better, and often they are substantially better than the older methods such as complete cases analysis (Graham 2009).

Graham et al. (1997) compared several different analysis methods with a mediation analysis using data related to the Adolescent Alcohol Prevention Trial (AAPT; Hansen and Graham 1991). A somewhat simplified version of the model tested is shown in Fig. 2.1. The variables on the left in the model represented three program

**Table 2.2** Results of analysis of a mediation model based on AAPT data

| | Effect | Amos | Mix | EM | CC |
|---|---|---|---|---|---|
| RT | → Skill | .365 (6.29) | .375 (6.36) | .365 (6.98) | .438 (4.56) |
| Comb | → Skill | .332 (5.49) | .330 (5.42) | .332 (5.10) | .354 (3.82) |
| Norm | → Percept | −.117 (3.31) | −.118 (3.22) | −.117 (3.73) | −.191 (2.31) |
| Comb | → Percept | −.270 (7.91) | −.273 (7.89) | −2.70 (8.13) | −.209 (2.90) |
| Skill | → Alc9 | −.019 (0.48) | −.021 (0.68) | −.019 (0.50) | −.034 (0.62) |
| Percept | → Alc9 | .143 (4.35) | .119 (3.26) | .143 (3.50) | .135 (1.89) |

*Note*: Table adapted from Graham et al. (1997). Regression coefficients are shown (with corresponding $t$-values shown in parentheses). Amos refers to the Amos Program (Arbuckle 1995); Mix refers to Schafer's (1997) Mix program (multiple imputation for mixed continuous and categorical data); EM refers to the EM algorithm; Standard errors ($t$-values shown) for EM estimates were based on bootstrap methods (Efron 1982); CC refers to complete cases analysis

group variables (variables were dummy coded so that each variable represented a comparison against an information-only control group). The programs were implemented in the seventh grade. The variables in the middle represented the hypothesized mediators of longer term effects. These measures were taken approximately 2 weeks after completion of the programs. The variable on the right represented the longer term outcome (ninth grade alcohol use). In NORM, students received a norms clarification curriculum designed to correct student misperceptions about the prevalence and acceptability of alcohol and other drug use among their peers. In RT, students received resistance skills training. In the COMBined program, students received the essential elements of both NORM and RT curricula. It was hypothesized that receiving the NORM (or COMBined) curriculum would decrease perceptions of peer use, which in turn would decrease ninth grade alcohol use. It was also hypothesized that receiving the RT (or COMBined) curriculum would increase resistance skills, which in turn would decrease ninth grade alcohol use.

Approximately 3,000 seventh grade students received the programs and completed the pretest survey. Approximately the same number completed the immediate posttest survey, which included questions about perceptions of peer use. At the same time as the immediate posttest survey administration, approximately one-third of the students were selected at random to be taken out of the classroom to complete an in-depth, role-play measure of drug resistance skills. Approximately 54 % of those present at the seventh grade pretest also completed the survey at the ninth grade posttest. Given all this, approximately 500 students had data for all measures.

The data described above were analyzed using several procedures, including MI with the MIX program for mixed categorical and continuous data (Schafer 1997), Amos, an SEM program with a FIML feature for handling missing data (Arbuckle 1995), EM algorithm (with bootstrap for standard errors; for example., Graham et al. 1996), and complete cases (CC) analysis. The results of these analyses appear in Table 2.2. The key point to take away from these results is that the results based on complete cases appears to be slightly biased. But more importantly, the mediator → outcome effects were both nonsignificant using complete cases analysis. Thus, had that been our approach, we would not have found significant mediation in this instance (MacKinnon et al. 2002).

## Pairwise Deletion

Pairwise deletion is a procedure that focuses on the variance-covariance matrix. Each element of that matrix is estimated from all data available for that element. In concept, pairwise deletion seems like it would be good, because it does make use of all available data. However, because different variances and covariances are based on different subsamples of respondents, parameter estimates may be biased unless missingness is MCAR. In addition, because the different parameters are estimated with different subsamples, it often happens that the matrix is not positive definite, and therefore cannot even be analyzed using most multivariate procedures. An odd by-product of pairwise deletion is that eigenvalues from principal components analysis are either positive (good) or *negative* (bad). With complete cases, eigenvalues are either positive (good) or zero (bad).

In practice, I have found the biggest limitation of pairwise deletion to be the fact that there is no obvious way to estimate standard errors. Estimation of standard errors requires specifying the sample size, and there is no obvious way to do that with pairwise deletion. Thus, with the one exception, outlined in Chap. 8, I do not use pairwise deletion. Even if parameter estimation is all that is needed, better parameter estimates are easily obtained with EM (see below; also see Chaps. 3 and 7).

## Mean Substitution

Mean substitution is a strategy in which the mean is calculated for the variable based on all cases that have data for that variable. This mean is then used in place of any missing value on that variable.

This is the worst of all possible strategies. Inserting the mean in place of the missing value reduces variance on the variable and plays havoc with covariances and correlations. Also, there is no straightforward way to estimate standard errors. Because of all the problems with this strategy, I believe that using it amounts to nothing more than pretending that no data are missing. I recommend that people should NEVER use this procedure. If you absolutely must pretend that you have no missing data, a much better strategy, and one that is almost as easy to implement, is to impute a single data set from EM parameters (see Chaps. 3 and 7) and use that.

## Averaging the Available Variables

This is the situation in which the mean for a scale is calculated based on partial data when the person does not have complete data for all variables making up the scale. I cover this topic thoroughly in Chap. 9 (coauthored by Lee van Horn and Bonnie

**Table 2.3** Missing data patterns

| $X_1$ | $X_2$ | $X_3$ | Y |
|---|---|---|---|
| 1 | 1 | 1 | 1 |
| 1 | 1 | 1 | 0 |

1 = value observed; 0 = value missing

Taylor). But I wanted also to mention here to distinguish it from mean substitution. The idea of using available variables to calculate a scale score is not at all the same as mean substitution. Rather, I think of it as being a variant of regression-based single imputation (see next section). And as such, this strategy, although not perfect, has much better statistical properties.

## *Regression-Based Single Imputation*

With this strategy, one begins by dividing the sample into those with a variable (Y), and those for whom Y is missing, as shown in Table 2.3. One then estimates a regression model in the first group ($X_1$, $X_2$, and $X_3$ predicting Y) and applies that regression equation in the second group.

For example, in the first group, the regression equation is:

$$\hat{Y} = b_0 + b_1 X_1 + b_2 X_2 + b_3 ?$$

And because all three X variables have data for the second group, the $\hat{Y}$ values are calculable in the second group. These values are the imputed values and are inserted wherever Y is missing.

Conceptually, this is a good way to impute values. It is good in the sense that a great deal of information from the individual is used to predict the missing values. And as I shall show throughout this book (especially see Chap. 11 on auxiliary variables), the higher correlation between the predictors and Y, the better the imputation will be. In fact, this is such a good way to impute values that it forms the heart of the EM algorithm for covariance matrices and normal-model MI procedures.

However, regression-based single imputation is not a great imputation procedure in and of itself. Most importantly, although covariances are estimated without bias with this procedure (when certain conditions are met), variances are too low. It is easy to see why this is. When Y is present, there is always some difference between observed values and the regression line. However, with this imputation approach, the imputed values always fall right on the regression line. It is for this reason that I do not recommend using this approach. The option available within the MVA package in SPSS (even as recent as version 20) for imputing data from the EM solution is this kind of single imputation (von Hippel 2004). I therefore cannot recommend using this imputed data set (however, please see Chaps. 3 and 7 for other options).

# Basics of the Recommended Methods

I have often said that the recommended methods for handling missing data fall into two general categories, model-based procedures and data-based procedures. Model-based approaches rewrite the statistical algorithms so as to handle the missing data and estimate parameters all in a single step. Data-based approaches, on the other hand, handle the missing data in one step, and then perform the parameter estimation in a second, distinct, step. The most common of the model-based procedures are the current crop of structural equation modeling (SEM) programs, which use a FIML feature for handling missing data. The most common of the data-based procedures is normal-model MI. However, with the EM algorithm, this distinction gets a little fuzzy (see below). When an EM algorithm is tailored to produce parameter estimates specific to the situation, EM is a model-based approach. However, when the EM algorithm produces more generic output, such as a variance-covariance matrix and vector of means, which is then analyzed in a separate step, it is more like a data-based procedure. The basics of these recommended approaches are presented below.

## *Full Information Maximum Likelihood (FIML)*

The most common of the model-based procedures are the SEM programs that use a FIML feature for handling missing data. As with all model-based approaches, these programs handle the missing data and parameter estimation in a single step. The FIML approach, which has sometimes been referred to as raw-data maximum likelihood, reads in the raw data one case at a time, and maximizes the ML function one case at a time, using whatever information is available for each case (e.g., see Graham and Coffman in press). In the end, combining across the individuals produces an overall estimate of the ML function. All of these SEM/FIML programs provide excellent (ML) parameter estimates for the model being studied and also provide reasonable standard errors, all in one step.

### Amos and Other SEM/FIML Programs

Several SEM programs have the FIML feature, including, in alphabetical order, Amos (Arbuckle 2010), EQS 6.1 (Bentler and Wu 1995), LISREL 8.5+ (Jöreskog and Sörbom 2006; also see Mels 2006), Mplus (Muthén and Muthén 2010), Mx (Neale et al. 2003), and SAS (v. 9.2) Proc CALIS. All of these programs allow ML estimation with missing data and provide good standard errors. Amos has the added advantage of being part of the SPSS package. Amos also has the advantage of being exceptionally intuitive and easy to use. For these reasons, and because SPSS users need more missing data tools, I emphasize Amos a little more here. A more detailed discussion of the workings of Amos can be found in Graham et al. (2003; also see Graham et al. in press).

## *Basics of the EM Algorithm for Covariance Matrices*

First, E and M stand for Expectation and Maximization. Also, please understand that it is not quite proper to refer to "the" EM algorithm. There are several EM algorithms. Collins and Wugalter (1992) described one for estimating LTA models, a type of latent class model. Rubin and Thayer (1982) described an EM algorithm for factor analysis. And early versions of the HLM program (Raudenbush and Bryk 2002) also made use of an EM algorithm (Raudenbush et al. 1991). In each case, the EM algorithm is tailored to produce the ML parameter estimates of interest. The version of the EM algorithm I am talking about in this chapter (and throughout this book) is what I refer to as the EM algorithm for covariance matrices.

As with all of these versions, the EM algorithm for covariance matrices first reads in, or calculates the sufficient statistics, the building blocks of the particular analysis being done, and reads out the relevant parameters. In this case, the relevant parameters are a variance-covariance matrix and vector of means. From here on, when I refer to "the EM algorithm," I am speaking of the version that produces a variance-covariance matrix and vector of means.

The EM algorithm is an iterative procedure that goes back and forth between the E-Step and the M-step.

**The E-Step**

The sufficient statistics for the EM algorithm are sums, sums of squares, and sums of cross products. The program reads in the raw data, and as each case is read in, it updates the sums, sums of squares, and sums of cross products. Where the data point is observed, it is used directly to update these sums. If the data point is missing, however, the best estimate is used in its place. The best estimate of the missing value is the $\hat{Y}$ from a regression equation using all other variables as predictors. For sums, the value is added directly whether it was observed or missing. For sums of squares and sums of cross products, if one or both values were observed, the value is added directly. However, if both values were missing, then the best estimate is added along with a correction term. This correction term is the residual from the regression with all other variables as predictors. Thus, it is like the error variance added to imputed values in multiple imputation (see below).

**The M-Step**

Once the sums, sums of squares, and sums of cross products have been estimated, the variance-covariance matrix (and vector of means) can simply be calculated. This concludes the first iteration.

From the variance-covariance matrix and means from the first iteration, one can calculate all of the regression equations needed to predict each variable in the model. During the next iteration, these equations are used to update the "best estimate" when the value is missing. After the sums, sums of squares, and sums of cross products have been calculated at this iteration, a new variance-covariance matrix and vector of means are calculated, and new regression equations are estimated for the next iteration.

This process continues until the variances, covariances, and means change so little from iteration to iteration that they are considered to have stopped changing. That is, when this happens, EM is said to have *converged*.

The variance-covariance matrix and vector of means from the last iteration are ML estimates of these quantities. Any analysis that requires only a variance-covariance matrix and vector means as input can be used with these EM estimates as input. If the new analysis is something that is simply calculated based on the input matrix, for example, a multiple regression analysis, then those estimates are also ML (note, e.g., that the EM and Amos parameter estimates from Table 2.2 are identical). However, if the analysis itself is an iterative procedure, such as a latent-variable regression model, then the estimates based on the EM variance-covariance matrix and means will be unbiased and efficient but technically will not be ML.

## Standard Errors

The one drawback with EM is that standard errors are not produced as a by-product of the parameter estimation. There are other approaches (e.g., see Yuan and Bentler 2000), but the most common approach to estimating standard errors with EM estimates is to use bootstrap procedures (e.g., Graham et al. 1997). Note that the $t$-values based on bootstrapping in Table 2.2 are reasonable, but are somewhat different from the those based on FIML and MI analysis. Although the EM + bootstrapping process is generally more time consuming than FIML or MI, one notable advantage of EM with bootstrapping is that this is a good approach when data are not normally distributed. In this instance, bootstrapping to yield direct estimates of the confidence intervals (which requires one or two thousand bootstraps) provides better coverage than does either MI or FIML with regular (i.e., not robust) standard errors.

## Implementations of the EM Algorithm

The EM algorithm for covariance matrices now has many implementations, including SAS Proc MI, Norm (Schafer 1997), and EMCOV (Graham and Hofer 1991). SPSS does have an EM algorithm routine within its MVA module. This is a stand-alone routine that does not interface with other parts of SPSS, but it can be very useful for estimating EM means, variances, and correlations. The latest versions of STATA also have EM capabilities.

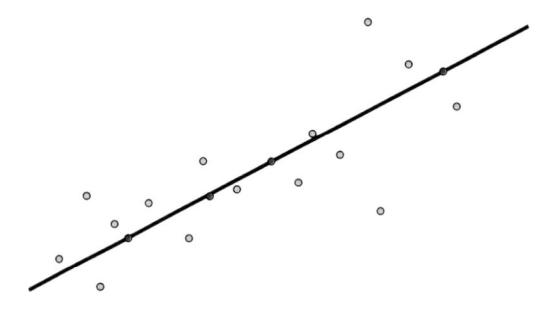

**Fig. 2.2** A bivariate distribution with the best-fitting straight line. Imputed values based on regression-based single imputation lie right on the regression line. Real (observed) data points deviate by some amount from the regression line

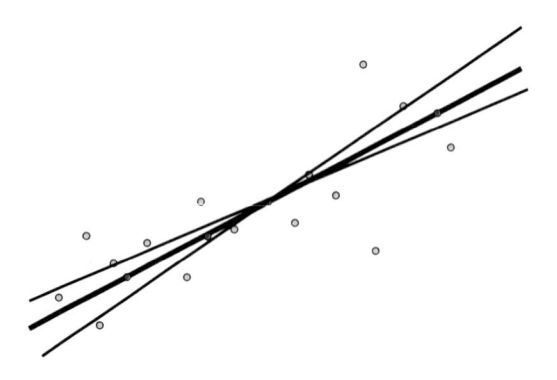

**Fig. 2.3** Regression lines are slightly different for different random draws from the population

## Basics of Normal-Model Multiple Imputation

In a previous section, I said that the regression-based, single imputation procedure formed the heart of EM and normal-model MI. I also said that regression-based single imputation underestimates variances. That is, there is too little variability in the imputed values. The first reason for this is that the imputed values have too little error variance. This problem is depicted in Fig. 2.2. The observed data points deviate from the regression line by some amount, but, of course, the imputed values lie right on the regression line. This problem is easily resolved simply by adding random normal error to each imputed value (this corresponds to adding the correction term in the E-step of the EM algorithm, as described above).[1]

The second reason there is too little variability relates to the fact that the regression equations used in single imputation are based on a single sample drawn from the population. As depicted in Fig. 2.3, there should be additional variability around

---

[1] It is this random error that is missing from the data set imputed from the EM solution in the MVA module of SPSS (von Hippel 2004; this remains the case at least through version 20).

the regression line itself to reflect what would occur if there were a different random draw from the population for each imputed data set. Of course, researchers seldom have the luxury of being able to make several random draws from the population of interest. However, bootstrap procedures (Efron 1982) can be used in this context. Or random draws from the population can be simulated using Bayesian procedures, such as Markov-Chain Monte Carlo (MCMC) or data augmentation (Tanner and Wong 1987; Schafer 1997) procedures.

It has been said that data augmentation (DA), which is used in Schafer's (1997) NORM program, is like a stochastic version of EM. DA is also a two-step, iterative process. In the I-step (imputation step), the data are simulated based on the current parameter values. In the P-step (posterior step), the parameters are simulated from the current data. On the other hand, DA converges in a way that is rather different from how EM converges. Whereas EM converges when the parameter estimates stop changing, DA converges when the distribution of parameter estimates stabilizes.

Recall that DA is used in order to simulate random draws from the population. However, as with all Markov Chain procedures, all information at one iteration comes from the previous iteration. Thus the parameter estimates (and imputed data) from two consecutive steps of DA are much more like one another than if they had come from two random draws from the population. However, after some large number of DA steps from some starting point, the parameter estimates are like two random draws from the population. The question is how many DA steps between imputed data sets is enough? The answer (described in more detail in Chaps. 3 and 7) is that the number of iterations for EM convergence is a good estimate of the number of DA steps one should use between imputed data sets.

## The Process of Doing MI

Analysis with MI is a three-step process. First, one imputes the data, generating $m$ imputed data sets. With each data set, a different imputed value replaces each missing value. Early writers suggested that very few imputed data sets were required. However, more recent work has suggested that more imputations (e.g., $m=20$–$40$ or more) are required to achieve the statistical power of equivalent ML procedures (Graham et al. 2007; see below for more details). The details for performing MI are given in Chaps. 3 and 7.

Second, one analyzes the $m$ data sets with usual, complete data, procedures (e.g., with SAS, SPSS, HLM, etc.), saving the parameter estimates and standard errors from analysis of each data set. Details for performing analyses are given in Chaps. 4, 5, 6, and 7.

Third, one combines the results to get ***MI inference***. Following what are commonly known as Rubin's rules (Rubin 1987), the two most important quantities for MI inference are the point estimate of the parameters of interest and the MI-based standard errors. These and other important quantities from the MI inference process are described below.

## Point Estimate of the Parameter

The point estimate for each parameter is simply the arithmetic average of that parameter estimate (e.g., a regression coefficient) over the $m$ imputed data sets. It is this average for each parameter of interest that is reported in the article you are writing.

## Standard Errors and $t$-Values

The MI inference standard error (SE) is in two parts. One part, *within-imputation variance* ($U$) reflects the regular kind of sampling variability found in all analyses. The other part, between-imputation variance ($B$), reflects the added variability, or uncertainty, that is due to missing data. The within-imputation variance is simply the average of the squared SE over the analyses from the $m$ imputed data sets, that is,

$$U = \Sigma \, SE^2 \, / \, m,$$

for each parameter being studied. The between-imputation variance is the sample variance of the parameter estimate (e.g., a regression coefficient) over the $m$ imputed data sets,

$$B = S^2_P,$$

where P is the parameter being studied. The total variance is a weighted sum of the two kinds of variance,

$$T = U + (1 + 1/m)B.$$

It should be clear that $B$ is the variance that is due to missing data. If there were no missing data, then the variance of the parameter over the $m$ imputed data sets would be 0 and the $B$ component of variance would be 0. The MI inference standard error is simply the square root of $T$.

## Degrees of Freedom (df)

The *df* associated with the *t*-value in Rubin's rules, adapted from Schafer (1997), is

$$df = (m-1) = \left[ 1 + \frac{U}{(1+m^{-1})B} \right]^2.$$

The *df* in MI analysis is different from *df* in other statistical contexts; for example, it has nothing to do with $N$. Just looking at the formula for *df* can give insights into its meaning. First, if there were very little missing data, $B$ would be very small. At the limit, $B$ would tend toward 0, and *df* would tend toward infinity. On the other hand, if there were much missing data and uncertainty of estimation due to missing data, then B would tend to be large in comparison to U, and the right-hand term in the brackets would tend to be very small. In that case, *df* would tend toward its lower limit ($m-1$). More conceptually, I think of *df* as indicating the stability of the MI estimates. If *df* is large, compared to *m*, then the MI estimates have stabilized and can be trusted. However, if *df* is small, for example, near the lower limit, it indicates that the MI estimates have not stabilized, and more imputations should be used.

**Fraction of Missing Information**

The fraction of missing information (*FMI*) in Rubin's rules, adapted from Schafer (1997), is

$$FMI = \frac{r + 2/(df+3)}{r+1}$$

where

$$r = \frac{(1+m^{-1})B}{U}.$$

*FMI* is an interesting quantity. Conceptually, it represents the amount of *information* that is missing from a parameter estimate because of the missing data. In its simplest form, the *FMI* is theoretically the same as the amount of missing data. For example, with a simple situation of two variables, X and Y, where X is always observed, and Y is missing, say 50 % of the time, $FMI=.50$ for $b_{YX}$, the regression coefficient for X predicting Y. However, when there are other variables in the model that are correlated with Y, *FMI* will theoretically be reduced, because, to the extent that those other variables are correlated with Y, some of the lost information is restored (see Chap. 11 for a detailed presentation of this issue).

It is important to note that in any analysis, the estimated FMI will differ from the hypothetical value. *FMI* based on the formulas given above is only an estimate. And it can be a rather bad estimate, especially when *m* is small. I do not trust the *FMI* estimate at all unless $m=40$ or greater. And even then, although I do look at the *FMI* to get a sense of its magnitude, I always bear in mind that the true *FMI* could be a bit different.

# What Analyses Work with MI?

It should be clear from reading this book that I believe strongly that normal-model MI is an exceptionally useful analytic tool. Normal-model MI, which is just one of the MI models that has been described in the literature, is (a) without doubt the best implemented of the available programs, and (b) able to handle an exceptionally wide array of analytic problems.

I think it helps to know that normal-model MI "preserves," that is, estimates without bias, means, variances, covariances, and related quantities. It does not, however, give unbiased estimates for the proportion of people who give a particular answer to a variable with more than two response levels. For example, normal-model MI (and the related EM algorithm) typically cannot be used to estimate the proportion of respondents who respond "none" to a variable asking about the number of cigarettes smoked in the person's lifetime. That proportion is really a categorical quantity, and unless the variable happens to be normally distributed, normal-model MI will get it wrong. The good news is that variables such as this can often be recast so that normal-model MI can handle them. With the lifetime cigarette smoking question, for example, if the variable were recoded to take on the values 0 (never smoked) and 1 (ever smoked), then normal-model MI (and EM) will produce unbiased estimates of the proportion. The reason it works in this instance is that the proportion of people responding "1" is the same as the mean for that recoded version of the variable, and the estimate of the mean is unbiased with normal-model MI.

## *Normal-Model MI with Categorical Variables*

Normal-model MI does not deal with categorical variables with more than two levels, unless they are first dummy coded; any categorical variable with $p$ levels must be recoded into $p-1$ dummy variables. When such variables have no missing data, that is all that needs to be done. When such variables have missing data, the values may be imputed with normal-model MI, but a minor ad hoc fix may be needed for certain patterns of imputed values (Allison 2002; also see Chaps. 3 and 7). Normal-model MI may also be used for cluster data (e.g., students within schools). I discuss this topic in much greater detail in Chap. 6, but suffice it to say here that normal-model MI does just ok with cluster data, and in this instance, other MI models (e.g., Schafer's PAN program; Schafer 2001; Schafer and Yucel 2002) are preferred.

## *Normal-Model MI with Longitudinal Data*

Schafer's (2001) PAN program was developed initially to handle the special longitudinal data problem depicted in Table 2.4. The data came from the AAPT study (Hansen and Graham 1991). The three variables shown were Alcohol (alcohol use), Posatt (beliefs about the positive social consequences of drinking alcohol), and Negatt (beliefs about the negative consequences of drinking alcohol). As shown in the table, students were asked about their alcohol consumption in each grade from fifth to tenth grades. However, the Posatt questions were not asked in eighth grade,

**Table 2.4** "Special" longitudinal missing data patterns

|         | Grade |   |   |   |   |    |
|---------|-------|---|---|---|---|----|
|         | 5     | 6 | 7 | 8 | 9 | 10 |
| Alcohol | 1     | 1 | 1 | 1 | 1 | 1  |
| Posatt  | 1     | 1 | 1 | 0 | 1 | 1  |
| Negatt  | 1     | 1 | 1 | 0 | 0 | 0  |

1 = data observed; 0 = data missing. Data for each case would normally appear in one long row

**Table 2.5** Typical longitudinal missing data patterns

|         | Alcohol in grade |   |   |   |   |    |     |
|---------|------------------|---|---|---|---|----|-----|
| Pattern | 5                | 6 | 7 | 8 | 9 | 10 | N   |
| 1       | 1                | 1 | 1 | 1 | 1 | 1  | 500 |
| 2       | 1                | 1 | 1 | 1 | 1 | 0  | 200 |
| 3       | 1                | 1 | 1 | 0 | 1 | 1  | 100 |
| 4       | 1                | 1 | 1 | 0 | 0 | 0  | 200 |

1 = data observed; 0 = data missing

but reappeared on the survey in ninth and tenth grades. The Negatt questions were not asked in any of the last three grades.

Normal-model MI cannot impute data such as those shown, because data for each case (which would normally appear in one long row) would be missing data for Posatt at eighth grade and Negatt at eighth, ninth, and tenth grades. However, PAN (short for panel) adds a longitudinal component (essentially a growth model) to the imputation procedure. Thus, Posatt data for fifth, sixth, seventh, ninth, and tenth grades can be used to make a good guess about the missing value for Posatt at eighth grade. Also, Negatt at fifth, sixth, and seventh grades can be used to make guesses about the missing Negatt scores for eighth, ninth, and tenth grades. Of course, we would be much more confident about imputing the missing Posatt score at eighth grade than we would about imputing the missing Negatt scores. But the point is that this kind of imputation is possible with PAN.

Many people believe, incorrectly, that programs such as PAN must also be used to impute longitudinal data under what I would refer to as typical circumstances (e.g., the pattern depicted in Table 2.5). The data shown in Table 2.5 differ significantly from the data shown in the previous example. With the data shown in Table 2.5, some people have complete data. More importantly, with these data, at least some cases have data for every variable and for every pair of variables. Under these circumstances, longitudinal models, for example, growth models, may be estimated based on a variance-covariance matrix and vector of means (e.g., using SEM procedures; see Willett and Sayer 1994). And because variances, covariances, and means are estimated without bias with normal-model MI (and the corresponding EM algorithm), these normal-model procedures are sufficient for imputing data in this longitudinal context.

## *Imputation for Statistical Interactions: The Imputation Model Must Be at Least as Complex as the Analysis Model*

Researchers are often interested in statistical interactions (e.g., see Aiken and West 1991; Jaccard and Turrisi 2003). One way to form a statistical interaction is simply to obtain a product of two variables, for example,

$$AB = A \times B$$

Suppose one is interested in testing a regression model with main effects and interaction terms, for example, A, B, and AB as predictors of Y. People often ask if they can go ahead and test this kind of interaction model if they did not address the interaction during imputation. The general answer is that the imputation model should be at least as complex as the analysis model. One way of thinking of this is that any variable that is used in the analysis model must also be included in the imputation model.[2]

If a variable is omitted from the imputation model, then imputation is carried out under the model in which the omitted variable is correlated $r=0$ with all of the variables included in the model. Thus, to the extent that there is missing data, the correlation between the omitted variable and any included variable will be suppressed, that is biased, toward zero. Interactions (product of two variables) are commonly omitted from the imputation model. And because the product is a nonlinear combination of two variables, it cannot simply be calculated after imputation. One solution, then, is to anticipate any interactions, and to include the appropriate products in the imputation model.

A more convenient approach to imputation with interactions is available for some classes of variables – categorical variables that fall naturally into a small number (e.g., just two or three) groups. This approach follows from the idea that interactions can also be conceived of as a correlation between two variables (e.g., $r_{AY}$) being different when some categorical third variable, B, is 0 or 1. With this approach, one simply imputes separately at the two (or more) levels of the categorical variable. The good news is that imputing in this manner allows one, after imputation, to test any interaction involving the categorical variable. For example, if one imputes separately for males and females, then any interaction involving gender can be tested appropriately after imputation. This strategy also works well for treatment membership variables. If one imputes separately within treatment and control groups, then any interaction involving that treatment membership variable can be tested appropriately after imputation.

---

[2] However, it is acceptable if variables are included in the imputation model that are not included in the analysis model.

## *Normal-Model MI with ANOVA*

The kind of analysis that works best with MI is the kind of analysis that produces a parameter estimate and standard error. Thus, virtually all analyses in the large family of regression analyses lend themselves very well to normal-model MI. Analyses that do not work so well are ANOVA-related analyses, specifically, analyses that focus on sums of squares, F-tests, and the like. Fortunately, it is generally possible to recast problems that are typically handled with some version of ANOVA into some kind of regression analysis.

## *Analyses for Which MI Is not Necessary*

Some analyses do not require the overhead associated with MI. For example, as I outline in Chaps. 4, 5, and 7, analyses (e.g., coefficient alpha analysis or exploratory factor analysis) that do not require hypothesis testing are more readily handled directly by analyzing the EM covariance matrix (see Chap. 7), or by imputing a single data set from EM parameters, and analyzing that (see Chaps. 4, 5, and 7).

Similarly, although one would definitely prefer to use MI for multiple regression analysis, certain quantities in those analyses do not necessarily involve hypothesis testing, and can be handled either by analyzing the EM covariance matrix directly (see Chap. 7), or by analyzing the single data set imputed from EM parameters (see Chaps. 4, 5, and 7). For example, standardized b-weights and $R^2$ values can theoretically be handled with MI. But it is much easier to estimate these quantities using the EM covariance matrix directly or by analyzing a single data set imputed from EM parameters.

## Missing Data Theory and the Comparison Between MI/ML and Other Methods

MI and ML methods for handling missing data were designed specifically to achieve unbiased estimation with missing data when the MAR assumption holds. Thus it is not surprising that when compared against older, ad hoc methods (e.g., listwise deletion, pairwise deletion, mean substitution), MI and ML methods yield unbiased parameter estimates. And regardless of whether the assumptions are met or not, MI and ML yield estimates that are at least as good as the older, ad hoc methods (Graham 2009). This does not mean that the MI/ML methods will always be better than, say, complete cases analysis. But they will always be at least as good, usually better, and often very much better than the older methods (Graham 2009).

An important point here is that missing data *theory* predicts that MI and ML will be better than the old methods. There are already numerous simulations to

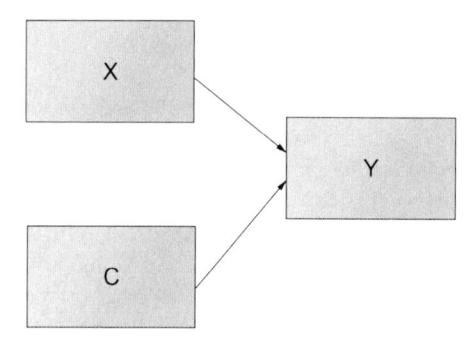

**Fig. 2.4** Simple regression model with X and C predicting Y

demonstrate that they are, in fact, better. An important point here is that we do not need more simulations to demonstrate this. What we do need are simulations and other studies that demonstrate the limits of the MI/ML advantage. My recommendation for future research in this area is that the researcher should acknowledge established missing data theory and articulate the reasons why it is either incorrect or incomplete. Here is one example.

## *Estimation Bias with Multiple Regression Models*

Consider the simple regression model depicted in Fig. 2.4. The regression coefficient of X predicting Y ($b_{YX}$) is of primary interest in the model, and the variable C is included as a covariate. In this instance, X and C are never missing. Y is sometimes missing, and C is the cause of missingness on Y. Graham and Donaldson (1993) demonstrated that under these circumstances, $b_{YX}$ is identical when based on the EM algorithm and on complete cases analysis.

Although this model is a very simple one, it is representative of a very common kind of model. That is, it is common to have a regression model such as that shown in Fig. 2.4, with perhaps several covariates. Even with several covariates, where the pattern of missingness among the covariates could be somewhat complex, complete cases analysis does tend to yield results that are similar to those given by EM and MI. What is important is that regardless of the type of missingness, these EM/MI and complete cases analysis yield similar results for regression coefficients under these circumstances (Graham and Donaldson 1993).

Note that this is not true of other parameters. For example, means and correlations based on complete cases are often substantially biased under the conditions described here. And with more complex models, such as that described in Fig. 2.1 and Table 2.2, the advantage of the MI/ML approach over complete cases analysis can be substantial.

Perhaps the biggest drawback with complete cases analysis is that it is not possible to make use of auxiliary variables. As noted above, with MI/ML methods, the information that is lost to missingness can be partially mitigated by adding auxiliary variables to the model (please see Chap. 11). However, this mitigation makes no sense when there are no missing data, as is the case with complete cases analysis.

## Missing Data Theory and the Comparison Between MI and ML

Missing data theory holds that MI and ML are asymptotically equivalent. We do not need new simulations to demonstrate this point. What we do need are studies to define the limits of this equivalence. Under such and such conditions, for example, ML or MI is better.

### *MI and ML and the Inclusion of Auxiliary Variables*

Collins et al. (2001) tested and found substantial support for the following proposition:

> *Proposition 1.* If the user of the ML procedure and the imputer use the same set of input data (same set of variables and observational units), if their models apply equivalent distributional assumptions to the variables and the relationships among them, if the sample size is large, and if the number of imputations, $M$, is sufficiently large, then the results from the ML and MI procedures will be essentially identical (p. 336).

Although their proposition was supported, Collins et al. (2001) noted that it holds in theory. But they also noted that, as typically practiced, MI and ML do have important differences. For example, as practiced, MI users have typically included variables in the imputation model that, although not intended for analysis, were included to "help" with the imputation (we now refer to these variables as auxiliary variables; see Chap. 11).

Users of ML methods, however, in usual practice, are much more likely to limit their models to include only those variables that will be part of the analysis model. Although strategies have been described for including auxiliary variables into some types of ML models (e.g., see Graham 2003, for strategies within a structural equation modeling context), it is not uncommon to see ML models that do not attempt to include auxiliary variables. The exclusion of important auxiliary variables from ML models violates the particulars of the Collins et al. proposition and leads to important differences between the models. An important extension of the concept of including auxiliary variables is that models are less well described for including auxiliary variables in ML approaches to latent class analysis.

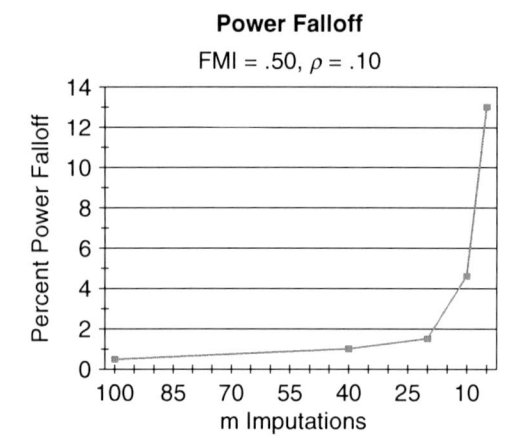

**Fig. 2.5** Power falloff with small number of imputations. Power falloff is in comparison to the comparable FIML model. FMI = Fraction of Missing Information; $\rho$ is the population correlation ($\rho = .10$ represents a small effect)

## MI Versus ML, the Importance of Number of Imputations

Missing data theorists have often stated that the number of imputations needed in MI in order to achieve efficient estimates was relatively small, and that $m = 3$–$5$ imputations were often enough. In this context the relative efficiency of the estimate is given by $(1 + \gamma / m)^{-1}$, where $\gamma$ is the fraction of missing information (Schafer and Olsen 1998). The point made in this context was articulated clearly by Schafer and Olsen:

> Consider … 30 % missing information ($\gamma = .3$), a moderately high rate for many applications. With $m = 5$ imputations, we have already achieved 94 % efficiency. Increasing the number to $m = 10$ raises the efficiency to 97 %, a rather slight gain for doubling of computational effort. In most situations, there is simply little advantage to producing and analyzing more than a few imputed datasets (pp. 548-549).

However, Graham et al. (2007) showed that the effect of number of imputations on statistical power gives a different picture. Graham et al. showed that although the relative efficiency difference might seem small in the context described by Schafer and Olsen (1998), MI with small $m$ could lead to an important falloff in statistical power, compared to the equivalent FIML model, especially with small effect sizes. The numbers below apply to a small effect size in Cohen's (1977) terms ($\rho = .10$). Under these conditions MI with $m = 5$ imputations yields statistical power that is approximately 13 % lower than MI with $m = 100$, and 13 % lower than the comparable FIML analysis (power is .682 for $m = 5$; .791 for $m = 100$; and .793 for the comparable FIML model). Figure 2.5 displays for power falloff compared to FIML for MI with various levels $m$ for $\gamma = .50$. Graham et al. agreed that an acceptable power falloff is a subjective thing, but that power falloff greater than 1 % would be

**Table 2.6** Recommended number of imputations needed for power falloff < .01 compared to FIML

| γ (Fraction of missing information) | | | | |
|---|---|---|---|---|
| .1 | .3 | .5 | .7 | .9 |
| 20 | 20 | 40 | 100 | >100 |

Effect size: $\rho = .10$

considered unacceptable to them. Given this judgment, their recommendations are shown in Table 2.6 for the number of imputations required to maintain a power falloff of less than 1 % compared to FIML.

## Computational Effort and Adjustments in Thinking About MI

In the Schafer and Olsen (1998) quote given above, the second to last sentence suggested that the increase in efficiency from .94 to .97 was "… a rather slight gain for doubling of computational effort." It is important to look carefully at this statement. I will go into more detail about this idea in later chapters, but let me say here that their doubling the number of imputations comes nowhere near doubling the computational effort. There are exceptions, of course, but with the latest versions of the common statistical software (especially SAS, but also SPSS to an important extent), and with the automation utilities described in later chapters, it often costs little in additional computational effort to increase from 5 to 40 imputations.

In the earliest days of MI, several factors conspired to make the computational intensity of the procedure undesirable. First, the procedure itself was brand new back in 1987 and was still relatively new even in 1998. Back then, it represented a radically new approach to handling missing data. Second, in 1987 computers were still very slow. With the computers available back then, the difference between 5 and 40 imputations would often have been very important in terms of computational effort. Third, software for performing multiple imputation was not generally available. Certainly, automation features for handling analysis and summary of multiple data sets were not available.

In this context, the MI theorists suggested the impute-once-analyze-many-times strategy. With this strategy, the computational costs of multiple imputation could be amortized over numerous analyses, thereby reducing the overall costs of the MI procedure. Along with the suggestion that perhaps just 3–5 imputations were enough for efficient parameter estimates, MI did not look so bad as an alternative to other possible approaches to handling missing data.

However, as the realities set in for performing multiple imputation in real-world data sets, it became clear that much of the original thinking regarding MI would not be feasible in large-scale research with missing data. In this context, I have begun to realize that the impute-once-analyze-many approach often does not work. Although it would certainly be desirable in many research contexts, it happens far too often that the researcher needs to make a change in analysis that requires a whole new set of imputations. In addition, pretty much everything is different now. Computers are now very much faster than they were in 1987, and they will continue to get faster. Perhaps more importantly, the software is catching up. The MI feature in SAS (Proc MI; see Chap. 7) is now a highly functional program. And SPSS, with versions 17+, (see Chap. 5) is not far behind. With a fast computer running SAS, it is very feasible to perform multiple imputation separately for each analysis.

# References

Aiken, L.S., & West, S.G. (1991). *Multiple regression: Testing and interpreting interactions.* Newbury Park, CA: Sage.
Allison, P. D. (2002). *Missing Data.* Thousand Oaks, CA: Sage.
Arbuckle, J. L. (1995). *Amos users' guide.* Chicago: Smallwaters.
Arbuckle, J. L. (2010). *IBM SPSS Amos 19 User's Guide.* Crawfordville, FL: Amos Development Corporation.
Bentler, P. M., & Wu, E. J. C. (1995). *EQS for Windows User's Guide.* Encino, CA: Multivariate Software, Inc.
Collins, L. M., Wugalter, S. E. (1992). Latent class models for stage-sequential dynamic latent variables. *Multivariate Behavioral Research, 27,*131–157.
Collins, L. M., Schafer, J. L., & Kam, C. M. (2001). A comparison of inclusive and restrictive strategies in modern missing data procedures. *Psychological Methods, 6,* 330–351.
Efron, B. (1982). *The jackknife, the bootstrap, and other resampling plans.* Philadelphia: Society for Industrial and Applied Mathematics.
Graham, J. W. (2003). Adding missing-data relevant variables to FIML-based structural equation models. *Structural Equation Modeling, 10,* 80–100.
Graham, J. W. (2009). Missing data analysis: making it work in the real world. *Annual Review of Psychology, 60,* 549–576.
Graham, J. W., Olchowski, A. E., & Gilreath, T. D. (2007). How Many Imputations are Really Needed? Some Practical Clarifications of Multiple Imputation Theory. *Prevention Science, 8,* 206–213.
Graham, J. W., and Coffman, D. L. (in press). Structural Equation Modeling with Missing Data. In R. Hoyle (Ed.), *Handbook of Structural Equation Modeling.* New York: Guilford Press.
Graham, J. W., Cumsille, P. E., and Elek-Fisk, E. (2003). Methods for handling missing data. In J. A. Schinka & W. F. Velicer (Eds.). *Research Methods in Psychology* (pp. 87–114). Volume 2 of *Handbook of Psychology* (I. B. Weiner, Editor-in-Chief). New York: John Wiley & Sons.
Graham, J. W., Cumsille, P. E., and Shevock, A. E. (in press). Methods for handling missing data. In J. A. Schinka & W. F. Velicer (Eds.). *Research Methods in Psychology* (pp. 000–000). Volume 3 of *Handbook of Psychology* (I. B. Weiner, Editor-in-Chief). New York: John Wiley & Sons.
Graham, J. W., & Donaldson, S. I. (1993). Evaluating interventions with differential attrition: The importance of nonresponse mechanisms and use of followup data. *Journal of Applied Psychology, 78,* 119–128.
Graham, J. W., & Hofer, S. M. (1991). EMCOV.EXE Users Guide. Unpublished manuscript, University of Southern California.
Graham, J. W., Hofer, S.M., Donaldson, S. I., MacKinnon, D.P., & Schafer, J. L. (1997). Analysis with missing data in prevention research. In K. Bryant, M. Windle, & S. West (Eds.), *The science of prevention: methodological advances from alcohol and substance abuse research.* (pp. 325–366). Washington, D.C.: American Psychological Association.

# References

Graham, J. W., Hofer, S.M., and MacKinnon, D.P. (1996). Maximizing the usefulness of data obtained with planned missing value patterns: an application of maximum likelihood procedures. *Multivariate Behavioral Research*, *31*, 197–218.

Hansen, W. B., & Graham, J. W. (1991). Preventing alcohol, marijuana, and cigarette use among adolescents: Peer pressure resistance training versus establishing conservative norms. *Preventive Medicine*, *20*, 414–430.

Jaccard, J.J. & Turrisi, R. (2003). *Interaction effects in multiple regression*. Newberry Park, CA: Sage Publications.

Jöreskog, K.G. & Sörbom, D. (2006). LISREL 8.8 for Windows [Computer software]. Lincolnwood, IL: Scientific Software International, Inc.

MacKinnon, D. P., Lockwood, C. M., Hoffman, J. M., West, S. G. & Sheets, V. (2002). A comparison of methods to test mediation and other intervening variable effects. *Psychological Methods*, *7*(1), 83–104.

Mels, G. (2006) *LISREL for Windows: Getting Started Guide*. Lincolnwood, IL: Scientific Software International, Inc.

Muthén, L. K., & Muthén, B. O. (2010). *Mplus User's Guide. (6th ed.)*. Los Angeles: Author.

Neale, M. C., Boker, S. M., Xie, G., and Maes, H. H. (2003). *Mx: Statistical Modeling*. VCU Box 900126, Richmond, VA 23298: Department of Psychiatry. 6th Edition.

Raudenbush, S. W., & Bryk, A. S. (2002). *Hierarchical Linear Models: Applications and Data Analysis Methods, Second Edition*. Newbury Park, CA: Sage.

Raudenbush, S. W., Rowan, B., and Kang, S. J. (1991). A multilevel, multivariate model for studying school climate with estimation via the EM algorithm and application to U.S. high-school data. *Journal of Educational Statistics*, *16*, 295–330.

Rubin, D.B. (1987). *Multiple imputation for nonresponse in surveys*. New York: Wiley.

Rubin, D. B., & Thayer, D. T. (1982). EM algorithms for ML factor analysis. *Psychometrika*, *47*, 69–76.

Schafer, J. L. (1997). *Analysis of Incomplete Multivariate Data*. New York: Chapman and Hall.

Schafer, J. L. (2001). Multiple imputation with PAN. In L. M. Collins and A. G. Sayer (Eds.) *New Methods for the Analysis of Change*, ed., (pp. 357–377). Washington, DC: American Psychological Association.

Schafer, J. L., and Olsen, M. K. (1998). Multiple imputation for multivariate missing data problems: A data analyst's perspective. *Multivariate Behavioral Research*, *33*, 545–571.

Schafer, J. L., and Yucel, R. M. (2002). Computational strategies for multivariate linear mixed-effects models with missing values. *Journal of Computational and Graphical Statistics*, *11*, 437–457.

Tanner, M. A., & Wong, W. H. (1987). The calculation of posterior distributions by data augmentation (with discussion). *Journal of the American Statistical Association*, *82*, 528–550.

von Hippel, P. T. (2004). Biases in SPSS 12.0 Missing Value Analysis. *American Statistician*, *58*, 160–164.

Willett, J. B., and Sayer, A. G. (1994). Using covariance structure analysis to detect correlates and predictors of individual change over time. *Psychological Bulletin*, *116(2)*, 363–381.

Yuan, K-H., & Bentler, P.M. (2000). Three likelihood-based methods for mean and covariance structure analysis with nonnormal missing data. *Sociological Methodology*, *30*, 165–200.

# Section 2
# Multiple Imputation and Basic Analysis

# Chapter 3
# Multiple Imputation with Norm 2.03

In this chapter, I provide step-by-step instructions for performing multiple imputation with Schafer's (1997) NORM 2.03 program. Although these instructions apply most directly to NORM, most of the concepts apply to other MI programs as well.

## Step-by-Step Instructions for Multiple Imputation with NORM 2.03

In this section, I describe in detail the use of the NORM software (version 2.03; Schafer 1997). For other descriptions of the workings of NORM, please see Graham et al. (2003), Graham and Hofer (2000), and Schafer and Olsen (1998).

### *Running NORM (Step 1): Getting NORM*

If you do not have NORM already, you can download it for free from the website, http://methodology.psu.edu. Click on "Free Software". Please note that you will be required to set up an account for access to the Methodology center web page. Once you have it downloaded, install the program. It is a self-extracting zip file that unzips, by default, to the folder, c:\winimp.

#### Installation Details

The defaults for downloading usually work well. However, there is one detail you should know. The NORM executable (norm.exe) and the library DLL (salflibc.dll) need to be in the same folder. If you always run NORM from the c:\winimp folder, or from any other folder containing both files, it will work fine. An alternative is to place the salflibc.dll file into a folder that is listed in the "path" statement. The folders listed there are searched any time a command or program is executed. I have found it useful to place the salflibc.dll file in the c:\windows folder.

Please contact me (at jgraham@psu.edu) if you are having difficulty negotiating this process.

## Running NORM (Step 2): Preparing the Data Set

### Select Variables that will be Included in NORM

A first step in running NORM is to prepare the data set that will be used as input to NORM. A key first step in this preparation is to select the variables that will be used in the MI analysis. It is crucial in selecting variables that you realize that it almost always happens that you cannot simply perform MI on all the variables in your data set. I usually say that in choosing your variables for MI analysis, you should

(a) Start with the analysis model of interest.
(b) Judiciously include a few auxiliary variables (variables that are highly correlated with the variables in your analysis model). If you have a longitudinal data set, the best auxiliary variables are variables that are the same as the variables in your analysis model, but that are not being used in this analysis. For example, if I were looking at a program effect at seventh grade on cigarette smoking at tenth grade, I might well include smoking at eighth and ninth grades as auxiliary variables, along with smoking at seventh grade (if it is not being used as a covariate in the analysis model). Similarly, for any mediating variable used in the model, good auxiliary variables would be that same mediating variable measured at other waves not otherwise included in the analysis. Especially important in this context is to include measures that were measured after the mediating variable to be used in the analysis. For example, suppose beliefs about the prevalence of cigarette smoking among peers, measured at the immediate posttest (late seventh grade) was the mediating variable. I might well include as auxiliary variables prevalence beliefs at eighth and ninth grades (along with prevalence beliefs in early seventh grade if that variable is not part of the analysis model).
(c) If multilevel analysis of cluster data is the analysis of choice, then cluster membership dummy variables should be included (Chaps. 6 and 7 present examples and important caveats to the strategy of including dummy variables to represent cluster membership).

The variables that are included in the MI analysis should all be continuous (or reasonably assumed to be continuous, including "ordered categorical" variables), or dichotomous categorical. Any categorical variables with more than two levels must be recast as dummy variables before the MI analysis ($p-1$ dummy variables must be used to represent the categorical variable with $p > 2$ categories).

Be sure to convert *all* missing values in the data set to −9 or some other negative number (positive numbers that are clearly out of range are also possible, but negative numbers work best in this context). In some data sets, multiple numbers are used to refer to the different reasons as the variables have missing values. This strategy will not be used here.[1] Be sure that all missing values have the same missing value indicator. Whatever this missing value indicator is, it should be well out of the range of legal values in all your variables. Thus, I prefer −9 or some other negative number (e.g., −99 or −999), because these values are typically out of range for all variables. It is crucial that the system missing code (typically a period) NOT be used. It is also important that the missing value not be a blank or space.

Finally, write the data out to an ASCII data set. Each value should be separated by a space (freefield format; space delimited), or a tab (tab delimited), and the data for each subject should be output to a single long line.

In naming the output data set, it is best if the name be broken into a "root" (e.g., mydata), followed by ".dat" as the suffix (e.g., mydata.dat). It is also highly useful to produce a second ASCII text file with the names of the variables appearing in the ".dat" file, in the order that they appear in that file. This variables names file should have the same "root" as the data file, but should have the ".nam" suffix (e.g., mydata.nam).

## *Writing Data Out of SPSS*

There are many acceptable ways to write SPSS data out to an ascii data set. This is one way.

(a) Create a version of your SPSS data set that contains only those variables you will include in the NORM analysis.
(b) Click on "Transform" and on "Recode into Same Variables".
(c) Select all of the variables on the left and transfer them to the "Variables" window on the right.
(d) Click on "Old and New Values".
(e) On the left, under "Old Value", click on "System-missing"; on the right, under "New Value", enter the value (use "−9" or some other number clearly out of range for all variables in the data set). Click on "Add" for the "Old −> New" window. Click on "Continue", and on "OK".
(f) While in the Data editor window, click on "File" and "Save As". For "Save as type", select "Tab delimited (*.dat)"; uncheck the box, "Write variable names to spreadsheet". Enter the desired "File name" (e.g., mydata.dat), and click on "Save".

---

[1] There has been some attempt to expand standard normal model MI for dealing with two missing data mechanisms in the same data set (e.g., see Harel 2003, 2007), but the usefulness of approaches such as this remains to be demonstrated.

## Writing a Variable Names File from SPSS

(a) Go to the Data Editor window. Click on the "Variable View" tab at the bottom left.
(b) Highlight and copy all of the variable names in the "Name" column.
(c) Open a Notepad window and paste the variable names.
(d) Click on File and on Save. Under "File name", enter the same root as you used in (f) above, but with the ".nam" suffix (e.g., mydata.nam). Be sure the new file is being saved to the same folder containing the data (mydata.dat).
(e) If you click on "Save" now, the file will be saved with the ".txt" suffix (e.g., mydata.nam.txt). So first click on "Save as type", and select "All Files". Click on "Save". Now the file will be saved with the ".nam" suffix (e.g., mydata.nam).

## Empirical Example Used Throughout this Chapter

In order to facilitate learning the procedures outlined in this chapter, I encourage you to download the data file, "ex3.dat", and the corresponding variable names file, "ex3.nam", from http://methodology.psu.edu.

The sample data set comes from a subset of one cohort of students ($N=2,756$) who took part in the Adolescent Alcohol Prevention Trial (AAPT; Hansen and Graham 1991). The sample data set includes a variable, *School*, indicating which of 12 schools the student was from. In addition, 19 substantive variables are included: Lifetime alcohol use at seventh, eighth, and ninth grades (*Alc7, Alc8, Alc9*); five variables making up a scale tapping relationship with parents at seventh grade (*Likepar71, Likepar72, Likepar73, Likepar74, Likepar75*); three variables making up a scale tapping beliefs about the positive social consequences of alcohol use at seventh grade (*Posatt71, Posatt72, Posatt73*); four variables tapping risk-taking and rebelliousness in grade 7 (*Riskreb71, Riskreb72, Riskreb73, Riskreb74*); and four variables tapping risk-taking and rebelliousness in eighth grade (*Riskreb81, Riskreb82, Riskreb83, Riskreb84*).

As you read through the steps for conducting imputation with Norm 2.03, I encourage you to try out each step with this sample data set.

## Running NORM (Step 3): Variables

NORM 2.03 is a Windows program, so users will recognize familiar aspects of the layout. Begin by clicking on "File" and starting a "new session." Locate your recently created datafile and read it into NORM. The data set appears in the main window. Verify that the number of cases, number of variables, and the missing data indicator are all correct.

▶ **Sample Data**. Find and click on the data set named ex3.dat.

Click on the "Variables" tab. In the left column are the default variable names. If you have included a root.nam file, the variables names in that file will appear here. If you are dealing with a small file, you can double-click on the variable name to change it.

▶ **Sample Data**. Because the file "ex3.nam" exists in that same folder, you will see the 20 variable names listed.

The second column from left ("In model") can be very valuable. It is sometimes useful to include variables (e.g., Subject ID codes) in the data set even if they are not intended for analysis. Such variables are easily removed from the imputation model by double-clicking to remove the asterisk for that variable. Sometimes it is also useful to retain in the data set certain categorical variables with $p>2$ categories, along with the dummy variables representing that variable (this makes sense only where there are no missing data on that categorical variable). In this case, remove the "In model" asterisk for the original variable, but leave the "In *.imp" asterisk (rightmost column).

▶ **Sample Data**. For these analyses, eliminate the variable "school" from the imputation model. Remove (double-click on) the asterisk for "In model". This will leave 19 variables in the imputation model.

Transformations (e.g., log transformations) can sometimes speed up the imputation process. But although Norm 2.03 does allow transformations to be made, it is usually better to perform any such transformations in the statistical program (e.g., SPSS) used to write the data out in the first place. If one wishes to transform one or more variables for imputation, but retain the original untransformed variables for analysis, it is relatively easy to back transform the variables (again with SPSS or whatever program one uses) after imputation (e.g., using the antilog after a log transformation).

An interesting exception to my rule of doing transformations in the regular statistical program you use relates to forming dummy codes for categorical variables for which there are no missing data. For such variables, one option is to leave those variables in the model in their original (categorical) format, and let Norm generate the dummy variables. An often useful example of this option is found with variables that indicate cluster membership, for example, for students within schools, this kind of variable would indicate school membership (see Chap. 6 for more detail on this strategy). To create dummy variables for such variables, double-click on the word "none" in the Transformations column, and click on Dummy variables at the bottom of the screen, and on OK.

Rounding is an interesting issue. My view is that rounding should be kept to a minimum. Multiple imputation was designed to restore lost variability in the data set as a whole. However, rounding after imputation is the same as adding a small amount of additional random error variance to the imputed values. This is easiest to see when calculating coefficient alpha when scale items have been rounded and unrounded. The rounded versions always have scale alpha that is one or two points lower (indicating more random error in the scale score).

So my rule for rounding is this. If the variable will be used in an analysis where the unrounded values will be no problem (e.g., using a variable as a covariate in a regression model), then leave it in its unrounded form. Of course, if the variable is to be used in an analysis where only certain values make any sense (e.g., using gender as a blocking variable or using a dichotomous smoking variable as the dependent variable in a logistic regression analysis), then by all means, round to the legal values (e.g., 0 and 1).

▶ **Sample Data.** Go ahead and leave the rounding alone for this example. But just to see how it is done, change one variable. Double-click on the word "integer" in the Rounding column corresponding to the variable *Alc9* (last variable in the data set). Click on the word "hundredth" in the right column, and click on OK. This will allow rounding of imputed values to the nearest hundredth.

## *Running NORM (Step 4): The "Summarize" Tab*

This is an important step in the imputation process. Click on the "summarize" tab and "run". The output from this summary is saved in the file, "summary.out". It appears automatically when Summarize is run, and can be reloaded at any time by clicking on "Display" and "Output file". Be sure to rename this file if you wish to save it, because it is overwritten each time you run Summarize.

The Summarize output is in two parts. The top section displays the number and percent missing for each variable in the missing data model. I find it useful to scan down the percent missing column and make sure that each percent missing makes sense based on what I already know about the data set. Be especially watchful when the percent missing is high. Does it make sense that some variables have 50 % (or more) missing data? This sometimes happens for the right reasons, for example, the data are missing due to a planned missing data design. But it is also possible that a high percent missing could be due to a simple coding error. It is important not to go forward until you have an adequate explanation.

▶ **Sample Data.** Information about the number and percent of missing data for each variable is presented in Table 3.1. Because you dropped the school variable from the MI analysis, you should have 2,756 observations and 19 variables. Note that a small percentage (6.42 %) of students had missing data for Alc7, alcohol use at seventh grade. Normally there is virtually no missing data in this cohort on this variable at seventh grade. The small amount of missingness seen here is due mainly to the fact that in this data set, I included new students who "dropped in" to the study beginning at eighth grade. Also note that about 40 % of students were missing on each of the other variables measured at seventh grade. This amount of missingness is due largely to the planned missingness design used in this study (see Chap. 12 for a discussion of this type of design). In this case, approximately a third of the students were not given these questions. Add to that the approximately 6 % not present at all at the seventh grade measure, and the

**Table 3.1** Number and percent missing information

```
NUMBER OF OBSERVATIONS  =        2756
NUMBER OF VARIABLES     =          19
                    NUMBER MISSING     % MISSING
alc7                     177              6.42
rskreb71                1111             40.31
rskreb72                1100             39.91
rskreb73                1100             39.91
rskreb74                1101             39.95
likepa71                1116             40.49
likepa72                1114             40.42
likepa73                1119             40.60
likepa74                1108             40.20
likepa75                1111             40.31
posatt71                1122             40.71
posatt72                1118             40.57
posatt73                1130             41.00
alc8                     224              8.13
rskreb81                1211             43.94
rskreb82                1191             43.21
rskreb83                1192             43.25
rskreb84                1199             43.51
alc9                     944             34.25
```

number is very close to the 40 % missingness observed. The 8.13 % missing on Alc8 represents approximately 8 % attrition between seventh and eighth grades. This is reasonable in this study. The somewhat higher rate of missingness on the riskreb8 items (43–44 %), compared to the seventh grade versions of these variables, is also reasonable. The 34.25 % missing on Alc9 reflects the somewhat greater attrition between eighth and ninth grades. This, too, makes sense given what I already know about these data.

The second part of the summarize output is the matrix of missing data patterns. When many variables are included in the model, and with large sample sizes, this section of output may be too complex to be of immediate usefulness. However, there is always some valuable information in this matrix. The top row of this matrix shows the number of cases (if any) with complete data. This is always useful information. It is good to know what proportion of the total sample has complete data (also see Step 5, below). The bottom row of this matrix also provides useful information. The bottom row displays the pattern with the least data. Occasionally, one finds that this bottom row has all "0" values, that is, some cases happen to have no data at all for this set of variables. Although NORM and other missing data procedures do handle this situation in an appropriate way, it is not good form to keep cases in the model when they have no data at all. If you are not convinced of this, imagine the sentences you must write in the Method section of your article describing

**Table 3.2** 23 largest patterns of missing and observed values

| Count | | | | | | | | | | | | | | | | | | |
|---|---|---|---|---|---|---|---|---|---|---|---|---|---|---|---|---|---|---|
| 386 | 1 | 1 | 1 | 1 | 1 | 1 | 1 | 1 | 1 | 0 | 0 | 0 | 1 | 1 | 1 | 1 | 1 | 1 |
| 58  | 0 | 0 | 0 | 0 | 0 | 0 | 0 | 0 | 0 | 0 | 0 | 0 | 1 | 1 | 1 | 1 | 1 | 1 |
| 10  | 1 | 1 | 0 | 0 | 0 | 1 | 1 | 1 | 1 | 1 | 1 | 1 | 1 | 0 | 1 | 1 | 1 | 1 |
| 351 | 1 | 0 | 1 | 1 | 0 | 0 | 0 | 0 | 0 | 1 | 1 | 1 | 1 | 0 | 1 | 1 | 1 | 1 |
| 11  | 1 | 1 | 1 | 1 | 1 | 1 | 1 | 1 | 1 | 0 | 0 | 0 | 1 | 0 | 1 | 1 | 1 | 1 |
| 58  | 0 | 0 | 0 | 0 | 0 | 0 | 0 | 0 | 0 | 0 | 0 | 0 | 1 | 0 | 1 | 1 | 1 | 1 |
| 369 | 1 | 1 | 0 | 0 | 0 | 1 | 1 | 1 | 1 | 1 | 1 | 1 | 1 | 1 | 0 | 0 | 0 | 1 |
| 36  | 0 | 0 | 0 | 0 | 0 | 0 | 0 | 0 | 0 | 0 | 0 | 0 | 1 | 1 | 0 | 0 | 0 | 1 |
| 29  | 1 | 1 | 0 | 0 | 0 | 1 | 1 | 1 | 1 | 1 | 1 | 1 | 1 | 0 | 0 | 0 | 0 | 1 |
| 47  | 1 | 0 | 1 | 1 | 1 | 0 | 0 | 0 | 0 | 1 | 1 | 1 | 1 | 0 | 0 | 0 | 0 | 1 |
| 36  | 1 | 1 | 1 | 1 | 1 | 1 | 1 | 1 | 1 | 0 | 0 | 0 | 1 | 0 | 0 | 0 | 0 | 1 |
| 66  | 1 | 1 | 0 | 0 | 0 | 1 | 1 | 1 | 1 | 1 | 1 | 1 | 0 | 0 | 0 | 0 | 0 | 1 |
| 63  | 1 | 0 | 1 | 1 | 1 | 0 | 0 | 0 | 0 | 1 | 1 | 1 | 0 | 0 | 0 | 0 | 0 | 1 |
| 48  | 1 | 1 | 1 | 1 | 1 | 1 | 1 | 1 | 1 | 0 | 0 | 0 | 0 | 0 | 0 | 0 | 0 | 1 |
| 216 | 1 | 1 | 1 | 1 | 1 | 1 | 1 | 1 | 1 | 0 | 0 | 0 | 1 | 1 | 1 | 1 | 1 | 0 |
| 10  | 1 | 1 | 1 | 0 | 0 | 1 | 1 | 1 | 1 | 0 | 0 | 0 | 1 | 1 | 1 | 1 | 1 | 0 |
| 217 | 1 | 0 | 1 | 1 | 1 | 0 | 0 | 0 | 0 | 1 | 1 | 1 | 1 | 0 | 1 | 1 | 1 | 0 |
| 12  | 1 | 0 | 1 | 1 | 1 | 0 | 0 | 0 | 0 | 1 | 1 | 0 | 1 | 0 | 1 | 1 | 1 | 0 |
| 218 | 1 | 1 | 0 | 0 | 0 | 1 | 1 | 1 | 1 | 1 | 1 | 1 | 1 | 1 | 0 | 0 | 0 | 0 |
| 13  | 1 | 0 | 0 | 0 | 0 | 0 | 0 | 0 | 0 | 0 | 1 | 1 | 1 | 1 | 0 | 0 | 0 | 0 |
| 25  | 1 | 1 | 0 | 0 | 0 | 1 | 1 | 1 | 1 | 1 | 1 | 1 | 1 | 0 | 0 | 0 | 0 | 0 |
| 23  | 1 | 0 | 1 | 1 | 1 | 0 | 0 | 0 | 0 | 1 | 1 | 1 | 1 | 0 | 0 | 0 | 0 | 0 |
| 22  | 1 | 1 | 1 | 1 | 1 | 1 | 1 | 1 | 1 | 0 | 0 | 0 | 1 | 0 | 0 | 0 | 0 | 0 |

the rationale for leaving these variables in. I recommend that you go back to the original program and delete these cases before proceeding.

▶ **Sample Data**. There are three key things to see here. First, there are no complete cases. I know this, because the top row, which will show the complete cases if there are any, have "0" values in columns 3, 4, and 5 (rebel72, rebel73, rebel74). This is expected because with the planned missingness design used in this study, the 3-form design (see Graham et al. 2006; also see Chap. 12), no one has complete data for all variables in the data set. Second, there are 232 different patterns of missing and nonmissing data. Third, because the bottom row of this matrix contains some "1" values, I know there are no cases with no data.

I also find it useful to scan the matrix of missing value patterns for the largest patterns. This also serves as a diagnostic tool. Does it make sense that many people have missing data for a particular block of variables?

▶ **Sample Data**. I often find it useful to provide a version of this matrix of missing data patterns in articles I write. However, with 232 patterns, such a table would most likely be more confusing than helpful. However, one thing I often do is to provide a table with the largest patterns. For example, in this data set, Table 3.2 shows all missing data patterns with at least ten cases.

## Running NORM (Step 5): EM Algorithm

Start by clicking on the "EM algorithm". Although it is often reasonable to accept all of the defaults when running EM, first click on the "Computing" button to view several options.

**Maximum Iterations**

I outlined the workings of the EM algorithm in Chap. 2. EM iterates (back and forth between the E and M steps) until in "converges", or until the "maximum iterations" have been reached. My rule of thumb here is to leave the maximum iterations at the default (1,000 iterations). If EM has not converged in 1,000 iterations, I can almost always make changes that will allow it to converge in fewer iterations. It is often a sign of a fundamental data problem when EM takes as many as 1,000 iterations to converge.

**Convergence Criterion**

In Chap. 2, I noted that EM converges when the elements of the covariance matrix stop changing appreciably from one iteration to the next. Of course, what constitutes "appreciable" change can vary. The default convergence criterion for NORM is 1E-04 (.0001). It is important to know that with NORM, convergence is reached when the largest absolute change in any of the variance-covariance parameters, divided by that parameter's value, is less than the criterion. With NORM, the variables are also in standardized form for the interim analyses (variables are back standardized to their original scales for imputation). But other criteria are possible. For example, with EMCOV (Graham and Donaldson 1993; Graham and Hofer 1992), convergence is reached when the largest change in any of the variance-covariance parameters is smaller than the criterion (without dividing by the parameter's value). Thus, what constitutes "appreciable" change is typically a little larger for EMCOV than it is for NORM.

**Maximum-Likelihood Estimate or Posterior mode**

The last decision to make in this window is whether to ask for the standard maximum-likelihood estimate or to use the Bayesian "posterior mode under ridge prior with hyperparameter". My view is that the ML solution is better if it works, so it is always best to try that first. But occasionally, the ML mode does not work well (e.g., EM takes more than 1,000 iterations to converge, or never converges). I have found that having few or no cases with complete data can often (but not always) produce this problem. The problem can also manifest itself when one or more variables have a very high percent missing data (see Chap. 8 for other examples).

The posterior mode under ridge prior is like ridge regression in some respects. Ridge regression (e.g., see Price 1977) has been used when the predictors in multiple regression are so highly correlated as to produce unstable results. In ridge regression, one adds a small constant to all of the diagonal elements of the input correlation matrix (e.g., making them all 1.01 rather than 1.00). It is easy to see that all correlations in this new input matrix are slightly biased toward 0. The result is that the regression results will be slightly biased, but the solution will also be more stable because the predictors are less correlated.

A similar thing happens with multiple imputation. The idea is to introduce a little bias in order to make the MI analysis more stable. Adding a ridge prior with hyperparameter is a little like adding some number of cases at the bottom of one's data set, such that all of the variables are uncorrelated. The number of cases added is similar to the value of the hyperparameter. So, if one sets the hyperparameter to 5, it is a little like adding five cases at the bottom of one's data set. It makes sense why this should work. If your data set has no complete cases, then adding these five cases means that your data set now has five complete cases. But the cost of doing this is that all correlations are biased slightly toward 0. This is why I say that I prefer using the ML mode if it works; I would like to avoid this bias if possible. Also, even if you must use the posterior mode, it is a good idea to use a hyperparameter as small as possible. My rule of thumb here is to use a hyperparameter no larger than 1 % of the overall sample size. In order to help keep that number as low as possible, think of the hyperparameter as adding "bogus" cases to the bottom of your data set. What reviewer will respond favorably to your adding a large number of bogus cases to your data set?

**Other Options**

Another option under the EM algorithm tab is whether to have the covariance matrix or correlation matrix output to the EM output file. Either is fine, but I generally find it more useful to have the correlation matrix output. The covariance matrix is always written to the file "em.prm" (default name) in case it is needed.

The other options here relate to input and output file names. By default, EM begins with values calculated from the data set itself. I do not remember when I have ever needed to change this, so I leave the input file name blank. The output file for EM parameters is "em.prm" by default. Again, I do not remember ever having to change this.

**EM Output: Iteration History**

Output from the EM run is saved in the file "em.out". This window appears automatically at the end of the EM run and can be retrieved at any time by clicking on "Display" and "Output file". Be sure to rename this file if you want to save it, because it is overwritten each time EM is run.

The top part of the EM output file contains basic information about the data set, any transformations that were used, and the means and standard deviations of the observed data (using available complete data). I typically skip all this information.

The next section of the EM output is the iteration history for the observed data loglikelihood function. This can be highly informative. Scan down the iterations. The function value should change monotonically over the iterations. When this has occurred, and the number of iterations is reasonably low (definitely some number less than 1,000), then I feel comfortable saying (e.g., in my article) that "EM converged normally in xxx iterations."

▶ **Sample Data**. In this instance, EM (ML mode) converged normally in 72 iterations. The iteration history is shown in Table 3.3. Scanning down the iterations, we can see that the fit function did indeed change monotonically. The function

**Table 3.3** Iteration history

| ITERATION # | OBSERVED-DATA LOGLIKELIHOOD |
|---|---|
| 1 | -16428.50000 |
| 2 | -12336.59596 |
| 3 | -11591.68956 |
| 4 | -11402.88252 |
| 5 | -11347.51545 |
| 6 | -11328.21002 |
| 7 | -11320.20358 |
| 8 | -11316.42661 |
| 9 | -11314.49253 |
| 10 | -11313.44867 |
| 11 | -11312.86328 |
| 12 | -11312.52409 |
| 13 | -11312.32136 |
| 14 | -11312.19641 |
| 15 | -11312.11702 |
| 16 | -11312.06510 |
| 17 | -11312.03021 |
| 18 | -11312.00619 |
| 19 | -11311.98930 |
| 20 | -11311.97721 |
| 21 | -11311.96843 |
| 22 | -11311.96197 |
| 23 | -11311.95718 |
| 24 | -11311.95358 |
| 25 | -11311.95088 |
| 26 | -11311.94883 |
| 27 | -11311.94727 |
| 28 | -11311.94607 |

(continued)

**Table 3.3** (continued)

| ITERATION # | OBSERVED-DATA LOGLIKELIHOOD |
|---|---|
| 29 | -11311.94516 |
| 30 | -11311.94446 |
| 31 | -11311.94391 |
| 32 | -11311.94349 |
| 33 | -11311.94317 |
| 34 | -11311.94292 |
| 35 | -11311.94273 |
| 36 | -11311.94257 |
| 37 | -11311.94246 |
| 38 | -11311.94237 |
| 39 | -11311.94229 |
| 40 | -11311.94224 |
| 41 | -11311.94220 |
| 42 | -11311.94216 |
| 43 | -11311.94213 |
| 44 | -11311.94211 |
| 45 | -11311.94210 |
| 46 | -11311.94208 |
| 47 | -11311.94207 |
| 48 | -11311.94207 |
| 49 | -11311.94206 |
| 50 | -11311.94206 |
| 51 | -11311.94205 |
| 52 | -11311.94205 |
| 53 | -11311.94205 |
| 54 | -11311.94205 |
| 55 | -11311.94204 |
| 56 | -11311.94204 |
| 57 | -11311.94204 |
| 58 | -11311.94204 |
| 59 | -11311.94204 |
| 60 | -11311.94204 |
| 61 | -11311.94204 |
| 62 | -11311.94204 |
| 63 | -11311.94204 |
| 64 | -11311.94204 |
| 65 | -11311.94204 |
| 66 | -11311.94204 |
| 67 | -11311.94204 |
| 68 | -11311.94204 |
| 69 | -11311.94204 |
| 70 | -11311.94204 |
| 71 | -11311.94204 |
| 72 | -11311.94204 |
| EM CONVERGED AT ITERATION 72 | |

value for the last 17 iterations did not change (to five decimal places). This is normal. Remember it is the change in parameter estimates that determines convergence, not the change in the function value. Note that, in this instance, EM (ML mode) converged normally in a reasonable number of iterations, despite the fact that there were no complete cases.

▶ **Important Note**. Everything to here, including EM (ML mode) converging in exactly 72 iterations is something you should expect to find when you run this example on your computer. However, when dealing with imputation steps that follow, any two people will get slightly different results (e.g., for specific imputed values and for results based on imputed data). This is because the error added to each imputed values is random. However, differences will not be large, provided the number of imputations is sufficiently large.

On the other hand, if the fit function value sometimes gets smaller, then larger, then smaller, etc., this is a sign of a serious problem with the data. You should NOT proceed with the EM solution when this happens. In these instances, it is important to troubleshoot the source of the problem. Please see Chap. 8 for strategies for troubleshooting problems of this sort.

But also watch for more subtle signs that the fit function value is not always changing in the same direction. I recently had a case where the absolute value of the fit function was getting smaller and smaller in what appeared to be a normal way for 267 iterations, but then it started getting larger again. Although EM eventually converged in 405 iterations, I was wary of the solution. (Note that this was a case with 43 variables and 517 cases – 62 complete cases. EM in ML mode converged normally in 664 iterations. The problem noted occurred in posterior mode with hyperparameter $r = 5$.)

A key bit of information from the iteration history is the final number of iterations it takes EM to converge. This information will be used later in the MI process, so it is a good idea to write it down. Also, as noted above, if it is true, I like to write this number in my article, for example, "EM converged normally in xxx iterations."

## EM Output: ML Estimates

The bottom section of the EM output contains the ML parameter estimates: means, standard deviations, and the correlation or covariance matrix (see Table 3.4). I believe these are the best point estimates for these parameters. If you want to report these quantities in your article, I believe they should come from this output. Your table (or text) should, of course, be clear that these means and standard deviations (and correlation matrix) are EM parameter estimates.

Table 3.4 EM parameter estimates

| | MEAN | ST.DEV. |
|---|---|---|
| alc7 | 2.93940 | 2.02527 |
| rskreb71 | 1.74012 | 0.904454 |
| rskreb72 | 2.03761 | 0.915954 |
| rskreb73 | 1.81162 | 0.892740 |
| rskreb74 | 2.67124 | 1.01144 |
| likepa71 | 3.07546 | 0.808821 |
| likepa72 | 3.33576 | 1.14970 |
| likepa73 | 2.73071 | 0.953776 |
| likepa74 | 4.12873 | 1.08177 |
| likepa75 | 3.71806 | 0.604865 |
| posatt71 | 1.56977 | 0.961201 |
| posatt72 | 1.50885 | 0.891302 |
| posatt73 | 1.28612 | 0.689568 |
| alc8 | 3.68106 | 2.34676 |
| rskreb81 | 2.07498 | 0.955559 |
| rskreb82 | 2.18698 | 0.958981 |
| rskreb83 | 1.99252 | 0.936962 |
| rskreb84 | 2.75440 | 1.01388 |
| alc9 | 4.38120 | 2.44073 |

**Speed of EM**

How long it takes EM to converge depends on many factors. The two biggest factors are the number of variables ($k$) in the model and the amount of missing information (related to the amount of missing data). EM estimates $k(k+1)/2$ variances and covariances and $k$ means. Table 3.5 shows how the number of parameters to be estimated increases exponentially with the number of variables. Because the EM algorithm works primarily with the variance-covariance matrix, and other matrices of the same size, the number of variables is far more important to the time to EM convergence than is the number of cases.

The second major factor in EM convergence rate is the amount of missing data. The more the missing data, the longer it takes EM to converge. Another factor is the correlation between other variables in the model and the variables with missing data (higher correlations mean faster convergence). The number of different missing data patterns also contributes to the convergence rate (more patterns take longer). I have also observed that EM with highly skewed variables also seems to take longer to converge.

## *Running NORM (Step 6): Impute from (EM) Parameters*

Imputing from EM parameters could not be easier. Just be sure you have just run EM (and that EM has converged "normally," as described above). Then simply click

Table 3.5 Increase in parameters estimated in EM as number of variables increases

| Variables $k$ | Parameters estimated $[(k(k+1)/2)+k]$ |
|---|---|
| 20 | 230 |
| 40 | 860 |
| 60 | 1,890 |
| 80 | 3,320 |
| 100 | 5,150 |
| 120 | 7,380 |
| 140 | 10,010 |
| 160 | 13,040 |
| 180 | 16,470 |
| 200 | 20,300 |

on "Impute from parameters" tab, and click on "Run". You will see a window: "use parameters from parameter (*.prm) file:" with the just-created "em.prm" listed. That is the default if you have just run EM; leave that as is. At the bottom of the window, you will also see a window "Imputed data set save to file:". The file name will be the root of your original data set, with "_0.imp" as the suffix (e.g., mydata_0.imp). This file may be read into any statistical analysis program. This file is particularly useful for data quality analyses such as coefficient alpha analysis and exploratory factor analysis. This file can be used to obtain certain parameter estimates from other analyses such as multiple regression analysis. Parameter estimates from any number of statistical analyses will be very useful. ***However, this file should NOT be used for any type of hypothesis testing.*** I typically create this imputed data set at this point in the process, even if I have no immediate plans for it. It is easiest to create at this point, and you may well discover later that you need it.

▶ **Sample Data.** Some things to note about the newly created single data set imputed from EM parameters. First, the output data set will have the name: "ex3_0.imp" and will appear in the same folder with "ex3.dat". Second, note that this imputed data set includes the original values for the cluster indicator variable, *School* (and not the dummy codes) even though it was omitted from the imputation model. Finally, note that all of the variables were imputed to the integer values, except the last variable. For that variable (Alc9), any imputed value was imputed to the nearest hundredth.

One caveat with NORM 2.03 is that this step sometimes fails, giving an error message that the covariance matrix is not positive-definite. This is an error, but a simple work-around is possible. Simply proceed to the next step, Data Augmentation (DA), but ask for just one iteration of DA. I have never seen this alternative strategy fail.

Imputed data sets from two adjacent steps of DA will be very similar. So this alternative data set will be very close to the single data set imputed from EM parameters. Both versions of this data set will provide unbiased parameter estimates. However, this alternative version will be very slightly less efficient than the data set imputed from EM parameters.

## *Running NORM (Step 7): Data Augmentation (and Imputation)*

The data augmentation (and imputation) part of this process is normally run immediately after running EM (and imputing from EM parameters). Begin this next step by clicking on the "Data augmentation" tab. Perform this part of the process in three steps, moving from right to left at the bottom of the screen.

First, click on the **Series** button. This is where you select information that will be used in the diagnostic plots (the diagnostics themselves will be described later). I usually select "Save all parameters at every $k$th cycle", where $k=1$. Although in some instances, it may be sufficient to select "Save only worst linear function of parameters at every $k$th cycle", I seldom use this option. Click on "OK".

Next, click on the **Imputation** button. Occasionally, I will choose "No imputation". I do this when I have doubts about my data. Seeing the diagnostic plots after, say, 1,000 steps of data augmentation will often help me see a problem I was unable to see in other ways.

It is also possible to select "Impute once at end of DA run". I occasionally have used this option when imputing a single data set from EM parameters failed. However, the most common option here is to select "Impute at every $k$th iteration". As described in Chap. 2, spacing imputations some largish number of DA steps apart is how one simulates random draws from the population. As I said in Chap. 2, a good number to choose for $k$ is the number of iterations it took EM to converge. This number (which will normally be less than about 200, but will certainly be less than 1,000) should be entered for the value of $k$. Click on OK.

▶ **Sample Data**. Because EM converged in 72 iterations, enter 72 for the value of $k$ in this screen.

Finally, click on the **Computing** button. If you used the ML version of EM, then "Standard noninformative prior" will already be selected (select it if that is not the case). If you used EM with the Ridge prior, then "Ridge prior with hyperparameter" will be selected, and the value of the hyperparameter will be the same as that used in EM.

The "No. of iterations" should be the number of steps of DA between imputations (the value of $k$ from the previous screen) times the number of imputed data sets you wish to create. As described in Chap. 2, the number of imputed data sets should be larger than previously thought. I typically use 40 imputations (and often more) for work I hope to publish, but, depending on how long the process takes, I sometimes use fewer imputations to help me draw tentative conclusions about a problem.

Step-by-Step Instructions for Multiple Imputation with NORM 2.03    89

In any event, the value to be entered here should be the product of these two numbers: $k \times m$. For example, if EM converged in 164 iterations, and you wish to produce 40 imputed data sets, then $k \times m$ would be $164 \times 40 = 6,560$. This is the value to enter in this window for "No. of iterations".

▶ **Sample Data**. In this case, impute 40 data sets. $40 \times 72 = 2,880$, so enter 2,880 in the "No. of iterations" box.

As NORM runs, it pauses after every $k$ DA steps to write out an imputed data set. If yours is a small problem, you may not see the pauses. The default names of the data sets are root_1.imp, root_2.imp, root_3.imp, and so forth up to the number of imputed data sets you specified. If you follow the strategies outlined in this book, the imputation phase itself is usually relatively quick (minutes at the longest). However, large problems do take longer.

▶ **Sample Data**. This problem took about 2.5 min with a Dell Latitude D620 laptop (2 GHz Core Duo processor with 1 GB RAM) and 51 s with a Dell Latitude E6320 laptop (Intel® Core(TM) i7-2,620 M CPU @ 2.70 GHz, with 4 GB RAM).

**Results of Imputation**

Once completed, there will be $m$ (e.g., 40) imputed data sets in the same folder as the original data. As noted above, the default names will be root_1.imp, root_2.imp, ... root_39.imp, root_40.imp.

▶ **Sample Data**. The imputed data files for this example will be "ex3_1.imp", "ex3_2.imp", ..., "ex3_40.imp".

## *Running NORM (Step 8): Data Augmentation Diagnostics*

The final step in the imputation process is to check the diagnostic plots. The goals of checking these plots are to verify (a) that the number of DA steps between imputed data sets was sufficient, and (b) that the imputation solution was "acceptable," and not "pathological."

In Norm 2.03, click on "Series" and on "Open". The default name for the diagnostic plots is "da.prs". Click on the file, and on "Open". When the message "Parameter series open" appears at the bottom of the window, you are ready to view the diagnostic plots. It may sometimes be useful to view the "Worst linear function" (WLF) as a shortcut for seeing the worst-case scenario. But it occasionally happens that the WLF plots appear to be acceptable, even when there is a clear problem with one or more individual parameters. Thus, I take the time to view the plots for all the individual means and covariances. It often means paging through rather a lot of

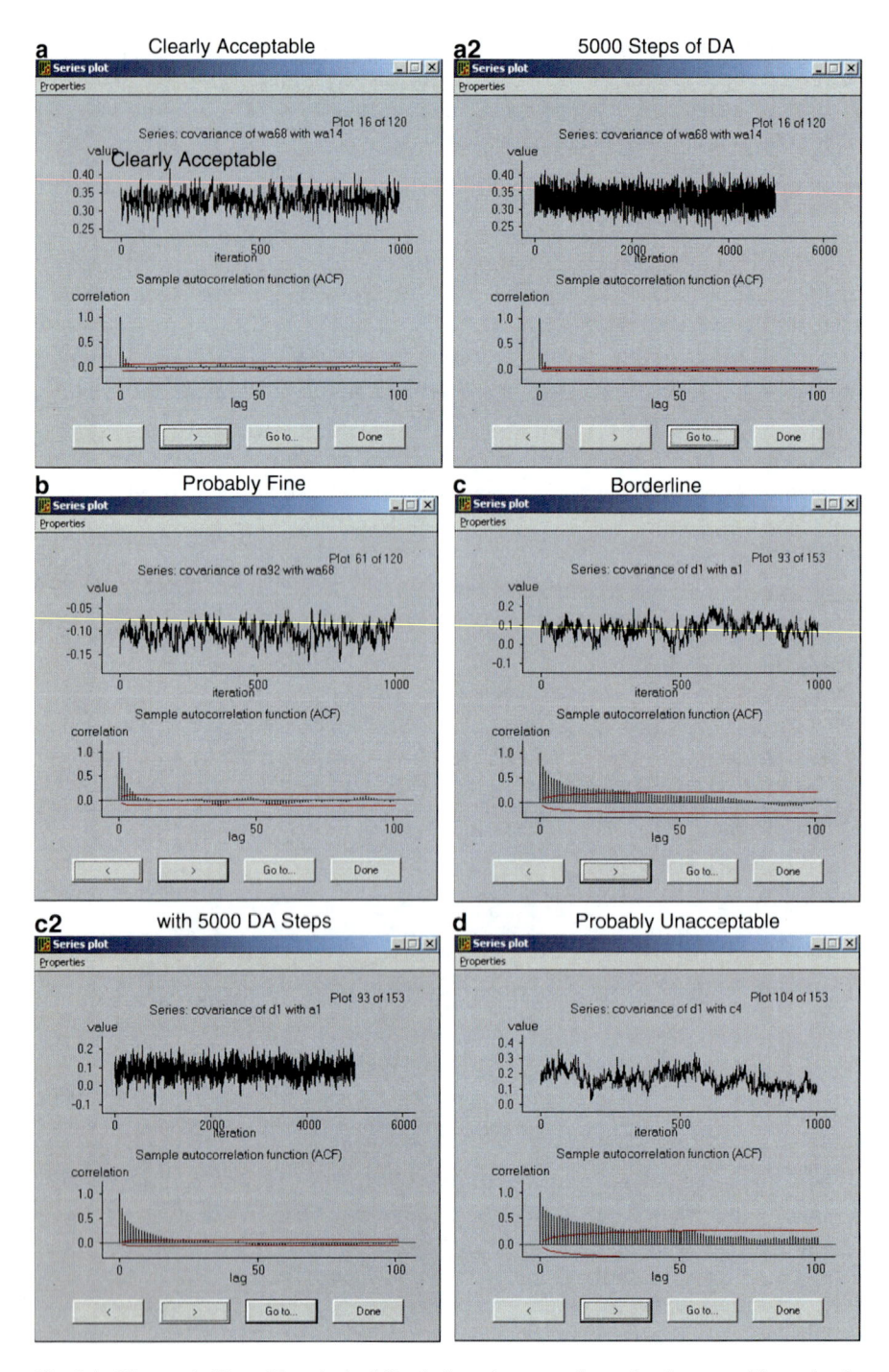

**Fig. 3.1** Diagnostic Plots. Plots depict MI solutions that range from clearly acceptable to clearly pathological

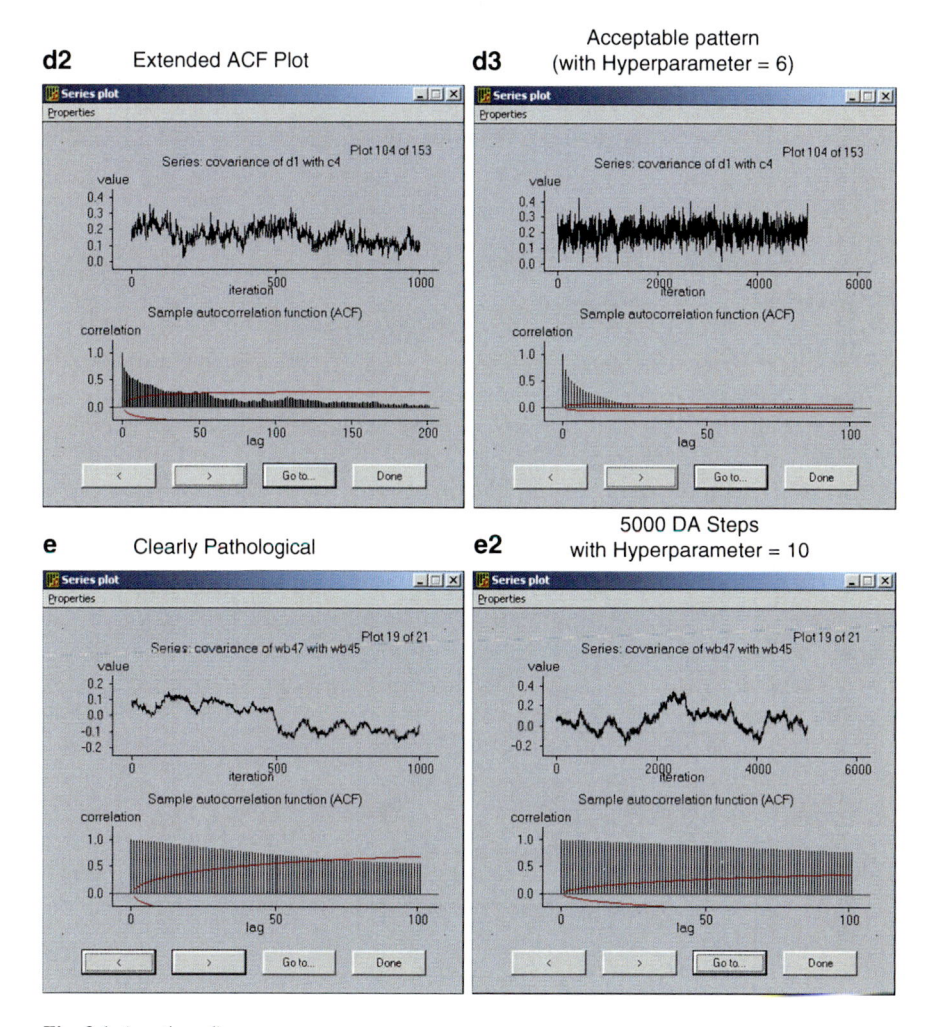

**Fig. 3.1** (continued)

plots, but it is worth it to be able to report in your article that "the diagnostic plots appeared normal for all parameters."

Click on "Series" again, this time clicking on "plot" and "means" or "covariances" (or "Worst linear function"). Sample plots appear in Fig. 3.1. The top plot in each Panel is the "series" plot for the parameter indicated. This plot displays the parameter value over the total number of DA steps requested. The bottom plot in each panel is for the Sample autocorrelation function (ACF). This plot gives the correlation of the parameter from one step of DA with the same parameter 1, 2, … 5, … 10, … 20, … 50, … 100 steps removed. The horizontal lines near the bottom of the plot indict the level of nonsignificant autocorrelations.

The top and bottom plots are related, but for the moment, focus on the bottom plots. Panel (a) in Fig. 3.1 shows that the autocorrelation falls below the (red) significance line between 5 and 10 steps of DA. That is, two imputed data sets separated by 10 steps of DA will simulate two random draws from the population. Panel (b) suggests we may need a few more (e.g., 15–20) steps of DA between imputed data sets. With the pattern shown in Panel (c), I might want as many as 75–100 steps of DA.

With the pattern shown in Panel (d), I might want even more (e.g., 100+) steps of DA. With a plot like this, it is useful to increase the lag for the ACF plot in order to get more information. To do this, click on Properties and on Plot options. Under ACF plot, change the Maximum lag to a larger value. The plot shown in Panel (d2) of Fig. 3.1 displays the same plot as in Panel (d), except that the ACF plot extends to a lag of 200. With a plot like this, I would start feeling comfortable with imputations separated with ~150 steps of DA.

Now focus on the top plots displayed in Fig. 3.1. These give a more direct sense of the acceptability of the DA analysis. Conceptually, it would be good if the parameter estimates at the beginning, in the middle, and at the end of the DA run all show a plausible range of values. Such a plot will typically resemble a rectangle, provided enough steps of DA have been requested. The plot in Panel (a) does not bear much resemblance to a rectangle, but Panel (a2) of Fig. 3.1 shows how that look can change simply by increasing the total number of DA steps, in this case from 1,000 to 5,000.

The plot in Panel (b) of Fig. 3.1 also displays an acceptable pattern. The pattern shown in Panel (c) could be ok, but it may also be indicative of a problem. Note how the plot tends to wander a bit over the 1,000 DA steps. This is a good example, however, of having too few total steps of DA. Panel (c2) of Fig. 3.1 shows a DA run on the same data, but with 5,000 rather than 1,000 steps of DA. Note how the upper plot looks much more rectangular, and the ACF plot seems to stabilize nicely by around lag of 50.

The top plot in Panel (d) of Fig. 3.1 is even more troubling. Note that in addition to wandering somewhat, this parameter estimate tends to be lower toward the end of the DA run; that is, the overall plot has a nonzero slope. An especially troublesome aspect of the DA analysis of these data is that I was not able to get it to perform 5,000 steps of DA. I tried several times, each time receiving the error message: "non-positive definite matrix or shape parameter." This is definitely a sign of trouble.

The pattern shown in Panel (d) of Fig. 3.1 came from a DA run using the standard noninformative prior (corresponds to ML option with EM). However, this is a good example of a case in which using the Ridge prior option (in this case with hyperparameter $r=6$, which was the smallest hyperparameter to yield normal, i.e., monotonic, EM convergence) yielded much better results. Panel (d3) of Fig. 3.1 shows the results of this latter run with 5,000 steps of DA. Those results much more clearly suggest an acceptable DA run.

Panel (e) of Fig. 3.1 displays a solution that is clearly pathological. In this case, the parameter estimate changes value throughout the DA run and has a clear

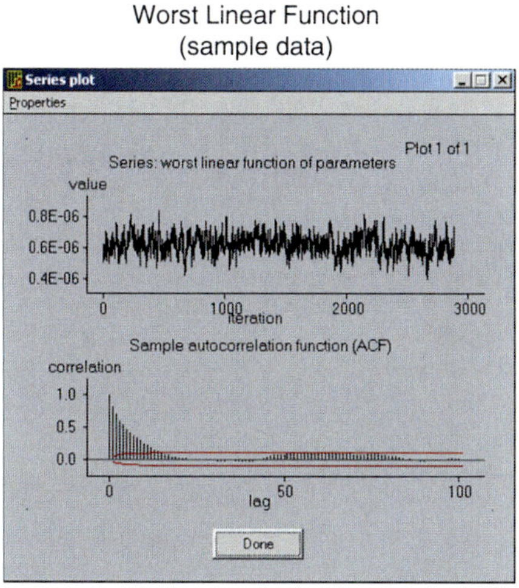

# Step-by-Step Instructions for Multiple Imputation with NORM 2.03

**Fig. 3.2** Diagnostic plots for sample data

nonzero slope. Also, although the ACF appears to drop below the significance level at lag of 100, the autocorrelation remains unacceptably high. This is also an instance in which 5,000 steps of DA did not solve the problem. It is also an instance when using the Ridge prior option with hyperparameter = 10 did not solve the problem. As shown in Panel (e2) of Fig. 3.1, the plot of parameter estimates remains clearly pathological, even with hyperparameter = 10, and 5,000 steps of DA. In general, the problem illustrated by the plot in Panel (e) of Fig. 3.1 can occur is that people with one level of a categorical variable are always missing on another variable in the imputation model. I discuss these and other troubleshooting issues in Chap. 8.

▶ **Sample Data.** Figure 3.2 presents the plots for the WLF for the sample data. In this instance, the WLF plot was not uncharacteristic of the plots for other parameters. The top plot shows a series plot that, although a bit ragged, appears to have a zero slope and is at least somewhat rectangular. The lower plot (ACF) suggests that with approximately 35 steps of DA, the plot goes beneath the significance lines. This suggests that the 72 steps of DA used between imputed values in this instance was fine.

Presenting all of the diagnostic plots for all parameters would be difficult (19 means; 190 variances and covariances). However, I have made the file, "da_ex3.prs" available on the website for ancillary information relating to this book. If you are interested, please go to: http://methodology.psu.edu.

Remember that the plots shown on this website will be different from those you obtain from your analysis of these same data. However, the general patterns will be the same.

# References

Graham, J. W., Cumsille, P. E., & Elek-Fisk, E. (2003). Methods for handling missing data. In J. A. Schinka & W. F. Velicer (Eds.). *Research Methods in Psychology* (pp. 87–114). Volume 2 of *Handbook of Psychology* (I. B. Weiner, Editor-in-Chief). New York: John Wiley & Sons.

Graham, J. W., & Donaldson, S. I. (1993). Evaluating interventions with differential attrition: The importance of nonresponse mechanisms and use of followup data. *Journal of Applied Psychology, 78,* 119–128.

Graham, J. W., & Hofer, S. M. (1992). EMCOV User's Manual. Unpublished manuscript, University of Southern California.

Graham, J. W., & Hofer, S. M. (2000). Multiple imputation in multivariate research. In T. D. Little, K. U. Schnabel, & J. Baumert, (Eds.), *Modeling longitudinal and multiple-group data: Practical issues, applied approaches, and specific examples.* (pp. 201–218). Hillsdale, NJ: Erlbaum.

Graham, J. W., Taylor, B. J., Olchowski, A. E., & Cumsille, P. E. (2006). Planned missing data designs in psychological research. *Psychological Methods, 11,* 323–343.

Hansen, W. B., & Graham, J. W. (1991). Preventing alcohol, marijuana, and cigarette use among adolescents: Peer pressure resistance training versus establishing conservative norms. *Preventive Medicine, 20,* 414–430.

Harel, O. (2007). Inferences on missing information under multiple imputation and two-stage multiple imputation. *Statistical Methodology, 4,* 75–89.

Harel, O. (2003). Strategies For Data Analysis With Two Types Of Missing Values. Technical Report, The Methodology Center, The Pennsylvania State University.

Price, B. (1977). Ridge regression: Application to nonexperimental data. *Psychological Bulletin, 84,* 759–766.

Schafer, J. L. (1997). *Analysis of Incomplete Multivariate Data.* New York: Chapman and Hall.

Schafer, J. L., and Olsen, M. K. (1998). Multiple imputation for multivariate missing data problems: A data analyst's perspective. *Multivariate Behavioral Research, 33,* 545–571.

# Chapter 4
# Analysis with SPSS (Versions Without MI Module) Following Multiple Imputation with Norm 2.03

In this chapter, I cover analyses with SPSS (v. 16 or lower) following multiple imputation with Norm 2.03. This chapter also applies to newer versions of SPSS that do not have the MI module installed. The chapter is split into three parts: (a) preliminary analyses for testing reliability, including exploratory factor analysis; (b) hypothesis testing analyses with single-level, multiple linear regression; and (c) hypothesis testing with single-level, multiple (binary) logistic regression (I also touch on other hypothesis testing analysis, such as multilevel regression with the Mixed routine).

The reliability and exploratory factor analyses make use of the single data set imputed from EM parameters. For these analyses, the output of interest comes directly from the SPSS output itself. The multiple regression and logistic regression analyses make use of the multiple imputed data sets. For the multiple regression analysis, the combining of results is handled by the MIAutomate utility, which is reasonably well automated and provides easy-to-read output outside of SPSS. For the logistic regression (and other SPSS) analysis, the combining of results is somewhat less automated, involving some copying and pasting to an external Notepad file, and the final results are provided by the Norm program. The worked examples provided in this chapter will help you master these procedures.

At the start of each section, I will first outline the use of my utility for creating an automated interface between the output from Norm 2.03 (i.e., the imputed data sets) and for achieving the goal of all analysis: to draw reasonable inferences from one's data.

## Analysis with the Single Data Imputed from EM Parameters

In this section, I describe the use of the MIAutomate utility, and then proceed to examining reliability of the scales with coefficient alpha, and exploratory factor analysis.

## Before Running MIAutomate Utility

Rather than jump right into use of the automation utility, I want to walk you through the process of reading raw (ascii text) data into SPSS. There are two reasons for this. First, I think it is valuable to understand at a conceptual level what is happening when you read data into SPSS. Second, I want you to appreciate that the process, which is conceptually very straightforward, is often a pain in the neck. That is, I want you appreciate what the automation utility is doing for you. On the other hand, after seeing what is involved, some readers may simply bypass use of the automation utility, especially for this first kind of analysis.

At a conceptual level, making use of the single data set imputed from EM could not be easier. This is, after all, a data set with no missing data. Unfortunately, most users do not routinely read "raw" (ascii text) data into SPSS. So the simple act of reading data into SPSS itself can often prove to be a challenge.

For this chapter, I used SPSS 15, but the process is the same for SPSS 16 and, from what I can remember, the procedure for reading in raw data has not changed appreciably as far back as SPSS 11, and possibly further. What I describe here also applies to newer versions of SPSS that do not have the MI module installed. So start SPSS. Click on File and on Read Text Data (fourth thing down on the File menu). Locate the recently created ***_0.imp file.

When you get to the right folder, remember that the file name ends with ".imp" and not ".txt", which is the default for SPSS. So either enter "*.imp" under File name (this may not work with SPSS 16), or click on Files of type, and choose "All Files". Click on the file you recently created.

▶ **Sample Data.** In Chap. 3, the single data set imputed from EM parameters was named, "ex3_0.imp", so for starters, look for that file.

The Text Import Wizard will walk you through the process of importing your data set. For this first example, just accept all the defaults. The result is that you will have an SPSS data set with $k=20$ variables and $N=2,756$ cases. The only problem is that the variables are named "V1" to "V20". If you are very familiar with your data set, this may be good enough. But it would be a lot better if you had the variable names at the top of your data file.

Conceptually, it is an easy matter to add the variable names to the SPSS file. But in practical terms, this simple task can also be a pain in the neck. One option is simply to switch to the Variable View of the data set and enter the variable names manually. This will certainly be acceptable for smallish data sets. But it is annoying to have to go through this process again if you decide to change something about the data set and redo the imputation. Entering the variable names manually also becomes more difficult as the number of variables increases. And with added difficulty comes more errors. One of the values of the automation utility, to be sure, is to make the process easier, but the more important value of the automation is that it cuts down on errors.

The second option for adding the variables to the SPSS file is to add them to the top of the input data before reading the data into SPSS. But how do you do that? The best way to do that is with an ascii editor, such as the Notepad utility that is part of

Analysis with the Single Data Imputed from EM Parameters    97

the Windows program. One drawback with Notepad is that it sometimes cannot handle the largest data sets. The bigger problem, however, is that within the Notepad window, you can have only one file open at a time. So you cannot read in the data set (ex3_0.imp) in one window and the variable names file (ex3.nam) in another. You can, on the other hand, open two Notepad windows: read ex3_0.imp into one and read ex3.nam into the other.

Note that using programs such as Word is not a good idea in this context. The main function of Notepad and other ascii editors is to handle ascii data sets. Programs such as Word do a poor job with this. Having a full-featured ascii text editor (I particularly like UltraEdit; see http://www.ultraedit.com) makes this process even easier, but some problems still remain (see below).

Regardless of how you do this, you must change the variable names from a single column, to be a single row, with the variable names *separated with exactly one space* (double spaces sometimes create problems for SPSS). If you do go this route, the process is almost as easy for reading this new data set into SPSS with the variable names as the first row of data. At the second screen of the Text Import Wizard, answer "yes" when asked if the variable names are included at the top of your file and accept all of the defaults after that.

Regardless of how you handle all this, it still requires some work on your part. More importantly, errors remain a possible problem. So consider using the automation utility.

## *What the MIAutomate Utility Does*

The automation utility takes care of all the steps I just described. It adds the names file in the appropriate way to the top of the file containing the data. It then generates the SPSS code needed for importing this data set into SPSS. Your task, then, after running the utility, is reduced to this running an SPSS syntax file generated by the MIAutomate utility.

## *Files Expected to Make Automation Utility Work*

The files listed below are expected to be in a single folder. I am giving the file names for the empirical example I am using throughout this chapter. Of course, the data set names will be different when you analyze your own data.

| | |
|---|---|
| ex3.dat | The original data file with missing values |
| ex3.nam | The variable names file. It is not absolutely necessary to have this file, but you are strongly encouraged to create one for the imputation process |
| ex3_0.imp | The single data set imputed from EM parameters (description of generating this file appears in Chap. 3) |

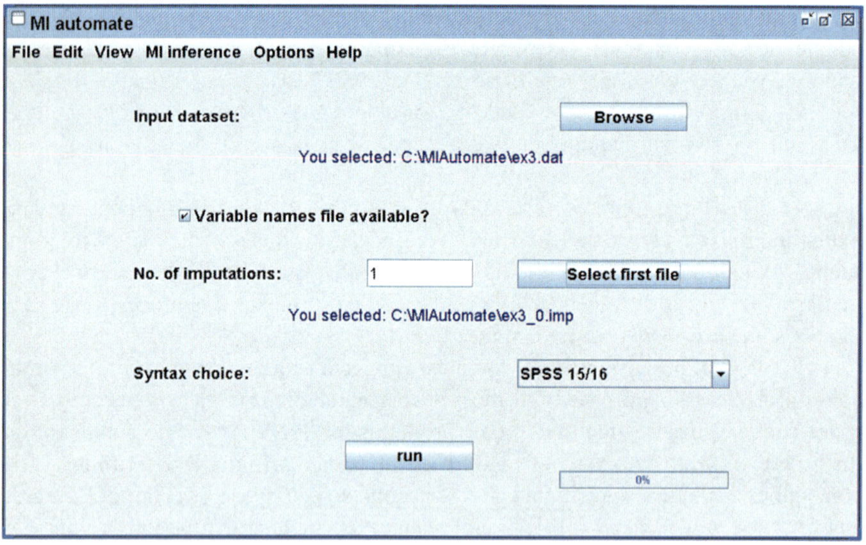

**Fig. 4.1** MIAutomate (automation utility) window translating NORM-imputed data into SPSS-read format: reading the single data set imputed from EM parameters

## *Installing the MIAutomate Utility*

The MIAutomate utility can be downloaded for free from http://methodology.psu.edu. The utility comes as a self-extracting zip file. The default location for installation is the folder, c:\MIAutomate, with the Java run-time library file located in c:\MIAutomate\lib. This will work fine, but I also find it useful to specify the desktop during this unzip process. In that case, the main executable file is unzipped to c:\...\desktop\MIAutomate, and the Java run-time library is unzipped to c:\...\desktop\MIAutomate\lib.

## *Running the Automation Utility*

Open a Windows Explorer window and locate the folder containing the Utility file. Double-click on MIAutomate.exe to start the utility. A picture of the window is shown in Fig. 4.1.

Click on the Browse button for "Input Dataset". Locate the folder containing the data and imputed files and locate "ex3.dat".
Click the check-box for "Variable names file Available?"
For "No. of Imputations" enter "1".
Click on the "Select First File" button and select "ex3_0.imp".
Finally, click on "Run".

## Products of the Automation Utility

After clicking on "Run", the automation utility completes its work by writing out three files:

| | |
|---|---|
| ex3all.imp | In this case, this file is the same as "ex3_0.imp" except that the variable names are at the top of the file (and the new variable, "imputation_" is added as the first variable) |
| spss1.sps | This is the SPSS syntax file you will use to read the raw data into SPSS |
| spss2.sps | This file is generated but is not used when analyzing the single data set imputed from EM parameters |

After you click on "Run", the MIAutomate utility normally takes just a few seconds to do its work. You will see the progress in the lower right-hand corner of the window. When the process is complete, the utility will prompt you to launch SPSS. Usually you will click on "Yes". This will launch SPSS, with the usual data editor window, along with a syntax window with SPSS1.SPS already loaded. Click on "Run" and "All" to complete the process of reading the imputed data into SPSS.

It occasionally happens that the SPSS window does not open automatically. In that case, start SPSS manually. When it opens, click on "File", "Open", and "Syntax", and locate the recently created syntax file, SPSS1.SPS. When that window opens, click on "Run" and "All" to proceed.

## Analysis with the Single Data Set Imputed from EM Parameters

The main thing to know about these analyses is that they will be performed and interpreted the same as you would perform and interpret them if you happened to have a data set with no missing data. The conclusions you draw are valid, and you should feel comfortable publishing results from these analyses. The one caveat is that you should make it clear that the results of these analyses were based on a single data set imputed from EM parameters (with error).

The single data set imputed from EM parameters is completely appropriate for addressing research questions for which hypothesis testing is not typically used (e.g., coefficient alpha analysis or exploratory factor analysis). This data set is not, however, appropriate for performing analyses for which hypothesis testing is common. For example, multiple regression analysis should NOT be performed with this data set.

I do have one caveat about using this data set for multiple regression analysis. Although it is best to perform hypothesis tests (standard errors, $t$-values, $p$-values) using multiple imputation, analysis of this single data set is very good for estimating standardized regression coefficients and $R^2$ values (which are commonly reported without significance levels).

## Analysis Following Multiple Imputation

Before describing the automation utility, it is important to be clear about the process of doing data analysis with any program following multiple imputation. As I pointed out in Chap. 2, the three-step process is (a) impute, (b) analyze, and (c) combine the results. I have already covered the imputation part in Chap. 3. In the analysis phase of the MI process, you simply perform the analysis just as you would if you had no missing data. For example, if the analysis of choice is SPSS regression, you would read the first imputed data set into SPSS and perform the regression analysis in the usual way. Then read the second imputed data set and perform the analysis on that, and so on.

The only problem is that, rather than using the results of these analyses for writing your article, you must save those results in a convenient form, so that the third step in the process (combining the results) can be done efficiently. For example, suppose you want to do multiple linear regression with a group of adolescents; you want to determine the extent to which the three seventh grade variables, rebelliousness (*Rebel7*), beliefs about the positive consequences of alcohol use (*Posatt7*), and relationship with parents (*Likepar7*), predict ninth grade alcohol use (*Alc9*), controlling for seventh grade alcohol use (*Alc7*). A simplified picture of the model appears in Fig. 4.2.

▶ **Sample Data.** Read into SPSS the data from the first imputed data set generated in Chap. 3 (i.e., from ex3_1.imp). For simplicity, for this analysis, use just one of the items from each scale to represent each of the scales. Use Alc9 as the dependent variable, and Alc7, Rebel71, Likepar72, and Posatt72 as predictors.

Such an analysis would have five parameter estimates: an intercept and a regression coefficient for each of the predictors. Further, a standard error would be associated with each of the five coefficients. These quantities can be organized as shown in the first two rows of Table 4.1. Now, if we read in the data from the second imputed data set (ex3_2.imp) and, conduct the same regression analysis, we see the regression coefficients and standard errors in the last two rows of Table 4.1. This process would be repeated over and over again, each time saving the regression coefficients and their standard errors.

At the conclusion of this process, we would perform the combining operation, using Rubin's rules, as described in Chap. 2. As outlined in Chap. 2, the regression

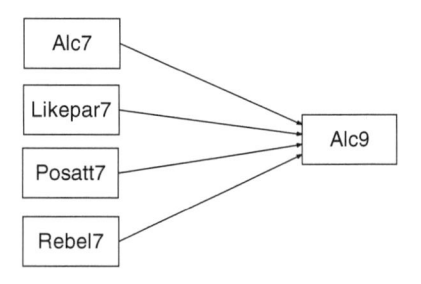

**Fig. 4.2** Example regression model for SPSS regression

**Table 4.1** Parameter estimates and standard errors for imputations 1 and 2

| Imputation | Quantity | Parameter | | | | |
| --- | --- | --- | --- | --- | --- | --- |
| | | Intercept | Alc7 | Likepar7 | Posatt7 | Rebel7 |
| 1 | b | 2.847 | .571 | −.215 | .242 | .102 |
| 1 | SE | .166 | .021 | .035 | .047 | .046 |
| 2 | b | 2.819 | .605 | −.182 | .030 | .153 |
| 2 | SE | .170 | .022 | .035 | .049 | .045 |

coefficient (e.g., for the effect of Likepar7 on Alc9) would be the simple mean of that b-weight over the results from the $m$ imputed data sets. Also as described in Chap. 2, the standard error for each parameter estimate is made up of the within-imputation variance and the between-imputation variance. The within-imputation variance, the normal kind of sampling variability, is the average of the squared standard error over the $m$ imputed data sets. The between-imputation variance, that is, the variance due to missing data, is the sample variance for the b-weight over the $m$ imputed data sets. The standard error is the square root of (weighted) sum of these two variances.

## Automation of SPSS Regression Analysis with Multiple Imputed Data Sets

It should be easy to see that going through this process "by hand," even with just a few imputed data sets, would be tedious and error prone. With the number of imputed data sets, I recommend ($m=40$ imputed data sets would be typical; see Graham et al. 2007), the work involved, and especially the high probability of errors, would render multiple imputation infeasible.

The automation utility for SPSS Regression accomplishes the same tasks as described above, except that the automation takes care of the tedium, and virtually eliminates the mistakes that are made when doing these analyses by hand. The steps for performing multiple linear regression in SPSS are virtually the same as the steps outlined above, with some obvious exceptions that relate to the regression analysis itself.

### *Running the Automation Utility*

Locate the MIAutomate utility and run it. A picture of the window for MI is shown in Fig. 4.3.

Click on the Browse button for "Input Dataset". Locate the folder containing the data and imputed files, and locate "ex3.dat".

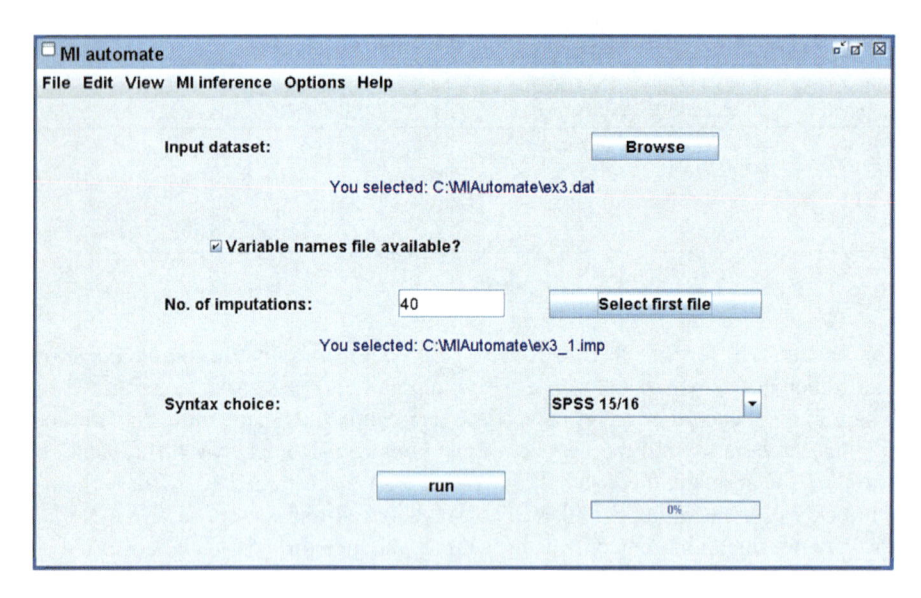

**Fig. 4.3** MIAutomate (automation utility) window translating NORM-imputed data into SPSS-read format: reading multiple imputed data sets

Click the check-box for "Variable names file Available?"
For "No. of Imputations" enter "40".
Click on the "Select First File" button and select "ex3_1.imp".
Finally, click on "Run".

## *Products of the Automation Utility*

After answering the last question, the automation utility completes its work by writing out three files:

| | |
|---|---|
| ex4all.imp | In this case, this file contains all 40 imputed data sets, stacked together. A new variable, "imputation_", has been added as the first variable. It takes on the value of 1, 2, 3, ..., 10, ..., 40, and indicates which of the 40 imputed data sets is which. This data set also has the variable names (including the new "imputation_" variable), added at the top of the data set |
| spss1.sps | This is the SPSS syntax file you will use to read the raw data into SPSS. This version of the syntax file also sorts the data by the new variable "imputation_", and performs the "split file" operation. This operation allows any analysis done (e.g., multiple regression) to be done automatically on each of the $m=40$ imputed data sets separately, producing $m$ separate sets of output |
| spss2.sps | This file is used after the regression analyses is complete, and it prepares the output for automated combining of results, which is completed by another part of the MIAutomate utility outside of SPSS |

Automation of SPSS Regression Analysis with Multiple Imputed Data Sets    103

After you click on "Run", the MIAutomate utility normally takes just a few seconds to do its work. You will see the progress in the lower right-hand corner of the window. When the process is complete, the utility will prompt you to launch SPSS. Usually you will click on "Yes". This will launch SPSS, with the usual data editor window, along with a syntax window with SPSS1.SPS already loaded. Click on "Run" and "All" to complete the process of reading the imputed data into SPSS.

It occasionally happens that the SPSS window does not open automatically. In that case, start SPSS manually. When it opens, click on "File", "Open", and "Syntax", and locate the recently created syntax file, SPSS1.SPS. When that window opens, click on "Run" and "All" to proceed.

## *Rationale for Having Separate Input and Output Automation Utilities*

You might wonder why the automation utility is divided. The main reason for that relates to how one typically performs data analysis. First you read in the data. Then you work with the data, for example, by performing transformations on skewed variables and by combining individual variables into scales for further analysis. Only then do you actually perform the intended multiple regression analysis. This process is no different when you have missing data. Although it is sometimes desirable to impute whole scales rather than individual items making up scales (e.g., see Chap. 9), it is often the case that one wants to impute the single items and then form scales after imputation. In any case, by dividing the input and output parts of the automation utility, you, the user, will be able to perform your data analyses with the greatest degree of flexibility.

## *Multiple Linear Regression in SPSS with Multiple Imputed Data Sets, Step 1*

After you have recoded or computed variables as needed, the data set is ready for the multiple regression analysis. Click on Analyze, Regression, and Linear.

▸ **Sample Data.** Find the variable Alc9 on the left and transfer it into the box labeled "Dependent". Find Alc7, Riskreb71, Likepar72, and Posatt72 on the left and transfer them into the box labeled "Independent(s)".

### A Crucial Step

Click on the "Save" button. Check the box (near the bottom) labeled "Create Coefficient Statistics" (Note that this crucial step may be slightly different in earlier versions of SPSS). Check the box labeled "Write a new data file". Click on the "File" button and write "**results.sav**" in the File Name window.[1] Be sure this file is being written to the same folder with the imputed data and click on Save. If a file named "results.sav" already exists, say "Yes" to overwrite it.

Click on "continue" and on "OK" to start the multiple regression analysis.

**Scan the Output**

In the output window, you should see evidence that SPSS did, indeed, run the regression analysis $m=40$ times (of course this number will depend on how many imputed data sets you actually have). It is important not to look too carefully at these analyses. Most of the reasons people do so come from what I sometimes refer to as "old" thinking. Remember, the imputed value does not represent what the subject would have said had the data actually been collected. Rather, the multiple imputed values are designed to preserve important characteristics of the data set as a whole, that is, to yield unbiased estimates of each parameter and to allow us to assess the variability around that estimate. The variability you see in the $m$ regression solutions are another part of this preserving important characteristics of the data set as a whole.

## *Multiple Linear Regression in SPSS with Multiple Imputed Data Sets, Step 2*

The analysis has been run (40 times in the data example for this chapter), and the results file has been stored conveniently in a SPSS system file called, "results.sav". However, we are not quite there. Some of the information must be trimmed from that data file, and the file must be written out as an ascii text file so the MIAutomate utility can finish its work.

From the data editor window, click on File, Open, and Syntax.[2] Find and double-click on the recently created syntax file, "spss2.sps".

Within the syntax window, click on Run and on All. This syntax has automatically stripped unneeded information from the results.sav file and has written the compact results out to the ascii text file, "output.dat".

Go back to the MIAutomate window, which should still be open. Click on MI inference and on SPSS 15/16. A window opens to give you an opportunity to browse

---

[1] It is best that this output file be named "results.sav". However, it also works to make this output file a temporary SPSS file, and give it an arbitrary name (e.g., "xxx"). After the analysis task is complete, be sure that the new file is the active screen and then load and run the syntax file, "spss2.sps". When you run that syntax file, there will be errors, but the correct actions are taken.

[2] Remember. If you named the output file, "results.sav", then you can load the syntax file, spss2.sps, and run it from any SPSS window. However, if you gave the results file another, temporary, name, then you must load the SPSS Data Editor window corresponding to that name, and load and run spss2.sps from that window.

**Table 4.2** Multiple imputation results for multiple linear regression in SPSS

| Parameter | EST    | SE     | t     | df  | % mis inf | p     |
|-----------|--------|--------|-------|-----|-----------|-------|
| CONST_    | 2.873  | 0.2474 | 11.62 | 131 | 55.2      | .0000 |
| alc7      | 0.610  | 0.0255 | 23.87 | 484 | 28.7      | .0000 |
| rskreb71  | 0.140  | 0.0672 | 2.08  | 134 | 54.6      | .0394 |
| likepa72  | -0.205 | 0.0513 | -4.01 | 125 | 56.4      | .0001 |
| posatt72  | 0.104  | 0.0735 | 1.42  | 113 | 59.3      | .1585 |

These results are based on $m=40$ imputations

for the newly created file, output.dat. In most instances, however, you can simply click "No". When you do, a Notepad window will open with the file "minfer.txt" (for MI Inference). This file contains the MI inference for the regression analysis just run.

▶ **Sample Data.** For the sample data used in this chapter, the final results of the multiple regression analysis appear in Table 4.2.

## Parameter Estimate (EST), Standard Error (SE), *t*- and *p*-Values

The parameter, as noted before, is simply the mean of the parameter estimate over the analyses of the *m* imputed data sets. The standard error is the square root of the weighted sum of the within- and between-imputation variances for that parameter estimate. The *t*-value for a parameter is the estimate divided by its SE. The *p*-value is calculated for that *t*-value and the df shown.

## Fraction of Missing Information (FMI/% mis inf)

The fraction of missing information, as discussed in Chap. 2, is related to the simple percent of missing data. But it is adjusted by the presence of other variables that are highly correlated with the variables with missing data. With multiple regression and with models that include auxiliary variables, the amount of missing information is less (in theory) than the amount of missing data, per se. However, as I noted in Chap. 2, even with *m* as high as 40, there remains some wobble in the FMI estimate. Thus, although I do present this information, it should be taken as a rough approximation of the true amount of missing information.

## Multiple Imputation Degrees of Freedom (DF)

As noted in Chap. 2, DF has unique meaning in multiple imputation. It is not related to the sample size, as in the common complete cases analysis. I like to think of it as an indicator of the stability of the estimates. When DF is low (the minimum value

**Table 4.3** Multiple imputation results based on 40 new imputed data sets

| parameter | EST | SE | t | df | % mis inf | p |
|---|---|---|---|---|---|---|
| CONST_ | 2.866 | 0.2647 | 10.82 | 107 | 60.9 | .0000 |
| alc7 | 0.608 | 0.0298 | 20.37 | 170 | 48.4 | .0000 |
| riskreb71 | 0.137 | 0.0690 | 1.99 | 122 | 57.2 | .0489 |
| likepar72 | -0.212 | 0.0557 | -3.81 | 99 | 63.2 | .0002 |
| posatt72 | 0.110 | 0.0699 | 1.58 | 135 | 54.4 | .1171 |

for DF is $m-1$), it indicates that $m$ was too low and that the parameter estimates remain unstable. When DF is high (substantially higher than $m$), it is an indicator that the estimation has stabilized. The bottom line is that whenever the DF is just marginally higher than $m$, it is an indication that more imputations are needed.

## *Variability of Results with Multiple Imputation*

Note that the table you construct based on multiple imputation of the data set ex3.dat will be different from what is shown in Table 4.2. Multiple imputation is based on simulated random draws from the population. Thus, just as each imputed data set is a little different to reflect that randomness, each set of imputed data sets produces slightly different results. To illustrate, I reran the multiple imputation analysis just described with 40 new imputed data sets. The results of that analysis appear in Table 4.3.

There are differences, to be sure, between the results shown in Tables 4.2 and 4.3. However, the differences between these two solutions is very small. Had I used $m=5$ or $m=10$ imputed data sets, the differences would have been larger (try it and see).

## *A Note About Ethics in Multiple Imputation*

With multiple imputation, each time you impute and repeat the analysis, you arrive at a somewhat different answer. For the most part, those differences are small. But occasionally, those small differences will happen to span the $p=.05$ level of significance. So what is the conclusion when this happens? Should we conclude that a particular predictor was significant or not?

In my mind, the answer to this question is clear only when you decide in advance of seeing the results how you are going to do to determine the answer. Normally, one would run just multiple imputation just once, and the problem would not arise. The significance level would be whatever one found in analysis of that one set of imputed data sets.

If I happen to stumble across a situation like the one just described (significant with one set, not quite significant with the other), then in my mind, the only acceptable solution is to run yet a third multiple imputation (this one could have $m=40$, or could make use of more imputed data sets, e.g., $m=100$). But the idea is that I would abide by the results no matter how they came out. It is absolutely inappropriate, of course, to do this more than once. That is, one cannot ethically keep producing new sets of $m=40$ imputed data sets until one gets the answer one was looking for.

One might also be tempted, after seeing the conflicting results, to switch to a comparable FIML analysis. But the same ethical problem exists. Sometimes the FIML analysis yields stronger results, and sometimes it yields weaker results. If you think FIML might solve your problems in this regard, I would say that you must decide before looking at the FIML results that you will go with them no matter what.

## Other SPSS Analyses with Multiple Imputed Data Sets

With newer versions of SPSS (version 17 and later) in which the MI module has been installed, performing other analyses with multiple imputed data sets (e.g., logistic regression or mixed-model regression; e.g., see Chap. 5) is very easy to do. However, if you happen to have an older version of SPSS, or a newer version that does not have the MI module, it is not as easy to do other analyses. The Regression program works reasonably well in older versions of SPSS because there is a built-in feature in the Regression program for saving the parameter estimates and standard errors. Unfortunately, this feature is not available with other similar programs like logistic regression.

If I were in the situation of having to perform such analyses, I would do the following. First, use the first part of the MIAutomate utility to read multiple imputed data sets into SPSS (as described above), except under "Syntax Choice", select SPSS 17+. The difference between the syntax choices is in how SPSS handles the split files process. With SPSS 15/16, SPSS splits the file using "separate by imputation_". This type of file splitting is needed for saving the parameter estimates and standard errors in the proper format for using MIAutomate to perform MI Inference.

However, with version 17+, SPSS splits the file using "layered by imputation_". The MI module uses this type of file splitting to perform the MI inference when the MI module is present. However, this type of file splitting also presents the output (e.g., for logistic regression) in more compact form. Sample output for logistic regression (first five imputations only) is shown in Table 4.4. With output in this compact form, it will be a relatively easy matter to copy all of the parameter estimates (from the column labeled "B" in Table 4.4) along with the SE values (from the "S.E." column in Table 4.4) and paste them into an ascii editor such as Notepad. This will produce two columns (B and SE) with the two elements on each row separated by a tab. This file can then be saved to an ascii text file (e.g., results.dat).

**Table 4.4** Sample logistic regression output from SPSS

| imputation_ | | | B | S.E. | Wald | df | Sig. | Exp(B) |
|---|---|---|---|---|---|---|---|---|
| 1 | Step 1[a] | alc7 | .504 | .028 | 314.467 | 1 | .000 | 1.655 |
| | | rskreb71 | .017 | .051 | .107 | 1 | .743 | 1.017 |
| | | likepa72 | −.219 | .040 | 30.626 | 1 | .000 | .804 |
| | | posatt72 | .242 | .054 | 20.240 | 1 | .000 | 1.274 |
| | | Constant | −1.326 | .195 | 46.240 | 1 | .000 | .266 |
| 2 | Step 1[a] | alc7 | .509 | .029 | 317.899 | 1 | .000 | 1.664 |
| | | rskreb71 | .199 | .053 | 14.248 | 1 | .000 | 1.220 |
| | | likepa72 | −.151 | .039 | 15.021 | 1 | .000 | .860 |
| | | posatt72 | .094 | .055 | 2.963 | 1 | .085 | 1.099 |
| | | Constant | −1.666 | .193 | 74.706 | 1 | .000 | .189 |
| 3 | Step 1[a] | alc7 | .544 | .031 | 299.929 | 1 | .000 | 1.723 |
| | | rskreb71 | .096 | .053 | 3.293 | 1 | .070 | 1.100 |
| | | likepa72 | −.099 | .039 | 6.323 | 1 | .012 | .906 |
| | | posatt72 | .210 | .056 | 14.306 | 1 | .000 | 1.234 |
| | | Constant | −1.361 | .197 | 47.687 | 1 | .000 | .256 |
| 4 | Step 1[a] | alc7 | .525 | .029 | 334.723 | 1 | .000 | 1.691 |
| | | rskreb71 | .125 | .052 | 5.660 | 1 | .017 | 1.133 |
| | | likepa72 | −.155 | .039 | 16.024 | 1 | .000 | .856 |
| | | posatt72 | .089 | .054 | 2.676 | 1 | .102 | 1.093 |
| | | Constant | −1.595 | .193 | 68.469 | 1 | .000 | .203 |
| 5 | Step 1[a] | alc7 | .512 | .029 | 319.202 | 1 | .000 | 1.669 |
| | | rskreb71 | .129 | .051 | 6.385 | 1 | .012 | 1.137 |
| | | likepa72 | −.167 | .039 | 17.977 | 1 | .000 | .847 |
| | | posatt72 | .120 | .054 | 4.913 | 1 | .027 | 1.128 |
| | | Constant | −1.528 | .192 | 63.083 | 1 | .000 | .217 |

MI inference may then be performed by reading the saved ascii file (e.g., results. dat) into NORM. Start NORM (as described in Chap. 3). Click on "Analyze" and on "MI inference: Scalar". Select the file (results.dat) and open it. For "File format", select "stacked columns". For "Number of estimands", select the number of predictor variables, plus one for the intercept (e.g., 5 if you have alc7, rskreb71, likepar72, posatt72, and the constant). For "Number of imputations", enter the number you used (e.g., 40). The results will be more meaningful if you copy from the output file the names of the predictors (in order), along with the intercept ("constant", if estimated), and paste them into another Notepad file, which should be saved as "results. nam". In NORM, you would then enter this file name (e.g., results.nam) under "Names for estimands", after clicking on "Get from file".

**Table 4.5** MI inference information as produced by NORM

```
*************************************************************
NORM Version 2.03 for Windows 95/98/NT
Output from MI INFERENCE: SCALAR METHOD
untitled
Monday, 22 August 2011
17:25:59


*************************************************************

Data read from file:
   C:\MIAutomate\results.dat
   Number of estimands = 5
   Number of imputations = 40
   File format: stacked columns


*************************************************************

QUANTITY      ESTIMATE      STD.ERR.       T-RATIO    DF  P-VALUE
alc7          0.524500      0.343787E-01   15.26      554 0.0000
rskreb71      0.138750      0.700222E-01    1.98      197 0.0489
likepa72      -.161200      0.569658E-01   -2.83      138 0.0054
posatt72      0.110475      0.755974E-01    1.46      172 0.1457
Constant      -1.44863      0.359952       -4.02       76 0.0001

CONFIDENCE LEVEL FOR INTERVAL ESTIMATES (%): 95.00

QUANTITY      LOW ENDPT.    HIGH ENDPT.    %MIS.INF.
alc7          0.456971      0.592029       26.8
rskreb71      0.660595E-03  0.276839       45.0
likepa72      -.273839      -.485614E-01   53.7
posatt72      -.387431E-01  0.259693       48.1
Constant      -2.16553      -.731719       72.1
```

When you click on "Run", NORM produces an MI inference table, much like that shown in Tables 4.2 and 4.3. The table itself will be saved in a file called "mi.out". It may need to be edited somehow to have it appear the way you want it for the table in your article, but all of the important information is there.

▶ **Sample Data.** Based on the data already imputed, I did a median split on the variable, Alc9, and used it in a logistic regression analysis in SPSS. The results from that analysis based on the first 5 imputed data sets appear in Table 4.4. The MI inference analysis, based on all 40 imputed data sets, and produced by NORM, appear in Table 4.5.

# Chapter 5
# Multiple Imputation and Analysis with SPSS 17-20

In this chapter, I provide step-by-step instructions for performing multiple imputation and analysis with SPSS 17-20. I encourage you to read Chap. 3 before reading this chapter.

Before launching into this chapter, I want to say that this version of the SPSS (version 20 was the current version as I wrote this) multiple imputation procedure has some excellent features. However, as an MI package, this product is still in its infancy, and remains seriously limited. To be fair, when Proc MI was first introduced in SAS version 8.1 (see Chap. 7), its usefulness was also seriously limited. However, in SAS version 8.2, Proc MI had matured substantially, and with SAS version 9, Proc MI is now a highly developed, and highly useful multiple imputation and analysis tool. So although this version of the SPSS multiple imputation procedure has some serious shortcomings, I am hopeful that future versions will be much more useful.

Because of the limitations in this version, this chapter will have two major focuses. First, in the pages that follow, I do describe multiple imputation and analysis with SPSS 17-20. Second, however, I describe procedures that are much like those described in Chap. 4 for using Norm-imputed data with SPSS 15-16 (and newer versions that do not have the MI module installed). These same procedures can be used largely unchanged for analysis with SPSS 17-20. Using (a) Norm for imputation, (b) the MIAutomate utility for reading Norm-imputed data into SPSS, and (c) the results-combining feature now built in to SPSS 17-20, analysis involving SPSS with missing data is now highly automated and exceptionally useful.

## Step-by-Step Instructions for Multiple Imputation with SPSS 17-20

Because of the limitations of this program, I strongly encourage you to consider using the procedure described a little later in this chapter for imputing with Norm 2.03 (see Chap. 3) and make use of the MIAutomate utility to import the Norm-imputed data into SPSS. If you must make use of the imputation procedure, remember that (a) it is very slow, and (b) there is no way of knowing if the few decisions available to you have indeed produced proper multiple imputations. For these reasons, if you must use SPSS 17-20 to do the imputation, you are encouraged to keep your models small, that is, limit the number of variables to some small number (e.g., 15–20 variables). Further, because of the shortcomings in this version, you will find describing the process in a paper meant for publication will be met with resistance from reviewers and editors.

In order to keep the material in this chapter as comparable as possible with the information presented in other chapters (especially Chaps. 3 and 7), the steps I present for imputing with SPSS 17-20 will have the same functions as those for doing multiple imputation with Norm (see Chap. 3).

## *Running SPSS 17-20 MI (Step 1): Getting SPSS MI*

Be sure that your version of SPSS 17-20 has the Multiple Imputation module. To see if your version does have it, click on "Analyze". If your version has the MI module, you will see "Multiple Imputation" near the bottom of the list. If your version does not have it, please see your system administrator to obtain it.

### Preparing SPSS

One option with SPSS should be modified before performing MI. When $m$ (the number of imputations) is large, SPSS may not display all of the results using the default display settings. You can correct this problem by clicking "Edit" and on "Options". Then click on the tab for "Pivot Tables". At the bottom left is a table labeled "Display Blocks of Rows". Check the box, "Display the table as blocks of rows". Be sure that the values in the next two boxes are sufficiently large. I use "1,000" for "Rows to Display" and "100,000" for Maximum Cells.

## *Running SPSS 17-20 MI (Step 2): Preparing the Data Set*

One of the best things about having an MI procedure built into a statistics package is that minimal work is required for preparing the data set. However, there are a few things you must do in this regard. First, you must be sure that the missing values in your SPSS file are displayed as "system missing" ("."), or that the missing value indicator (e.g., "−9") has been identified as a missing value (see the "Variable View"). This, of course, is a required step for any analysis with SPSS. If you wish to perform any other RECODE or COMPUTE operations prior to running MI, that should be done at this stage as well.

## Scale

An important bit of preparation is to set the scale of measurement for all variables to be involved in the MI analysis to "scale" (do this in the rightmost column in Variable view). Note that this must be done even for two-level categorical variables, such as gender or any dummy variable generated to represent 3+ level categorical variables.

## *Empirical Example Used Throughout this Chapter*

In order to facilitate learning the procedures outlined in this chapter, I encourage you to download the data file, 'ex3.sav' from our website (http://methodology.psu.edu). The file may be stored in any folder of your choosing.

The sample data set comes from a subset of one cohort of students ($N=2,756$) who took part in the Adolescent Alcohol Prevention Trial (AAPT; Hansen and Graham 1991). The sample data set includes a variable, School, indicating which of 12 schools the student was from. In addition, 19 substantive variables are included: Lifetime alcohol use at seventh, eighth, and ninth grades (Alc7, Alc8, Alc9); five variables making up a scale tapping relationship with parents at seventh grade (Likepar71, Likepar72, Likepar73, Likepar74, Likepar75); three variables making up a scale tapping beliefs about the positive social consequences of alcohol use at seventh grade (Posatt71, Posatt72, Posatt73); four variables tapping risk-taking and rebelliousness in grade 7 (Riskreb71, Riskreb72, Riskreb73, Riskreb74); and four variables tapping risk-taking and rebelliousness in eighth grade (Riskreb81, Riskreb82, Riskreb83, Riskreb84). As you read through the steps for conducting imputation with SPSS 17-20, I encourage you to try out each step with this sample data set.

## *Running SPSS 17-20 MI (Step 3): Variables*

Begin the MI analysis by clicking on "Analyze" and on "Multiple Imputation". The MI procedure in SPSS 17-20 is set up a little different from Norm 2.03, so you will need to select variables twice, once during the missing data summary process, and again for the MI process itself. Variable selection is described briefly below for each of these steps.

## *Running SPSS 17-20 MI (Step 4): Missingness Summary*

In order to summarize the missingness patterns, click on "Analyze", "Multiple Imputation", and "Analyze Patterns". Select variables in the usual way by clicking on a variable name in the window on the left, and hitting the arrow button to transfer it to the window on the right.

▶ **Sample Data**. For this example, select the following variables for inclusion: alc7, riskreb71, likepar71, posatt71, alc8, riskreb81, alc9.

Under "output", be sure that all three boxes are checked. It is a good idea to have information displayed for all variables. So for "maximum number of variables displayed", be sure the number is some large number, at least as large as the number of variables being analyzed. Also, for "Minimum percentage missing for variable to be displayed", enter 0.

The SPSS output from this analysis is presented in Fig. 5.1. SPSS did a nice job of presenting the missingness summary information. Figure 5.1 (panel A) shows three pie charts indicating the percentage of variables, cases, and values having missing and observed values. The "variables" chart may not be all that useful, but the other two are very valuable, allowing the user to capture the relevant information quickly. The "cases" chart indicates the number of complete cases (presented in blue) for the variables selected. The "values" chart indicates the number of individual values that are missing (green) and observed (blue).

▶ **Sample Data**. In our example, as shown in the "Cases" chart, only 381 cases (13.8 %) have complete data. On the other hand, the "values" chart indicates that only 30.6 % of the total, individual values are missing.

Figure 5.1 (panel B) shows, in very compact form, the number and percent missing for each variable selected. I find it useful to scan down the percent missing column and make sure that each percent missing makes sense based on what I already know about the data set. Be especially watchful when the percent missing is high. Does it make sense that some variables have 50 % (or more) missing data? This sometimes happens for the right reasons, for example, the data are missing due to a planned missing data design. But it is also possible that a high percent missing could be due to a simple coding error. It is important not to go forward until you have an adequate explanation.

▶ **Sample Data**. Note also that a small percentage (6.4 %) of students had missing data for Alc7, alcohol use at seventh grade. Normally there is virtually no missing data in this cohort on this variable at seventh grade. The small amount of missingness seen here is due mainly to the fact that in this data set, I included new students who "dropped in" to the study beginning at eighth grade. Also note that about 40 % of students were missing on each of the other variables measured at seventh grade. This amount of missingness is due to the planned missingness design used in this study (see Chap. 12 for a discussion of this type of design). In this case, approximately a third of the students were not given these questions. Add to that the approximately 6 % do not present at all at the seventh grade measure, and the number is very close to the 40 % missingness observed. The 8.1 % missing on Alc8 represent approximately 8 % attrition between seventh and eighth grades. This is reasonable in this study. The somewhat higher rate of missingness on the riskreb8 item (44 %), compared to the seventh grade version, is also reasonable. The 34.3 % missing on Alc9 reflects the somewhat greater attrition between eighth and ninth grades. This, too, makes sense given what I already know about these data.

# Step-by-Step Instructions for Multiple Imputation with SPSS 17-20   115

**a**  Overall Summary of Missing Values

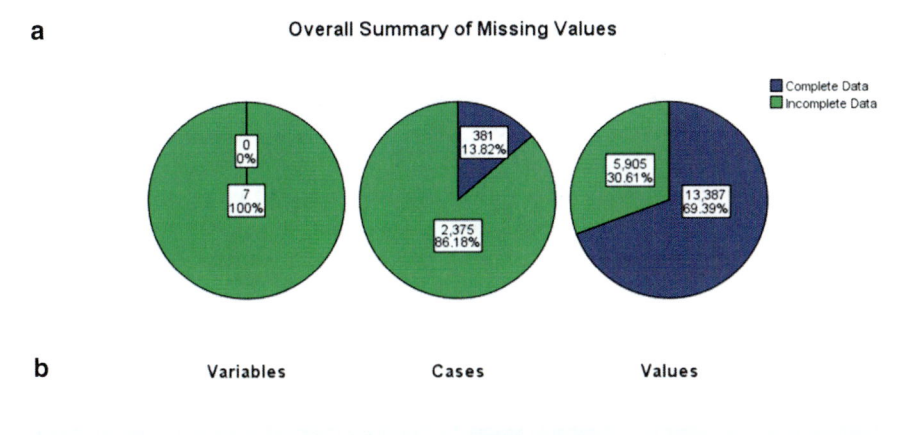

[Three pie charts: Variables — 7 (100%) Incomplete; Cases — 381 (13.82%) Complete, 2,375 (86.18%) Incomplete; Values — 5,905 (30.61%) Incomplete, 13,387 (69.39%) Complete]

**b**  Variable Summary

|  | Missing N | Missing Percent | Valid N | Mean | Std. Deviation |
|---|---|---|---|---|---|
| riskreb81 | 1211 | 43.9% | 1545 | 2.08 | .947 |
| posatt71 | 1122 | 40.7% | 1634 | 1.57 | .964 |
| likepar71 | 1116 | 40.5% | 1640 | 3.07 | .809 |
| riskreb71 | 1111 | 40.3% | 1645 | 1.75 | .902 |
| alc9 | 944 | 34.3% | 1812 | 4.29 | 2.419 |
| alc8 | 224 | 8.1% | 2532 | 3.67 | 2.342 |
| alc7 | 177 | 6.4% | 2579 | 2.96 | 2.028 |

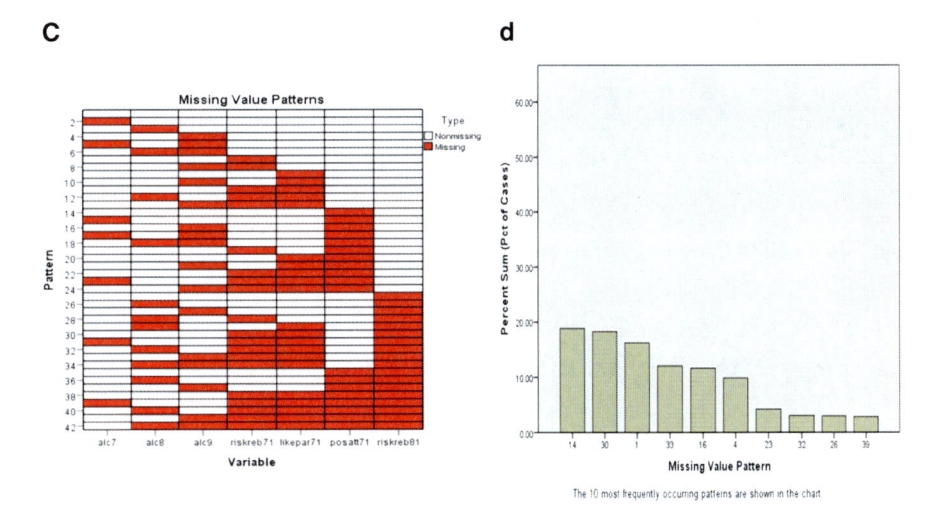

**c**  Missing Value Patterns (by variable: alc7, alc8, alc9, riskreb71, likepar71, posatt71, riskreb81)

**d**  Percent Sum (Pct of Cases) by Missing Value Pattern — The 10 most frequently occurring patterns are shown in the chart.

**Fig. 5.1** SPSS MI module: description of missing values

Figure 5.1 (panel C) presents a matrix of missing data patterns. The one thing missing from this part of the output is the number of cases with each pattern. However, this omission is a minor one, especially given that SPSS also shows the percent missing for the 10 most common patterns (see Fig. 5.1, panel D). When many variables are included in the model, and with large sample sizes, this section of output may be too complex to be of immediate usefulness anyway. And the most important information can be found in this matrix and elsewhere in the output. The top row of this matrix shows the pattern of complete data (if it exists). We already know from the middle pie chart (Fig. 5.1, panel A) that $N=381$ cases (13.8 %) have this pattern.

Taken together with the pie chart for "cases" at the top of the output, one has all the necessary information. It is always useful to know the number and percentage of complete cases in the analysis. The bottom row of this matrix also provides useful information. The bottom row displays the pattern with the least data. Occasionally, one finds that this bottom row has all red (missing) values, that is, some cases happen to have no data at all for this set of variables. Although MI procedures do handle this situation in the appropriate way, it is not good form to keep cases in the model when they have no data at all. If you are not convinced of this, imagine the sentences you must write in the Method section of your article describing the rationale for leaving these variables in. I recommend that you go back and delete these cases before proceeding.

▶ **Sample Data.** There are three key things to see here. First, there are 381 (13.8 %) complete cases. This information comes from the pie chart labeled "cases". Second, there are 42 different patterns of missing and nonmissing data. Third, because the bottom row of this matrix contains some white values, I know there 0 cases with no data. I like to keep any case having valid data for even one substantive variable.

I also find it useful to scan the matrix of missing value patterns for the largest patterns. This also serves as a diagnostic tool. Does it make sense that many people have missing data for a particular block of variables? The bottom panel of the SPSS output (see Fig. 5.1, panel D) shows the percent of cases with the 10 most frequently occurring patterns of missing and nonmissing values. Although this information can be useful when paired with the patterns themselves, the mode of presentation makes it difficult to put these bits of information together. An example of how such a table might look is given in Table 5.1. (Note also that the percents of missing values shown in Table 5.1 do not line up perfectly with the percents shown in Fig. 5.1, panel D; it could be that the denominator used in the percent calculations shown in the figure is 2349, the number of cases with the 10 most common patterns).

## *Running SPSS 17-20 MI (Step 5): EM Algorithm*

Norm 2.03 and SAS Proc MI both obtain EM algorithm estimates of the variance-covariance matrix as starting values for the MCMC (Data Augmentation) process (simulating random draws from the population and writing out imputed data sets).

**Table 5.1** Ten most common patterns of missing and nonmissing values

| Count | | | | | | | | Percent |
|---|---|---|---|---|---|---|---|---|
| 443 | 1 | 1 | 1 | 0 | 1 | 1 | 1 | 16.1% |
| 429 | 1 | 0 | 0 | 1 | 1 | 0 | 1 | 15.6% |
| 381 | 1 | 1 | 1 | 1 | 1 | 1 | 1 | 13.8% |
| 283 | 1 | 0 | 0 | 1 | 1 | 0 | 0 | 10.3% |
| 273 | 1 | 1 | 1 | 0 | 1 | 1 | 0 | 9.9% |
| 232 | 1 | 1 | 1 | 1 | 1 | 1 | 0 | 8.4% |
| 99  | 0 | 0 | 0 | 0 | 1 | 1 | 1 | 3.6% |
| 72  | 1 | 0 | 0 | 1 | 0 | 0 | 1 | 2.6% |
| 70  | 1 | 1 | 1 | 1 | 0 | 0 | 1 | 2.5% |
| 67  | 0 | 0 | 0 | 0 | 1 | 0 | 1 | 2.4% |

*Note*: 1=non-missing; 0=missing. Variable order: s1-s11, alc7, riskreb71, likepar71, posatt71, alc8, riskreb82, alc9

SPSS 17-20 may do the same thing. However, documentation with SPSS 17-20 is thin, and there is no indication that this is, in fact, part of the process with this version.

Whether or not EM is actually run to provide starting values for the MCMC process, it is a serious omission that information about EM is not presented. It is important to see the results of EM (a) to verify that EM has converged normally, and (b) to get an estimate of the number of steps of MCMC required between imputed data sets. It is also valuable to have an EM solution on which to base a single imputed data set (plus error; see Chaps. 3, 4, and 7). Given that SPSS 17-20 also does not include MI diagnostics (parameter estimate plots and autocorrelation plots; see Chaps. 3 and 7), there is no way of knowing whether the MI solution is an acceptable one. This is an omission that will make it difficult to publish results from imputation with SPSS 17-20.

Because of these omissions and because this version of the MI procedure is very slow (roughly 12 times slower than Norm 2.03), I cannot recommend this procedure as one's main multiple imputation program. However, provided that the problem (i.e., the number of variables) is small (e.g., no more than about 20), this version of the MI procedure should be good for preliminary analyses, provided the number of imputations is high enough (e.g., at least 20), and the number of iterations of MCMC between imputations is also high enough (e.g., at least 30; see Step 7, below).

## EM Algorithm with the MVA Procedure

One valuable use of the EM algorithm output is simply to see the EM estimates of means, variances, and correlations in the missing data case. Although EM analysis is missing from the Multiple Imputation procedure in SPSS 17-20, it is available in the MVA procedure. To run this analysis, click on "Analyze" and "Missing Value

Analysis". Select the same variables as quantitative variables. Check the box for "EM" and click on the EM button. Select "Normal" under Distribution and select some large number of iterations (e.g., 200) under Maximum Iterations. Do not check the box for "Save completed data" (see next section). The results of this analysis give you the EM estimates you seek. These are excellent parameter estimates for means, standard deviations, and correlations if you need to report these values in your article.

## *Running SPSS 17-20 MI (Step 6): Impute from (EM) Parameters*

This option is missing from the Multiple Imputation procedure in SPSS 17-20. This is a big omission. Please see Chaps. 3, 4, and 7 for examples of analyses that follow from imputing a single data set from EM parameters (plus error). It is important to understand that the MVA (Missing Value Analysis) routine in SPSS 17-20 is not a solution in this regard. It is possible to write out a single imputed data set based on EM parameters, but this data set is known to be flawed in that the imputed values are written without adding a random error term. Thus, any variable with imputed values has variances that are too small (von Hippel 2004; Graham 2009).

## *Running SPSS 17-20 MI (Step 7): MCMC (and Imputation)*

Click on "Analysis", on "Multiple Imputation", and on "Impute Missing Data Values". Click on the "Variables" tab and select variables in the usual way.

▶ **Sample Data**. For this example, select the following variables for inclusion: alc7, riskreb71, likepar71, posatt71, alc8, riskreb81, alc9.

**(Number of) Imputations**

Early MI theorists often suggested that analysis of multiple-imputed data sets could be adequately efficient with just 3–5 imputations. More recent work, however, has suggested that many more imputations are required, especially with small effect sizes, and when the fraction of missing information (FMI) is 20 % or higher. For example, Graham et al. (2007) showed that with FMI = 50 %, 40 imputations were needed to guarantee that the falloff in statistical power (compared to the equivalent FIML procedure) was less than 1 %. For this reason, I recommend that one consider using 40 imputations routinely.

Unfortunately, because the SPSS 17-20 MI procedure is so slow (approximately 12 times slower than Norm), asking for 40 imputations, especially with larger problems, will be daunting.

▶ **Sample Data.** Using the recommended settings of 40 imputations, 50 iterations of MCMC between imputed data sets (see below), SPSS 19 took 1 min 35 s to perform the 40 imputations. By comparison, Norm 2.03 took 8 s to perform 40 imputations. Norm was 95/8 = 11.9 times faster.

However, if you accept my recommendation that this procedure be used only for preliminary analyses, then it may sometimes be acceptable to run the MI procedure with many fewer imputations (e.g., 10 or 20), just to get a sense of the significance levels.

### Imputation Method

Next click on the "Method" tab. Normally, I would recommend checking "Custom", and checking "Fully conditional specification (MCMC)". Unfortunately, there is no way of knowing, based on SPSS alone, what value should be entered for "Maximum Iterations". I know from running Norm 2.03 that this value should be set at 42 (but I used 50 to be conservative), but there is no way to know this with SPSS alone. And because there are no diagnostics with SPSS 17-20, there is no way of knowing whether this value is adequate.

Nevertheless, if you follow my suggestion to use this procedure only for quick and dirty (i.e., preliminary) analyses, then what this value is will be less important, it may even be acceptable simply to select the "Automatic" option. Leave the "Include two-way interactions ..." option unchecked.

▶ **Sample Data.** Under the "Variables" tab, select "5" Imputations. Under "Create a new data set", enter something descriptive, such as "Impute5". Under the "Methods" tab, select "Custom", and "Fully conditional specification (MCMC)". Enter 20 for "Maximum Iterations". Click on the "OK" button to start imputations.

Remember that each time this analysis is run, a different set of randomly determined imputed values are used. So results will vary slightly from one set of imputations to the next. If the number of imputations is large (e.g., $m=40$), the differences from one set to the next will be small. However, with a smaller number of imputations (e.g., $m=5$), the differences from one set of imputations to the next could be considerable.

## *Running SPSS 17-20 MI (Step 8): MCMC Diagnostics*

This step is missing from SPSS 17-20. Please see Step 8 in Chap. 3 or 7 to get a sense of the value of these diagnostics.

## Analysis of Multiple Data Sets Imputed with SPSS 17-20

### Split File

This is where SPSS 17-20 really shines. One preliminary step is required for these analyses. Click on "Data" and on "Split File". Click on the middle option, "Compare Groups", and move the special SPSS variable "imputation_" from the left box to the right box. Click on OK. Your data set is now ready.

### Multiple Linear Regression in SPSS with Multiple Imputed Data Sets

After you have recoded or computed variables as needed, the data set is ready for the multiple regression analysis. Click on Analyze, Regression, and Linear.

▶ **Sample Data.** Find the variable Alc9 on the left and transfer it into the box labeled "Dependent". Find Alc7, Riskreb71, Likepar72, and Posatt72 on the left and transfer them into the box labeled "Independent(s)". Note that after multiple imputation, all variables are conditioned on variables included in the imputation (including alc8 and riskreb81). The nice thing about this is that one need include only the variables of interest in the analysis model.

Click on "continue" and on "OK" to start the multiple regression analysis.

#### Scan the Output

In the output window, you should see evidence that SPSS did, indeed, run the regression analysis $m=5$ times (of course, this number will depend on how many imputed data sets you actually have). It is important not to look too carefully at the analyses from the individual analyses. Most of the reasons people do so comes from what I sometimes refer to as "old" thinking. Remember, the imputed value does not represent what the subject would have said had the data actually been collected. Rather, the multiple imputed values are designed to preserve important characteristics of the data set as a whole, that is, to yield unbiased estimates of each parameter, and to allow us to assess the variability around that estimate. The variability you see in the $m$ regression solutions is another part of this preserving important characteristic of the data set as a whole.

**Table 5.2** MI inference for linear regression

|        |           | B      | SE    | t     | p     | FMI   |
|--------|-----------|--------|-------|-------|-------|-------|
| Pooled | Constant  | 2.951  | 0.369 | 8.00  | 0.000 | 0.770 |
|        | alc7      | 0.623  | 0.026 | 23.91 | 0.000 | 0.417 |
|        | riskreb71 | 0.187  | 0.112 | 1.68  | 0.146 | 0.869 |
|        | likepar71 | −0.257 | 0.080 | −3.22 | 0.009 | 0.684 |
|        | posatt71  | 0.034  | 0.119 | 0.28  | 0.788 | 0.910 |

**MI Inference Output**

The MI inference information – the information you will include in your article – is found in the bottom row (labeled "Pooled") of the "Coefficients" output table.

▶ **Sample Data**. Table 5.2 displays the key results for this analysis. Remember that your results may look rather different from those shown in Table 5.2.

Relevant information in this output (what might go in a table in your article) is: Parameter name, unstandardized regression coefficient (B), Standard Error, $t$-value, and $p$-value (Sig). Also relevant for multiple imputation is the first column to the right of the $p$-value: the estimate of the fraction of missing information (FMI). Remember that the FMI values are only estimates, and these estimates are rather unstable until one has 40 or more imputations. Still, the fact that the FMI estimate for three of the four regression coefficients are above .60, which means that more imputations (possibly 50 or more) are needed for key hypothesis tests when effect sizes are small.

An important omission in the SPSS 17-20 output for MI inference is the MI estimate of degrees of freedom (DF). Although the $p$-value shown in the output is correct for the correct DF, it would be better to able to see it.

## *Binary Logistic Regression in SPSS with Multiple Imputed Data Sets*

A major improvement in SPSS 17-20 is the ability to automate analysis with procedures other than linear regression. Many other procedures allow MI inference pooling, including Independent-Samples T Test, One-Way ANOVA, GLM Univariate, GLM Multivariate, and GLM Repeated, Linear Mixed Models, Generalized Linear Models and Generalized Estimating Equations, Binary Logistic Regression, Multinomial Logistic Regression, and Ordinal Regression. For illustration, I present briefly here an example with binary logistic regression. In the next chapter, I present an example with Linear Mixed Models.

**Table 5.3** MI inference for binary logistic regression

|  |  | B | SE | t* | df* | p | Exp(B) | FMI |
|---|---|---|---|---|---|---|---|---|
| Pooled | alc7 | 0.6752 | 0.0553 | (12.21) | (26) | 0.000 | 1.964 | 0.430 |
|  | riskreb71 | 0.1375 | 0.1297 | (1.06) | (6) | 0.325 | 1.147 | 0.813 |
|  | likepar71 | −0.2063 | 0.0974 | (−2.12) | (12) | 0.055 | 0.814 | 0.630 |
|  | posatt71 | −0.0131 | 0.0748 | (−0.18) | (18) | 0.863 | 0.987 | 0.519 |
|  | Constant | 0.1166 | 0.4860 | (0.24) | (7) | 0.816 | 1.124 | 0.765 |

*Note*: *t-values and MI df, shown in parentheses, were not given in the SPSS output. However, the significance level (p) is based on these quantities. t-values shown above in parentheses were calculated (t = B/SE). df values, also shown in parentheses, were calculated from the results of the five imputations using Norm 2.03

▶ **Sample Data.** Using the same data already imputed in the previous example, create a dichotomous version of the dependent variable, Alc9, using syntax such as this[1]:

```
DATASET ACTIVATE Impute5.
RECODE alc9 (MISSING=SYSMIS) (Lowest thru 2.5=0)
            (2.500000001 thru Highest=1) INTO xalc9.
EXECUTE.
```

Click on "Analyze", "Regression", and "Binary Logistic".[2] Choose the newly created binary variable, Xalc9, as the dependent variable. Choose Alc7, riskreb71, likepar71, posatt71 as Covariates. Click on OK to run the analysis.

▶ **Sample Data.** The key output appears in Table 5.3. Shown in the table is a copy of the last row of the SPSS output for the "Variables in the Equation" table.

The relevant information for your article appears in Table 5.3. As with multiple regression analysis, the MI DF is omitted from the SPSS output. Also omitted from the SPSS output for logistic regression is the *t*-value on which the significance level is based. The *t*-value is easily calculated simply by dividing each parameter estimate (B) by its standard error.

## SPSS 17-20 Analysis of Norm-Imputed Data: Analysis with the Single Data Imputed from EM Parameters

In this section, I describe the use of the MIAutomate utility for importing Norm-imputed data into SPSS, and then proceed to examining reliability of the scales with coefficient alpha, and exploratory factor analysis. Chapter 3 details the use of Norm

---

[1] Please note that I am suggesting creating a dichotomous variable (xalc9) from the previously "continuous" variable, alc9. I suggest that here merely to illustrate the use of the logistic regression analysis with MI. For a variety of reasons, it is generally not acceptable simply to dichotomize continuous variables for this purpose, especially when the continuous variable has been imputed.

[2] I do not consider myself to be an expert with binary logistic regression. This example is meant to be a simple example of using this procedure with multiply-imputed data sets.

2.03 for multiple imputation. Chapter 4 details the use of Norm-imputed data for analysis with earlier versions of SPSS. The strategies described in Chap. 4 may also be used, virtually unchanged, with SPSS 17-20, except that the utility as described here takes advantage of the new analysis combining features in SPSS 17-20.

## *Before Running MIAutomate Utility*

Rather than jump right into use of the automation utility, I want to walk you through the process of reading raw (text) data into SPSS. There are two reasons for this. First, I think it is valuable to understand at a conceptual level what is happening when you read data into SPSS. Second, I want you to appreciate that the process, which is conceptually very straightforward, is often a pain in the neck. That is, I want you appreciate what the automation utilities are doing for you. On the other hand, after seeing what is involved, some readers may simply bypass use of the automation utilities, especially for this first kind of analysis.

At a conceptual level, making use of the single data set imputed from EM could not be easier. This is, after all, a data set with no missing data. Unfortunately, most users do not routinely read "raw" (ascii text) data into SPSS. So the simple act of reading data into SPSS itself can often prove to be a challenge.

For this chapter, I used SPSS 19, but the process is the same for SPSS 17-20, and, from what I can remember, the procedure for reading in raw data has not changed appreciably as far back as SPSS 11, and possibly further. So start SPSS. Click on File and on Read Text Data (fourth thing down on the File menu). Locate the recently created \*\*\*_0.imp file.

When you get to the right folder, remember that the file name ends with ".imp" and not ".txt" or ".dat", which are the defaults for SPSS 19. So either enter "\*.imp" under File name, or click on Files of type, and choose "All Files". Click on the file you recently created.

▶ **Sample Data**. In Chap. 3, the single data set imputed from EM parameters was named, "ex3_0.imp", so for starters, look for that file.

The Text Import Wizard will walk you through the process of importing your data set. For this first example, it could not be easier; just accept all the defaults. The result is that you will have an SPSS data set with $k = 20$ variables and $N = 2{,}756$ cases. The only problem is that the variables are named "V1" to "V20". If you are very familiar with your data set, this may be good enough. But it would be a lot better if you had the variable names at the top of your data file.

Conceptually, it is an easy matter to add the variable names to the SPSS file. But in practical terms, this simple task can also be a pain in the neck. One option is simply to switch to the Variable View of the data set and enter the variable names manually. This will certainly be acceptable for smallish data sets. But it is annoying to have to go through this process again if you decide to change something about the data set and redo the imputation. Entering the variable names manually also becomes more difficult as the number of variables increases. And with added difficulty come mistakes. One of the values of the automation utility, to be sure, is to make the process easier, but the more important value of the automation is that it cuts down on errors.

The second option for adding the variables to the SPSS file is to add them to the top of the input data before reading the data into SPSS. But how do you do that? The best way to do that is with an ascii editor, such as the Notepad utility that is part of the Windows program. One drawback with Notepad is that it sometimes cannot handle the largest data sets. The bigger problem, however, is that within the Notepad window, you can have only one file open at a time. So you cannot read in the data set (ex3_0.imp) in one window and the variable names file (ex3.nam) in another. You can, on the other hand, open two Notepad windows: read ex3_0.imp into one and read ex3.nam into the other.

Note that using programs such as Word is not a good idea for this task. The main function of Notepad and other ascii editors is to handle ascii data sets. Programs such as Word do a poor job with this. Having a full-featured ascii text editor (I particularly like UltraEdit; see http://www.ultraedit.com) makes this process even easier, but some problems still remain (see below).

Regardless of how you do this, you must change the variable names from a single column, to be a single row, with the variable names *separated with exactly one space* (double spaces sometimes create problems for SPSS). If you do go this route, the process is almost as easy for reading this new data set into SPSS with the variable names as the first row of data. At the second screen of the Text Import Wizard, answer "yes" when asked if the variable names are included at the top of your file, and accept all of the defaults after that.

Regardless of how you handle all this, it still requires some work on your part. More importantly, errors remain a possible problem. So consider using the automation utility.

## *What the MIAutomate Utility Does*

The automation utility takes care of all the steps I just described. It adds the names file in the appropriate way to the top of the file containing the data. It then generates the SPSS code needed for importing this data set into SPSS. Your task, then, after running the utility, is reduced to this running an SPSS syntax file generated by the MIAutomate utility.

## *Files Expected to Make the MIAutomate Utility Work*

The files listed below are expected to be in a single folder. I am giving the file names for the empirical example I am using throughout this chapter. Of course, the data set names will be different when you analyze your own data.

SPSS 17-20 Analysis of Norm-Imputed Data...   125

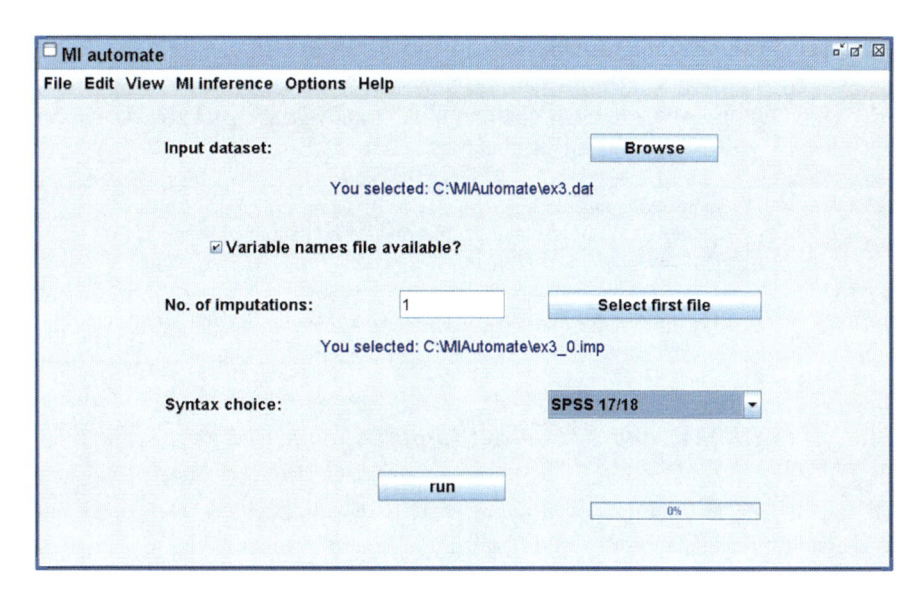

**Fig. 5.2** MIAutomate (automation utility) window translating NORM-imputed data into SPSS-read format: reading the single data set imputed from EM parameters

| | |
|---|---|
| ex3.dat | The original data file with missing values |
| ex3.nam | The variable names file. It is not absolutely necessary to have this file, but I strongly encourage you to create one for the imputation process |
| ex3_0.imp | The single data set imputed from EM parameters (description of generating this file appears in Chap. 3) |

## Running the Automation Utility

Locate MIAutomate.exe and start it in the usual way (e.g., by double-clicking on its icon). A picture of the window is shown in Fig. 5.2.

Click on the Browse button for "Input Dataset". Locate the folder containing the data and imputed files, and locate "ex3.dat".

Click the check-box for "Variable names file Available?"

For "No. of Imputations" enter "1".

Click on the "Select First File" button, and select "ex3_0.imp".

Finally, click on "Run"

**Products of the Automation Utility**

After clicking on "Run", the automation utility completes its work by writing out three files:

| | |
|---|---|
| ex3all.imp | In this case, this file is the same as "ex3_0.imp" except that the variable names are at the top of the file (and the new variable, "imputation_" is added as the first variable) |
| spss1.sps | This is the SPSS syntax file you will use to read the raw data into SPSS 17-20 |
| spss2.sps | This file is generated, but is not used with SPSS 17-20 (with MI module installed) |

## *Analysis with the Single Data Set Imputed from EM Parameters*

The main thing to know about these analyses is that they will be performed and interpreted the same as you would perform and interpret them if you happened to have a data set with no missing data. The conclusions you draw are valid, and you should feel comfortable publishing results from these analyses. The one caveat is that you should make it clear that the results of these analyses were based on a single data set imputed from EM parameters (with error).

The single data set imputed from EM parameters is completely appropriate for addressing research questions for which hypothesis testing is not typically used (e.g., coefficient alpha analysis or exploratory factor analysis). This data set is not, however, appropriate for performing analyses for which hypothesis testing is common. For example, multiple regression analysis should NOT be performed with this data set.

I do have one caveat about using this data set for multiple regression analysis. Although it is best to perform hypothesis tests (standard errors, $t$-values, $p$-values) using multiple imputation, analysis of this single data set is very good for estimating standardized regression coefficients and $R^2$ values (which are commonly reported without significance levels).[3]

## **SPSS 17-20 Analysis of Norm-Imputed Data: Analysis of Multiple Data Sets Imputed with Norm 2.03**

Before describing the automation utility for multiple imputation, it is important to be clear about the process of doing data analysis with any program following multiple imputation. As I pointed out in Chap. 2, the three-step process is (a) impute, (b) analyze, and (c) combine the results. I have already covered the imputation part in

---

[3] Note that although the meaning of the $R^2$ is the same in this context as it is for complete cases analysis (i.e., percent of variance accounted for), you should not use complete cases procedures for testing the significance of this $R^2$ or $R^2$-related quantities (e.g., $R^2$-improvement).

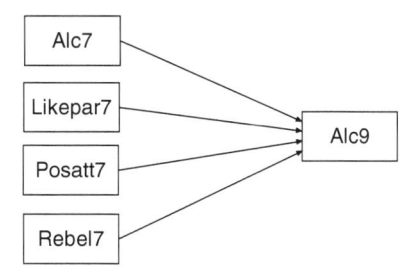

**Fig. 5.3** Example regression model for SPSS regression

Chap. 3. In the analysis phase of the MI process, you simply perform the analysis just as you would if you had no missing data. For example, if the analysis of choice is SPSS regression, you would read the first imputed data set into SPSS, and perform the regression analysis in the usual way. Then read the second imputed data set and perform the analysis on that, and so on.

The only problem is that, rather than using the results of these analyses for writing your article, you must save those results in a convenient form, so that the third step in the process (combining the results) can be done efficiently. For example, suppose you want to do multiple linear regression with a group of adolescents, and you want to determine the extent to which the three seventh grade variables, rebelliousness (*Rebel7*), beliefs about the positive consequences of alcohol use (*Posatt7*), and relationship with parents (*Likepar7*), predict ninth grade alcohol use (*Alc9*), controlling for seventh grade alcohol use (*Alc7*). A simplified picture of the model appears in Fig. 5.3. We could read into SPSS the data from the first imputed data set.

▶ **Sample Data.** Read into SPSS the data from the first imputed data set generated in Chap. 3 (i.e., from ex3_1.imp). For simplicity, for this analysis, use just one of the items from each scale to represent each of the scales. Use Alc9 as the dependent variable, and Alc7, Rebel71, Likepar72, and Posatt72 as predictors.

Such an analysis would have five parameter estimates: an intercept and a regression coefficient for each of the predictors. Further, a standard error would be associated with each of the five coefficients. These quantities can be organized as shown in the first two rows of Table 5.4. Now, if we read in the data from the second imputed data set (ex3_2.imp), and conduct the same regression analysis, we see the regression coefficients and standard errors in the last two rows of Table 5.4. This process would be repeated over and over again, each time saving the regression coefficients and their standard errors.

At the conclusion of this process, we would perform the combining operation, using Rubin's rules, as described in Chap. 2. As outlined in Chap. 2, the regression coefficient (e.g., for the effect of Likepar7 on Alc9) would be the simple mean of that b-weight over the results from the $m$ imputed data sets. Also as described in Chap. 2, the standard error for each parameter estimate is made up of the within-imputation variance and the between-imputation variance. The within-imputation variance, the normal kind of sampling variability, is the average of the squared

**Table 5.4** Parameter estimates and standard errors for imputations 1 and 2

| Imputation | Quantity | Parameter | | | | |
|---|---|---|---|---|---|---|
| | | Intercept | Alc7 | Likepar7 | Posatt7 | Rebel7 |
| 1 | b | 2.847 | .571 | −.215 | .242 | .102 |
| 1 | SE | .166 | .021 | .035 | .047 | .046 |
| 2 | b | 2.819 | .605 | −.182 | .030 | .153 |
| 2 | SE | .170 | .022 | .035 | .049 | .045 |

standard error over the $m$ imputed data sets. The between-imputation variance, that is, the variance due to missing data, is the sample variance for the b-weight over the $m$ imputed data set. The standard error is the square root of (weighted) sum of these two variances.

## Automation of SPSS Regression Analysis with Multiple Imputed Data Sets

It should be easy to see that going through this process "by hand," even with just a few imputed data sets, would be tedious and error prone. With the number of imputed data sets I recommend ($m=40$ imputed data sets would be typical; see Graham et al. 2007), the work involved, and especially the high probability of errors, would render multiple imputation infeasible.

The automation utility for SPSS Regression accomplishes the same tasks as described above, except that the automation takes care of the tedium, and eliminates the mistakes that are made when doing these analyses by hand. The steps for performing multiple linear regression in SPSS are virtually the same as the steps outlined above, with some obvious exceptions that relate to the regression analysis itself.

### Running the Automation Utility

Locate MIAutomate.exe and start the utility. A picture of the window for MI is shown in Fig. 5.4.

Click on the Browse button for "Input Dataset". Locate the folder containing the data and imputed files, and locate "ex3.dat".

Click the check-box for "Variable names file Available?"
For "No. of Imputations" enter "40".
Click on the "Select First File" button and select "ex3_1.imp".
Finally, click on "Run"

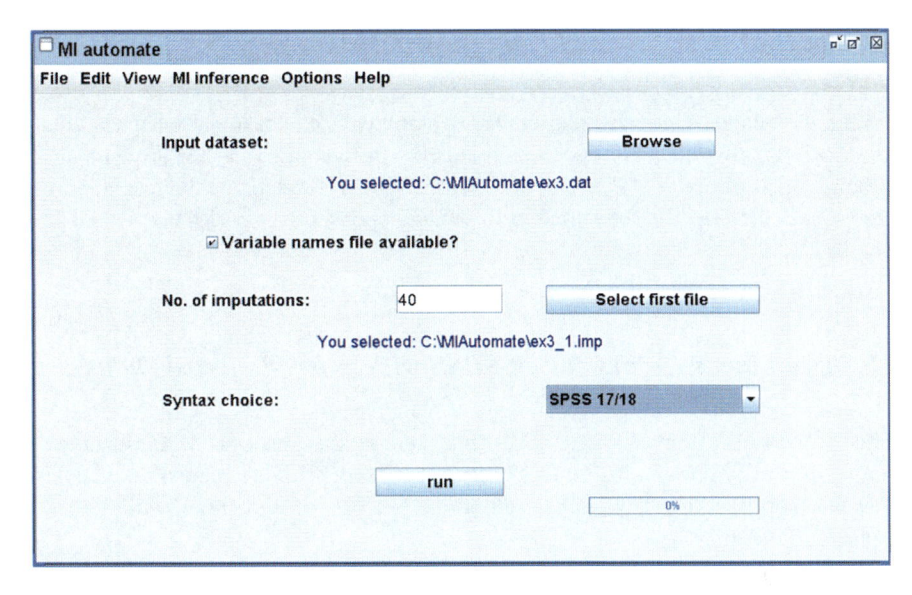

**Fig. 5.4** MIAutomate (automation utility) window translating NORM-imputed data into SPSS-read format: reading multiple imputed data sets

## Products of the Automation Utility

After clicking on "Run", the automation utility completes its work by writing out three files:

| | |
|---|---|
| ex3all.imp | In this case, this file contains all 40 imputed data sets, stacked together. A new variable, "imputation_", has been added as the first variable. It takes on the value of 1, 2, 3, ..., 10, ..., 40, and indicates which of the 40 imputed data sets is which. This data set also has the variable names (including the new "imputation_" variable), added at the top of the data set |
| spss1.sps | This is the SPSS syntax file you will use to read the raw data into SPSS. This version of the syntax file also sorts the data by the new variable "imputation_", and performs the "split file" operation. This operation allows any analysis done (e.g., multiple regression) to be done automatically on each of the $m=40$ imputed data sets separately, producing $m$ separate sets of output |
| spss2.sps | This file is generated by the MIAutomate utility, but is not used when using SPSS 17-20 with the MI module installed |

When the automation process is complete, you are asked, "Do you wish to start SPSS now with this syntax file?" Answering this question with "Yes" automatically starts SPSS 17-20 and automatically loads the newly created syntax file, "spss1.sps".

## Setting Up Norm-Imputed Data for Analysis with SPSS 17-20

Within the syntax window, click on "Run" and "All". It occasionally happens that the SPSS window does not open automatically. In that case, start SPSS manually. When it opens, click on "File", "Open", and "Syntax", and locate the recently created syntax file, SPSS1.SPS. When that window opens, click on "Run" and "All" to proceed.

## Multiple Linear Regression in SPSS with Norm-Imputed Data Sets

This process is exactly as described above under the heading, *Multiple Linear Regression in SPSS with Multiple Imputed Data Sets*. Run the regression analysis however you like. The key results will be the last part of the output, with the row heading "Pooled".

## Binary Logistic Regression in SPSS with Norm-Imputed Data Sets

This process is also exactly as described above under the heading, *Binary Logistic Regression in SPSS with Multiple Imputed Data Sets*.

## Other Analyses in SPSS with Norm-Imputed Data Sets

I do not describe other analysis procedures in detail here (except that linear mixed modeling will be described in Chap. 6). SPSS documentation indicates that the following procedures allow MI inference pooling: Independent-Samples T Test, One-Way ANOVA, GLM Univariate, GLM Multivariate, and GLM Repeated, Linear Mixed Models, Generalized Linear Models and Generalized Estimating Equations, Binary Logistic Regression, Multiple Linear Regression, Multinomial Logistic Regression, and Ordinal Regression.

Although these procedures are not described here, they follow same basic pattern described for multiple linear regression and binary logistic regression. Rubin's rules (Rubin 1987) for combining results of analysis of multiple-imputed data sets require that there be a parameter estimate and a standard error from the complete-cases analysis of each data set. These quantities are then combined, as described in Chap. 2. In SPSS 17-20, the key output based on this combining, is presented at the bottom of one of the output matrices, and has the row label "Pooled". Not all quantities can be pooled in this way, but it is generally possible to work out a good method for obtaining all necessary quantities.

# References

Graham, J. W. (2009). Missing data analysis: making it work in the real world. *Annual Review of Psychology, 60*, 549–576.

Graham, J. W., Olchowski, A. E., & Gilreath, T. D. (2007). How Many Imputations are Really Needed? Some Practical Clarifications of Multiple Imputation Theory. *Prevention Science, 8*, 206–213.

Hansen, W. B., & Graham, J. W. (1991). Preventing alcohol, marijuana, and cigarette use among adolescents: Peer pressure resistance training versus establishing conservative norms. *Preventive Medicine, 20*, 414–430.

Rubin, D.B. (1987). *Multiple imputation for nonresponse in surveys*. New York: Wiley.

von Hippel PT. 2004. Biases in SPSS 12.0 Missing Value Analysis. *Am. Stat.* 58:160–64

# Chapter 6
# Multiple Imputation and Analysis with Multilevel (Cluster) Data

In this chapter, I provide a little theory about multilevel data analysis and some basic imputation strategies that match up with the desired analysis. I then describe the automation utility for performing multilevel (mixed model) analysis with SPSS 15/16 and SPSS 17-20 based on Norm-imputed data. Finally, I describe the automation utility for using HLM 6/7 with Norm-imputed data.

When I say "multilevel" data, I mean "cluster" data. That is, I am thinking of situations in which data are collected from many individuals (e.g., students) within naturally occurring clusters (e.g., schools; see Raudenbush and Bryk 2002). Although many people like to use the term "multilevel" analysis to refer to the situation in which data are collected from a single individual at many points in time, I would prefer to think of that kind of analysis as "growth modeling," or more generally, modeling change over time. This chapter has nothing to do with growth modeling but everything to do with analysis of cluster data.

Throughout this chapter, I will make use of the example of students within 12 schools. The empirical example I will use throughout will come from the Adolescent Alcohol Prevention Trial (AAPT; Hansen and Graham 1991), in which students were pretested, and received an intervention as seventh graders, and were then given follow-up measures in eighth and ninth grades. In this chapter, I will also deal mainly with 2-level data (e.g., students within schools). The procedures described do generalize, to an extent, to multilevel models with three or more levels (e.g., students within classrooms within schools). I will spend a little time at the end of the chapter discussing special issues relating to missing data imputation in multilevel data situations.

One last caveat – I am writing this chapter in the hopes that people will be able to perform appropriate imputation analyses with multilevel data. This chapter is not designed to provide instruction or any new insights about multilevel analysis per se, except as it relates to multiple imputation. In brief, I write this chapter with the assumption that the reader already has multilevel data and already knows how to perform the appropriate multilevel analysis when there are no missing data. I assume that you are already familiar with the few equations I present. I will try to stay at least close to the typical notation for this kind of model.

## Imputation for Multilevel Data Analysis

Multilevel analysis is often presented as analysis at two levels: (1) between individuals (level-1 units) within each cluster, and (2) between clusters (level-2 units). I begin with a simple model of a pretest score (e.g., alcohol use at seventh grade; Alc7) predicting a posttest score (e.g., alcohol use at ninth grade; Alc9) within each school.

$$\text{Alc9}_j = \mathbf{b}_{0j} + \mathbf{b}_{1j} \text{ Alc7}_j + e_j \tag{6.1}$$

In (6.1), the subscript, $j$, refers to the school. In this case, this equation is repeated 12 times, once for each school.

The level-2 equations, then, look something like this:

$$\mathbf{b}_0 = \gamma_0 + \gamma_1 \text{ Program} + \varepsilon_0 \tag{6.2}$$

$$\mathbf{b}_1 = \gamma_0 + \gamma_1 \text{ Program} + \varepsilon_1 \tag{6.3}$$

The variable "Program", in (6.2) and (6.3) is defined at level 2 (it is a constant for everyone within each school). In this case, six schools were randomly assigned to receive the intervention program, and six other schools were randomly assigned to serve as controls (no program).

The idea is that the dependent variables, $\mathbf{b}_0$ in (6.2) and $\mathbf{b}_1$ in (6.3) are allowed to vary across schools. That is, they are *random effects*. In many instances, researchers are interested in a *random intercepts* model. In these models, the intercepts (the $\mathbf{b}_0$ in 6.2) are allowed to vary across schools, but the slopes (the $\mathbf{b}_1$ in 6.3) are *fixed effects*, that is, they are (assumed to be) the same across schools. Random intercepts models are very common in program evaluation research, where the researcher simply wants to account for the effect of the intraclass correlation (ICC) on the estimate of the standard error of the estimate.

On the other hand, researchers might be interested in a random intercepts and random slopes model, in which case both the $\mathbf{b}_0$ and $\mathbf{b}_1$ are allowed to vary across schools. The imputation model you use should match up with the analysis model of choice. As with any imputation model, it is always important that the imputation model be at least as complex as the analysis model. In this case, if your analysis of choice is a single-level analysis (ignoring the multilevel structure), then the imputation model may also ignore the multilevel structure. If you are correct that the multilevel structure is not important in your analysis, using an imputation model that takes the multilevel structure into account will not hurt you (however, see the caveat described below in section "Problems with the dummy-coding strategy").

However, the reverse is not true. If your analysis of choice is a random intercepts model, then imputing without taking multilevel structure into account will bias your results. As explained previously (see Chap. 2), if a variable is omitted from the

Imputation for Multilevel Data Analysis

Table 6.1 Dummy variables for representing school membership

| School | S1 | S2 | S3 | S4 | S5 |
|---|---|---|---|---|---|
| 1 | 1 | 0 | 0 | 0 | 0 |
| 2 | 0 | 1 | 0 | 0 | 0 |
| 3 | 0 | 0 | 1 | 0 | 0 |
| 4 | 0 | 0 | 0 | 1 | 0 |
| 5 | 0 | 0 | 0 | 0 | 1 |
| 6 | 0 | 0 | 0 | 0 | 0 |

imputation model, the all imputations are produced under the model that the correlation is $r=0$ between that variable and all variables that are in the imputation model. In this instance, not taking the multilevel structure into account during imputation means that you are imputing under the model that the means (and variances and covariances) are all equal across clusters. This means that the imputation will tend to suppress differences in these quantities toward 0 across clusters. Given that you were interested in a random intercepts model, it may well be the case that variances and covariances are reasonably equal across clusters, so this will not be a problem. But if you were interested in a random intercepts model, it is because you believe that the means do vary across clusters, and the suppression of mean differences across clusters will bias your results to the extent that the cluster means really are different.

## *Taking Cluster Structure into Account (Random Intercepts Models)*

I have written previously that cluster data can reasonably be imputed using dummy variables to represent the cluster membership. That is, represent the $p$ clusters with $p-1$ dummy variables as shown in Table 6.1. Ignoring the cluster membership during imputation forces the means toward the grand mean during imputation, thereby suppressing the ICC. In theory, the presence of the dummy variables in the imputation model allows the cluster means to be different during imputation, thereby allowing the ICC to be estimated properly.

### Program Variable in Group Randomized Trials

In group randomized intervention trials, whole groups or clusters (e.g., schools) are assigned to treatment conditions (e.g., treatment and control; see Murray 1998). If such a variable exists, it is important that it be omitted from any imputation model that includes the cluster membership dummy variables described above. The information contained in such a program variable is completely redundant with the dummy variables. However, one definitely wants the program variable for analyses. The most convenient strategy is to omit the program variable from the imputation model, but to include it in the imputed data sets.

## Problems with the Dummy-Coding Strategy

Very recent work by Andridge (2011) has shown that this dummy-coding strategy overcompensates for school structure. Andridge showed that ignoring the cluster structure during imputation does, indeed, produce an artificially low ICC, but she also showed that including cluster membership dummy variables in the normal model MI analysis produces an artificially high ICC. The explanation for this latter effect is that including the dummy variable represents a fixed effect for cluster in the multilevel imputation model. However, in the corresponding multilevel analysis model, the effect for cluster is a *random* effect. In short, including the dummy variables in the normal model MI analysis has the effect of increasing the between-cluster variance, thereby producing an inflated ICC.

Andridge (2011) found that the biasing effects of the dummy variable strategy increases as the ICC gets small. The bias also increases as the cluster size gets small. It is difficult to know exactly what the biasing effects there will be on the ICC of ignoring cluster membership or using the dummy code strategy in any particular empirical study. In one empirical study, Andridge showed that without covariates (the "unconditional" model), using the dummy-coding strategy produced ICC estimates that were 55 %, 78 %, and 26 % too high for three measures whose true ICCs were .032, .016, and .038, respectively. The true ICC was calculated using PAN (Schafer 2001; Schafer and Yucel 2002), an MI method that allows a random intercept for cluster membership. With covariates in the model, she showed that the dummy code strategy produced ICCs that were 32 %, 80 %, and 37 % too high for these same three measures. Andridge also showed that without covariates, ignoring cluster membership during imputation produced ICCs that were 63 %, 109 %, and 50 % too low for these same three measures. For models with covariates, ignoring cluster membership during imputation produced ICCs that were 53 %, 89 %, and 80 % too low for these same three measures.

I conducted a small simulation involving one of my data sets from the AAPT project, which involves cluster data (students within schools). I imputed data with and without the cluster membership dummy variables. When I omitted the dummy variables (ignoring school membership) in the imputation model, a model with one covariate (seventh grade smoking) and one outcome (eighth grade smoking) produced an ICC (.0027) that was 73 % too small. When I imputed the same data, including the dummy variables to represent school, the ICC (.0184) was 82 % too large (I judged the true ICC to be .0101 in this case).

## PAN: Best Solution for Imputing Cluster Data

The best solution for imputing cluster data is to use an imputation model that matches the multilevel analysis model. That is, one must employ an imputation model that, at the very least, allows random effects for cluster membership. PAN (Schafer 2001; Schafer and Yucel 2002) is such a program. PAN is a FORTRAN program that must be executed within the R package. Unfortunately, I can give you no guidance for this solution, beyond suggesting (a) that you obtain a copy of the PAN program on the Internet (I suggest you begin by entering "pan multiple imputation" – without quotes – in Google), and (b) that you find an expert in R who can help you get started.

## A Partial Solution for Imputing Cluster Data: A Hybrid Dummy Code Strategy

A partial solution is possible for performing multiple imputation with cluster data. Earlier, I described briefly results reported from the Andridge (2011) study and results from the AAPT study. The data from both of these studies show (a) that ignoring cluster membership during imputation produces ICCs that are generally too small, and (b) that using the dummy code strategy produces ICCs that are too large. My solution, then, is simply to combine these two approaches. For example, if you are imputing $m=40$ data sets, you would impute 20 data sets omitting the dummy variables and 20 data sets including the dummy variables. The results of analyses based on this approach will have ICCs that are between the two extremes. My brief simulation work to date suggests that the resulting ICCs will still tend to be somewhat too high, but not nearly as high as the ICCs produced using the dummy code approach alone. For example, with the AAPT data I described above, the true ICC was judged to be .0101. The dummy code strategy produced ICC=.0184 (82 % too high), and ignoring school membership produced ICC=.0027 (73 % too small). My hybrid dummy code strategy, which combined these imputed data sets, produced ICC=.0128, which was only 27 % too high. In program effects analyses for cluster-randomized trials, this procedure will provide a conservative estimate of program effects.

### Details for Combining the Imputed Data Sets

About the only issue with using this hybrid solution for cluster data relates to how one combines the two sets of imputed data sets. In this chapter (see below), I describe a strategy for doing this combining with the NORM program. In the next chapter, I describe a strategy for implementing this strategy with SAS PROC MI.

## *Limitations of the Random Intercepts, Hybrid Dummy Coding, Approach*

Because each dummy variable is a variable to be analyzed in the imputation model, one limitation is that the number of clusters in one's data set cannot be huge. Given my rule of thumb that the number of variables in the imputation should never exceed about 100, there are practical limits in the number of clusters that can be represented by dummy variables. I have seen imputation models with as many as about 35 cluster-membership dummy variables. A few more than this might also work, provided that the sample size within clusters as rather large.

Cluster size can be a limitation with this approach. The key issue here is that small clusters are more likely, by chance alone, to have little or no variance on one or more variables. Also, it is more likely with small clusters, that some variable might be completely missing within the cluster. These problems can limit how well the models work.

It is sometimes possible to get around problems caused by small clusters simply by combining the problem cluster with another cluster that is similar on important dimensions. If this is done, it is critical that the combined clusters belong to the same program group. It is also desirable that the clusters have similar means on variables critical to the study. This combining of clusters does, indeed, give up some information. But if the imputation model does not work with all the information intact, then some compromise is required.

## *Normal Model MI for Random Intercepts and Random Slopes Models*

The hybrid dummy code strategy just described works well when a random intercepts model is the analysis of choice. However, when one wishes to test a random intercepts and random slopes model, then a different imputation strategy must be employed. The strategy in this case is to perform a separate imputation within each of the clusters. This strategy preserves (i.e., estimates without bias) the mean, variances, and covariances within each cluster. In short, this strategy imputes under a model that allows each of these quantities to be different across clusters. Thus any analysis that specifically examines differences in these quantities across clusters produces unbiased estimates.

## *Limitations with the Impute-Within-Individual-Clusters Strategy*

### Cluster Size

The biggest limitation of this strategy is the cluster size. Because imputation is done within each cluster, the sample size for each cluster is like the sample size for the whole study with regular (1-group) imputation. With $N=200$ per cluster (or in the smallest cluster), you may be successful imputing, say, $k=40$ variables.[1] One benefit

---

[1] This estimate of $k=40$ variables is just a ballpark figure. With your data, you may be able to impute only $k=25$ variables. Or you may find that the imputation model is well behaved with as many as $k=60$ variables.

of doing the imputation this way is that the dummy codes for cluster membership need not (should not) be included in the model. So $k=40$ variables in this model can be compared against $k=60$ in a larger model that includes 20 dummy variables for cluster membership.

Note that when cluster membership is smaller (e.g., $N=50$ per cluster), the number of variables possible will be small. For certain kinds of multilevel models (e.g., examination of individual family members within families or individuals within couples), the N per cluster is so small as to preclude the use of this approach to imputation.

**Tedium and Error-Proneness**

Another issue that comes up with this approach to imputation is that the process itself is somewhat tedious and error prone.[2] For example, when imputing within, say, $p=12$ different clusters with Norm 2.03, one must have 12 original data sets, and, say, $m=40$ imputed data sets per cluster. That is 408 data sets that must be handled. After imputation, the 12 data sets labeled \*\*\*_1.imp must all be combined; those labeled \*\*\*_2.imp must all be combined, and so on. If you are considering making use of this approach with Norm 2.03, then some automation will be highly desirable.

**Problems with the ICC**

The hybrid dummy-coding strategy described above will not work for this type of model. Although it seems like a great solution for many problems, imputing within clusters does NOT solve the problems of ICCs that are too high. My preliminary simulation work suggests that ICCs with this model are comparable to ICCs calculated with the dummy variables only (not the hybrid strategy). Thus, it would seem that this strategy addresses one issue (random slopes), but it fails to address another important issue (random intercepts).

# Multilevel Analysis of Norm-Imputed Data with SPSS/Mixed

Chapter 3 details multiple imputation with Norm 2.03. The only addition from what was described in Chap. 3 is the use of the hybrid dummy-coding strategy for representing cluster (e.g., school) membership in the imputation process. During the

---

[2] Note that this limitation does not apply to imputing within clusters using Proc MI in SAS (see next chapter).

imputation phase (described in detail in Chap. 3), impute, say, 20 data sets with the dummy variables. Then impute another 20 data sets omitting the dummy variables. Then just continue as described in Chap. 3 to impute, say, $m=20$ data sets.

▶ **Sample Data** (Part 1).[3] Multiple imputation with Norm 2.03 is the same as described in Chap. 3, except that we add the 11 dummy variables to represent school membership. Let us start from the beginning. Open Norm, click on File and New Session. Find and open the file "ex6.dat" in the folder containing examples for Chap. 6. Click on the Variables tab. Double-click on the word "none" for the *School* variable, and click on "Dummy variables" at the bottom of the screen. Norm will warn you that "this will create a large number of dummy variables (11)," but do so anyway in order to take the cluster (school) membership into account during the imputation. This will be especially important if later analyses will be used that take cluster membership into account (e.g., random intercepts regression models).

Now select the following eight variables for the imputation model by leaving the asterisk in the "In model" column for those variables: *school, alc7, riskreb7, likepar7, posatt7, alc8, riskreb8,* and *alc9.* Exclude the variable, program, by double-clicking on, and removing the asterisk in the "In model" column for that variable. Remember you cannot have both the school membership variables and a school-level program variable in the same model.

Click on the Summarize tab and on Run.

Click on the EM Algorithm tab and on Run. Note that EM converged normally (function changed monotonically) in 37 iterations.

Click on the Impute from Parameters tab. Click on Run to impute a single data set from EM parameters (recall that I generally do this step even if I have no immediate plans for analyses involving this imputed data set).

Click on the Data Augmentation tab. I will skip the Series button for this example. Normally you would include it. Rest assured that the diagnostic plots for this analysis all looked fine.

Click on the Imputation button, and on "Impute at every *k*th iteration", and set $k=37$. Click on OK.

Click on the computing tab. Multiply 37 (number of iterations to EM convergence) by the number of imputations (use 20 in this example): $37 \times 20 = 740$. Enter 740 in the "No. of iterations" box and click on OK.

Click on Run to begin the Data Augmentation/Imputation process.

▶ **Sample Data** (Part 2). After you have the first 20 imputed data sets, start over. This time be sure that the "school" variable is NOT included in the MI analysis. Do this by removing the asterisk just to the right of the variable name "school". However, you should include the variable, program, in this second imputation

---

[3] I describe the imputation process in somewhat less detail here, focusing on what is different between this example and the example presented in Chap. 3. For greater detail about performing multiple imputation with Norm 2.03, please refer to Chap. 3.

model. For this second imputation model, when you get to the imputation phase (as described in Chap. 3), you need to make only one small change. Click in the "Imputation" button. In the middle of that window, leave the default data set name in the window labeled "Name imputed data file(s):". However, in the window immediately below that ("adding extension *_n.imp, starting at ") enter "21" in the window. The first imputation model produced data sets with names ending with 1–20. This second imputation model will then produce data sets with names ending with 21–40. Everything else about this process is as described elsewhere in this book.

## *Preparation of Data Imputed with Another Program*

Use of the hybrid dummy-coding strategy for imputing cluster data is a compromise solution. The only reason for using this strategy is that finding a way to use a better program, such as PAN and the R package, is just too difficult. However, many readers will want to make use of PAN, or some other imputation program that accomplishes the goal of imputing with a random effect for cluster membership. With PAN, the imputed files will be in the same form as with NORM, so use of the MIAutomate utility with PAN-imputed data will be the same as that described for NORM. Any imputation program that writes out one large file containing all the *m* imputed data sets, already stacked, will be relatively easy to handle. Simply import the data set into SPSS as described in Chap. 4. Any imputation program that writes out the m imputed data sets to individual data sets, but with a different naming convention than used by NORM and PAN will be somewhat more involved. Probably the easiest thing (although somewhat tedious) would be to rename the individual imputed files using the same naming convention used by NORM and PAN.

## *Multilevel Analysis of Norm-Imputed Data with SPSS 17-20/Mixed*

Chapter 5 details the use of Norm-imputed data for analysis with versions of SPSS that have the new MI module. The strategies described in Chap. 5 may also be used, virtually unchanged with these analyses. The operation of the MIAutomate utility is the same as described in Chap. 5 (the relevant part of Chap. 5 begins with section headed ***SPSS 17-19 Analysis of Norm-Imputed Data: Analysis of Multiple Data Sets Imputed with Norm 2.03***.) The steps described below begin after you have run the MIAutomate utility as described in Chap. 5. These steps include much the same information as described in Chap. 5 for performing Multiple Regression and Logistic Regression analysis.

## Setting Up Norm-Imputed Data for Analysis with SPSS 17-20

When the MIAutomate process is complete, you are asked, "Do you wish to start SPSS now with this syntax file?" Answering this question with "Yes" automatically starts SPSS 17-19, and automatically loads the newly created syntax file, "spss1.sps" (if SPSS does not load automatically, you will need to start SPSS and open the "spss1.sps" file manually). Within the syntax window, click on "Run" and "All".

## Multiple Linear Mixed Regression in SPSS 17-20 with Norm-Imputed Data Sets

Analysis with the Mixed procedure in SPSS 17-20 is much like that described in Chap. 5 for analysis with multiple linear regression. Click on Analyze, on Mixed Models, and on Linear. Test the multilevel (mixed) model of interest.

As with multiple regression and binary logistic regression analyses described in Chap. 5, one section (or more) of the output will contain, in addition to the output for the *m* imputed data sets, a row of results titled "Pooled". In this instance, the output matrix "Estimates of Fixed Effects" contains the key output for MI inference. Like the output for linear regression, this matrix contains pooled results for these effects. You may also be interested in the results appearing in the next output matrix, titled "Covariance Parameters." The last row of this matrix presents the pooled estimates.

▶ **Sample Data.** For this example, load the syntax file "mixed.sps", and click on "Run" and "All". The key results of the analysis appear in Table 6.2.

### DF with MI for Cluster Data

There is a question about what the appropriate DF should be for level-2 effects, for example, the effect of "Program" on the outcome. Most software, including SAS PROC MIXED and SPSS MIXED, use the standard estimate for DF, as shown in Table 7.3. However, current thinking is that this value should be much smaller; the upper bound for this DF should be the complete cases DF (10 for the example used here; Andridge 2011; Barnard and Rubin 1999; Little and Rubin 2002).

For comparison, Table 6.3 presents the MI inference based on 40 imputations when the school membership variables were omitted from the imputation model. Although some differences are always found from analysis to analysis, even with as many as 40 imputations, differences like this illustrate the undesirable effect of omitting the cluster membership variables from the imputation model. Focus especially on the *t*- and *p*-values for the variable *Program*. The *t* was 28 % too large when the dummy variables for school membership were omitted. Note, too, that the parameter estimate itself was in the ballpark in the second analysis (only 3 % too large), but the StdErr in the second analysis was substantially too small (20 % smaller than when the dummy variables were included).

**Table 6.2** MI inference for random intercepts model (school membership variables included in imputation model)

| | Parameter | Estimate | Std. Err. | MI df | t | p | FMI |
|---|---|---|---|---|---|---|---|
| Pooled | Intercept | 3.207 | 0.292 | (164) | 11.00 | .0000 | .493 |
| | Program | −0.449 | 0.143 | (1995) | −3.15 | .0017 | .141 |
| | alc7 | 0.630 | 0.025 | (308) | 24.84 | .0000 | .360 |
| | riskreb7 | 0.179 | 0.069 | (113) | 2.58 | .0111 | .595 |
| | likepar7 | −0.279 | 0.073 | (110) | −3.80 | .0002 | .601 |
| | posatt7 | 0.025 | 0.064 | (106) | 0.39 | .7000 | .612 |

*Note*: The MI *df* is not presented as part of the MI inference (pooled) SPSS 17-19 output. However, the MI *df* values (shown in parentheses as calculated manually using Norm) are used in SPSS 17-19 to determine the significance levels of each *t* statistic. With *df* = 10 for the program variable, *p* = .0103. Estimated ICC = .0087 for these data

**Table 6.3** MI inference for random intercepts model (school membership dummy variables omitted from imputation model)

| | Quantity | Estimate | Std. Err. | MI df | t | p | FMI (%) |
|---|---|---|---|---|---|---|---|
| Pooled | Intercept | 3.191 | 0.297 | (129) | 10.75 | .0000 | 55.6 |
| | Program | −0.464 | 0.115 | (380) | −4.02 | .0001 | 32.4 |
| | alc7 | 0.625 | 0.026 | (272) | 24.24 | .0000 | 38.3 |
| | riskreb7 | 0.184 | 0.071 | (108) | 2.60 | .0106 | 60.7 |
| | likepar7 | −0.272 | 0.073 | (113) | −3.72 | .0003 | 59.4 |
| | posatt7 | 0.033 | 0.068 | (91) | 0.48 | .6314 | 66.1 |

*Note*: The MI *df* is not presented as part of the MI inference (pooled) SPSS 17 output. However, the MI *df* values (shown in parentheses as calculated manually using Norm) are used in SPSS 17-19 to determine the significance levels of each *t* statistic. With *df* = 10 for the program variable, *p* = .0024. Estimated ICC = .0024 for these data

The results appearing in Table 6.4 are for the compromise solution using the hybrid dummy variable strategy. For this strategy, I used the first 20 imputed data sets from the analysis with dummy variables and the last 20 imputed data sets from the analysis that omitted the dummy variables. Note that the simple combining of imputed data sets was possible because the same variables appeared in the same order in both sets of imputed data sets. The results shown in Table 6.4 are more realistic, but are likely to be slightly conservative (e.g., *t*-value for the variable, program, is probably slightly too small) compared to results based on imputation procedure such as PAN.

## *Multiple Linear Mixed Regression in SPSS 15/16 with Norm-Imputed Data Sets*

The strategy described for performing mixed linear regression for SPSS 17-20 applies almost exactly to mixed linear regression analysis with older versions of SPSS and to newer versions of SPSS that do not have the MI module installed.

**Table 6.4** MI inference for random intercepts model (school membership dummy variables included for 20 data sets; omitted from 20 data sets)

|        | Quantity  | Estimate | Std. Err. | MI df  | t     | p     | FMI (%) |
|--------|-----------|----------|-----------|--------|-------|-------|---------|
| Pooled | Intercept | 3.210    | 0.277     | (186)  | 11.59 | .0000 | 46.4    |
|        | Program   | −0.462   | 0.127     | (1004) | −3.64 | .0003 | 19.9    |
|        | alc7      | 0.628    | 0.025     | (351)  | 25.14 | .0000 | 33.7    |
|        | riskreb7  | 0.181    | 0.066     | (135)  | 2.76  | .0066 | 54.3    |
|        | likepar7  | −0.281   | 0.069     | (133)  | −4.05 | .0001 | 54.8    |
|        | posatt7   | 0.034    | 0.067     | (95)   | 0.50  | .6166 | 64.9    |

*Note*: The MI *df* is not presented as part of the MI inference (pooled) SPSS 17 output. However, the MI *df* values (shown in parentheses as calculated with SAS) are used in SPSS 17-19 to determine the significance levels of each *t* statistic. With $df = 10$ for the program variable, $p = .0045$. ICC = .0052 for these data

The main difference is that these versions of SPSS will not have the "pooled" estimates given at the bottom of the key output matrix. You may then use the NORM program to perform the combining of results, or MI Inference. However, if you specify SPSS 17-20 for syntax choice with the MIAutomate utility, the output for SPSS/Mixed will be sufficiently compact that it is reasonable in this case to perform the MI Inference analyses using NORM.

By "compact," I mean that the parameter estimates and standard errors for *m* imputed data sets are printed side-by-side in two columns. The results for the *m* imputed data sets are stacked, making it a rather straightforward task simply to cut and paste the two columns for all imputed data sets into a separate ascii text file (Notepad works well for this). I find that it works best if you first copy the entire output matrix (Estimates of Fixed Effects) to a Word document, and then copy and paste the two key columns into Notepad. You should save this ascii file with a convenient name, such as "results.dat". Then copy the predictors labels (including "Intercept") and paste these labels into a second ascii file which you give the same name as the results file, except with the ".nam" suffix (e.g., results.nam). These two files may then be read by NORM 2.03 for MI inference.

## MI Inference with Norm 2.03

Open Norm 2.03, and click on "analyze", and on "MI Inference: Scalar". Locate your results file (e.g., "results.dat") and open it. Click on the "Stacked Columns" option. Enter the number of estimands (predictors; do not forget to count the intercept). An easy way to figure this is to count the number of labels in the parameter names file. Enter the number of imputations (e.g., 40). Click on Run.

The results appear in the NORM screen. The MI inference file is also saved in the same folder under the name "mi.out". That file may be edited to get the values into a form that is suitable for presentation in your article.

# Multilevel Analysis of Norm-Imputed Data with HLM 7

The MIAutomate Utility also has the capability of preparing files for use with HLM 6 or HLM 7. Note that this utility does NOT make use of the built-in HLM feature for combining results based on multiply-imputed data sets.[4]

There are five parts to the total task: (a) Impute multiple data sets using Norm 2.03; (b) run the MIAutomate program to locate all relevant files (same as described for SPSS); (c) locating the HLM executable file; (d) build the 2-level HLM model by answering questions about the status in the model of each variable included in the imputed data sets; and (e) run HLM and view the MI Inference results.

## *Step 1: Imputation with Norm 2.03*

Impute multiple (say 40) data sets using Norm 2.03. I describe this process in more detail above and in Chap. 3. As I have said before, you are STRONGLY encouraged to include a variable names file. This ***ascii text file*** should have all variable names in your data set, in the order in which they appear in the data set, one name per line. The name of the variable names file should be root.nam. For example, if your original data set is named "abc12.dat", then the variable names file should be "abc12.nam". This step is described briefly above in this chapter and in considerable detail in Chap. 3.

## *Step 2: Run MIAutomate Utility*

Launch the MIAutomate utility as described in Chaps. 4 and 5, and earlier in this chapter. I find it best to address all questions on the main MIAutomate window before making your syntax choice. First locate the original data file (e.g., mydata. dat). The name of the file, and the file, along with its folder location will appear in blue below the Browse button. Check the box for "Variable names file available?". Indicate the No. of imputations (e.g., 40). Click on "Select first file", and locate the first imputed file (usually named something like, mydata_1.imp) and click on Open. The name of the first imputed file, along with its folder location will appear in below the Select first file button. Now click on the Syntax choice window, and select HLM. This last step opens a new window, "Enter HLM information".

---

[4] The feature built in to HLM6 for combining results from multiply-imputed data sets is limited in some important ways and will not be used here. First, the feature works with only 10 imputed data sets. Although this does give reasonable preliminary results, it is often desirable to have more than ten imputed data sets (see Graham et al. 2007). Second, the built-in feature in HLM 6 does not calculate the Fraction of Missing Information. This is not a huge omission, but it would be better to have it.

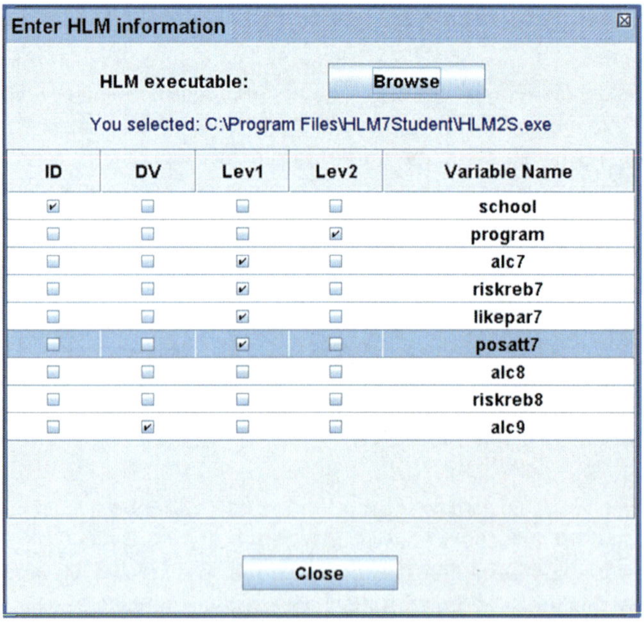

**Fig. 6.1** Enter HLM information window. ID = the cluster membership variable; DV = dependent variable in the regression analysis; Lev1 = Level 1 predictors; Lev2 = Level 2 predictors. One ID variable, and one DV must be selected. One or more variables may be indicated as Lev1 and Lev2 predictors

## *Step 3: Enter HLM Information Window: Executable Information*

A sample "Enter HLM information" window appears in Fig. 6.1. First click on the Browse button for "HLM executable", and locate the executable for the version you are using. Whichever version of HLM you are using, it is likely to be in the "c:\Program Files\" folder, so click on that first, and then look for folders beginning with "H". For example, the student version of HLM6 is located in c:\Program Files\HLM6S. The student version of HLM7 is located in c:\Program Files\HLM7Student. This executable itself begins with "HLM2", and ends with ".exe". The student versions of HLM6 and HLM7 are both named HLM2s.exe. The trial version may be named HLM2R.exe. The regular version may be named HLM2.exe. Locate the executable for your version of HLM and click on Open. The executable name, along with its folder location, will appear in blue below the Browse button.

## *Step 4: Enter HLM Information Window: HLM Model Information*

The HLM model possible with this version of the MIAutomate utility is a simple, 2-level model. The model is specified by selecting variables (from those listed in the rightmost column) for each of the columns describing the HLM model. The **ID** variable is the variable describing cluster membership (e.g., "school"). Check the box in the ID column for exactly one variable. Next check the box in the **DV** column for exactly one variable. This is the dependent variable in your regression analysis. Next, check the boxes in the **Lev1** column for any variable that will be a level-1 predictor. Finally, check the box in the **Lev2** column for any variable that will be a level-2 predictor. Note that the boxes for some variables listed on the right (e.g., auxiliary variables) may not be checked in any of the columns. This is fine.

When all model information has been given, click on "Close", and on "Run" at the bottom of the main MIAutomate window. The progress of HLM analyses will be shown in the lower right-hand corner of the main MIAutomate window. Note that this process can be rather slow. It is slow, first because HLM must be run twice for each imputed data set: once to set up the data (creating the MDM file) and a second time to perform the 2-level HLM analysis. This process is also slow because HLM itself is rather slow.

## *Step 5: MI Inference*

When the process is complete, "100 %" shows in the progress window in the lower right-hand corner of the main MIAutomate window. Also, two Notepad windows automatically open. One Notepad window shows the file, minfer1.txt, which displays the MI inference results based on regular (multilevel) standard errors. The second Notepad window shows the file minfer2.txt, which displays the MI inference results based on robust standard errors.

▶ **Sample Data.** For this example, the input data file is the same as used above for SPSS: ex6.dat (and ex6.nam). The Enter HLM Information screen for this example appears in Fig. 6.1. The $m=40$ imputations used for this example are based on the hybrid dummy code strategy described above (20 data sets imputed with the dummy variables, 20 data sets imputed without the dummy variables). Thus, these results correspond to the SPSS/Mixed results appearing in Table 6.4. The HLM analysis of $m=40$ imputed data sets took several minutes and produced the output displayed in Table 6.5 (copied from "minfer1.txt", based on regular standard errors). Note that the results in Table 6.5 are virtually identical in every respect to those shown above in Table 6.4, except for df for the level-2 variable, program. Note that df given here was based on the simple formula, $N-2=10$, where the N is for level-2 units (there were 12 schools in this example). It was $N-2$ because there was just one level-2 predictor (program). This value for df is not quite correct. The value for df described by Barnard and Rubin (1999; also see Andridge 2011; Little and Rubin 2002) will generally be very slightly smaller than this. However, using this formula will provide statistical inference that is very close to what is correct (and much closer than using the df estimate based on traditional MI theory). The *p*-value given in these tables is correct for $df=10$.

**Table 6.5** MI inference for random intercepts model in HLM 7 S: regular standard errors

| Parameter | EST | SE | t | df | % mis inf | p |
|---|---|---|---|---|---|---|
| Intrcpt2 | 3.210 | 0.2770 | 11.59 | 186 | 46.3 | .0000 |
| program | -0.462 | 0.1268 | -3.64 | 10 | 19.8 | .0045 |
| alc7 | 0.628 | 0.0250 | 25.13 | 350 | 33.7 | .0000 |
| riskreb7 | 0.181 | 0.0656 | 2.76 | 135 | 54.3 | .0066 |
| likepar7 | -0.281 | 0.0694 | -4.05 | 133 | 54.8 | .0001 |
| posatt7 | 0.034 | 0.0672 | 0.50 | 94 | 64.9 | .6166 |

*Note*: The results shown above came from the output file minfer1.txt. These results, which are virtually identical to those presented above in Table 6.4 for the SPSS/Mixed procedure, are based on "regular" standard errors. These results were based on 40 imputed data sets: 20 were imputed with dummy variables representing school membership; 20 were imputed omitting the dummy variables

**Table 6.6** MI inference for random intercepts model in HLM 7: robust standard errors

| Parameter | EST | SE | t | df | % mis inf | p |
|---|---|---|---|---|---|---|
| Intrcpt2 | 3.210 | 0.2558 | 12.55 | 135 | 54.3 | .0000 |
| Program | -0.462 | 0.1180 | -3.91 | 10 | 22.9 | .0029 |
| alc7 | 0.628 | 0.0215 | 29.24 | 191 | 45.7 | .0000 |
| riskreb7 | 0.181 | 0.0617 | 2.93 | 105 | 61.4 | .0041 |
| likepar7 | -0.281 | 0.0691 | -4.06 | 131 | 55.2 | .0001 |
| posatt7 | 0.034 | 0.0666 | 0.51 | 91 | 66.1 | .6134 |

*Note*: The results shown above came from the output file minfer2.txt. These results were based on "robust" standard errors. These results were based on 40 imputed data sets: 20 were imputed with dummy variables representing school membership; 20 were imputed omitting the dummy variables

The results shown in Table 6.6 were copied from the file "minfer2.txt". The difference between these results and those shown in Table 6.5 is that the standard errors from these results were described in HLM as "robust standard errors" (e.g., robust to deviations from the normal distribution assumption).

## *Limitations of the MIAutomate Utility for HLM*

This version of the MIAutomate utility works with HLM 6 and HLM 7.
This version of the utility works with 2-level HLM models.
This version of the utility works with random intercepts models.

# Special Issues Relating to Missing Data Imputation in Multilevel Data Situations

## Number of Level-2 Units

I have already discussed the limitations relating to MI when the number of level-2 units is large, even for random intercepts models. The problem with such models is that the number of variables relating to level-2 unit membership becomes so large as to severely limit the number of substantive variables that can be included in the model. On the other hand, it may be possible to combine level-2 units (within experimental conditions, if that is relevant) that already have similar means on key variables. One approach here might be to perform a k-means cluster analysis on the level-2 units (e.g., at the school level) on key variables. Even if the number of clusters is large compared to what is typically considered desirable for this kind of analysis, it will represent a big reduction in the number of level-2 units used with MI.

## Random Slopes Models

This issue was discussed briefly earlier in this chapter. The best inferences are made with this type of model if imputation is carried out within each level-2 unit. This allows all correlations to vary across level-2 units. Imputing once with the overall sample suppresses correlations to be equal across level-2 units. When level-2 units have relatively few (e.g., 50) cases, it will be possible to impute separately within each level-2 unit, but the number of variables in such models will be small. As I pointed out above, one bit of good news for this approach is that the dummy coding for level-2 group membership is not required.

Unfortunately, it much more complicated with random slopes models to combine groups that are similar with respect to their correlation matrices. However, it may be possible to do something unusual such as treating the correlations themselves as the data for a cluster analysis. As long as relatively few variables were involved, this might be a possibility.

Finally, imputing within clusters does not solve the problem of inflated ICC. Thus, although this approach does allow covariances (slopes) to differ across clusters during imputation, the inflated ICC seems to be an important limitation of this approach. When one wishes to impute under a random slopes model, it is advisable to invest in the PAN program for imputation.

## 3-Level Models

The analyses and utilities described in this chapter are limited to 2-level models. For example, the data illustrations in this chapter have related to students within schools. But it would be possible to examine the 3-level model: students within classes within schools. The structure of MI for 3-level models is the same as that for 2-level models. The only difference is that the number of groups that must be dummy coded increases geometrically with each new level. For example, in the AAPT example used in this chapter, rather than concerning ourselves with 12 schools, we would need to take 120 classes-within-schools combinations into account. Even with a sample size of over 3,000, this reduces to roughly 25 cases per class-within-school combination. It might still be feasible with such a model to do a random intercepts model by clustering the level-2 × 3 combinations into a much smaller number of like units. It might even be possible to estimate correlations within each of the 120 class-within-school combinations, and cluster analyze based on those correlations. But in this case, the stability of correlations and means with $N=25$ is very questionable.

## Other MI Models

In this chapter, I have described handling MI with multilevel data using normal model MI software. The main reason for this is the accessibility of normal model MI software, and the inaccessibility of software designed to handle cluster data. For example, Schafer's PAN software (2001; Schafer and Yucel 2002) will, among other things, handle MI with cluster data. The problem with PAN is that it was never implemented as a mainstream package (as was Norm). Although programs such as PAN will very likely be the wave of the future, the future is not yet here.

## References

Andridge, R. R. (2011). Quantifying the impact of fixed effects modeling of clusters in multiple imputation for cluster randomized trials. *Biometrical Journal, 53*, 57–74.
Barnard, J., and Rubin, D. B. (1999). Small-sample degrees of freedom with multiple imputation. *Biometrika, 86*, 948–955.
Graham, J. W., Olchowski, A. E., & Gilreath, T. D. (2007). How Many Imputations are Really Needed? Some Practical Clarifications of Multiple Imputation Theory. *Prevention Science, 8*, 206–213.
Hansen, W. B., & Graham, J. W. (1991). Preventing alcohol, marijuana, and cigarette use among adolescents: Peer pressure resistance training versus establishing conservative norms. *Preventive Medicine, 20*, 414–430.
Murray, D. M. (1998). *Design and Analysis of Group-Randomized Trials*. New York: Oxford Univ. Press.
Little, R. J. A., & Rubin, D. B. (2002). *Statistical analysis with missing data: Second Edition*. New York: Wiley.
Raudenbush, S. W., and Bryk, A. S. (2002). *Hierarchical Linear Models*. Thousand Oaks, CA: Sage. 2nd ed.
Schafer, J. L. (2001). Multiple imputation with PAN. In L. M. Collins & A. G. Sayer (Eds.), *New methods for the analysis of change* (pp. 357–377). Washington, DC: American Psychological Association.
Schafer, J. L., & Yucel, R. M. (2002). Computational strategies for multivariate linear mixed-effects models with missing values. *Journal of Computational and Graphical Statistics, 11*, 437–457.

# Chapter 7
# Multiple Imputation and Analysis with SAS

In this chapter, I provide step-by-step instructions for performing multiple imputation and analysis with SAS version 9. I describe the use of PROC MI for multiple imputation but also touch on two other ways to make use of PROC MI for handling missing data when hypothesis testing is not the issue: (a) direct use of the EM algorithm for input into certain analysis programs, and (b) generating a single data set imputed from EM parameters.

Although virtually all analyses can be handled using multiple imputation or one of the other missing data approaches, in this chapter I will focus on these analyses: Coefficient alpha analysis with PROC CORR; exploratory factor analysis with PROC FACTOR; multiple linear regression with PROC REG; logistic regression with PROC LOGISTIC; and multilevel linear regression with PROC MIXED. The purpose of discussing these Procs is not to give readers a grounding in the statistical procedures. I make the assumption that readers already know how to use these procedures. Rather, my goal here is provide readers with the grounding necessary to carry out these analyses in the missing data case.

The MI product I know most about is NORM 2.03. Despite some of its limitations and quirks, I would almost always rather be working with that program, especially when I am in the process of getting to know my data. However, I must say that I have been very impressed with PROC MI. Over the years, I have gained substantial confidence in this program. It is fast, efficient, and I am able to do pretty much everything with PROC MI that I can do with NORM, and more. PROC MI is an incredibly useful product. I will not say that the interface between PROC MI and the analysis procedures is seamless – this remains one of its weaknesses, but it is very good, nonetheless. At this point in time, it is my opinion that with PROC MI and the interface between it and the various analysis procedures, SAS offers the best combination of MI and analysis features available for dealing with missing data.

Help documentation with SAS is excellent. I have the following link in with my "bookmarks" ("favorites"). I refer to it constantly for help with SAS syntax.

http://support.sas.com/documentation/index.html

# Step-by-Step Instructions for Multiple Imputation with PROC MI

Although it is not absolutely necessary, I do encourage SAS users to read Chap. 3 on MI with Norm. There is considerable theoretical overlap between the two approaches, given that the PROC MI was based on Schafer's (1997) algorithms. However, it is important to have a good conceptual feel for the process before applying it with PROC MI, and I believe it is a little easier to see the process with Norm.

In order to keep things straight between the chapters, I stay with the same eight steps to describe the operation of PROC MI that I used to describe the operation of NORM 2.03. Also, as in Chap. 3, I will conduct each step with an empirical data set, reporting the interim results as I go along. I encourage you to conduct these analyses as you read and compare your results with mine.

## *Running PROC MI (Step 1): Getting SAS*

This is an easy one. You either have SAS or you do not. SAS is an expensive program. If your organization does not have a site license for the latest version of SAS, the chances are you do not have a copy of it. So I will assume that you do have a copy of SAS, version 9. Most of what I describe here also applies to SAS version 8.2, but PROC MI is much better developed in SAS version 9, and I encourage you to upgrade to that if possible.

## *Empirical Example Used Throughout This Chapter*

In order to facilitate learning the procedures outlined in this chapter, I encourage you to download the data file, "ex7.sas7bdat" from our website:

http://methodology.psu.edu

The sample data set comes from a subset of one cohort of students ($N=2,756$) who took part in the Adolescent Alcohol Prevention Trial (AAPT; Hansen and Graham 1991). The sample data set includes a variable, *School*, indicating which of 12 schools the student was from. In addition, 19 substantive variables are included: Lifetime alcohol use at seventh, eighth, and ninth grades (*Alc7*, *Alc8*, *Alc9*); five variables making up a scale tapping relationship with parents at seventh grade (*Likepar71*, *Likepar72*, *Likepar73*, *Likepar74*, *Likepar75*); three variables making up a scale tapping belief about the positive social consequences of alcohol use at seventh grade (*Posatt71*, *Posatt72*, *Posatt73*); four variables tapping risk-taking and rebelliousness in grade 7 (*Riskreb71*, *Riskreb72*, *Riskreb73*, *Riskreb74*); and four variables tapping risk-taking and rebelliousness in eighth grade (*Riskreb81*, *Riskreb82*, *Riskreb83*, *Riskreb84*).[1]

As you read through the steps for conducting imputation with PROC MI, I encourage you to try out each step with this sample data set.

## Running PROC MI (Step 2): Preparing the Data Set

This is one of the best features of conducing MI within SAS. The data set is already prepared in some respects. I will assume that you already have a SAS system file to work with.

Not surprisingly, SAS handles MI differently from NORM. This stems from the fact that the data structure itself (the DATA step) is carried along with the imputation. With NORM, one selects variables for imputation, and the data set produces typically has those variables, and not much more. With SAS, one begins with a possibly rather large data set (e.g., 500 variables), and from that number, performs MI with a much smaller subset (e.g., 50 variables). The data set output from PROC MI will include imputed values for the 50 selected variables, and the multiple-imputed data sets will be stacked, but the stacked, multiple-imputed data set will also contain unimputed versions of the variables not included in the PROC MI analysis. So if you have 500 variables, 50 of which were analyzed with PROC MI, and if you asked for $m=40$ imputations, the resulting output data set will be rather large. It will contain 40 versions of the 50 variables, with different imputed values for each version, plus 40 copies of the original 450-variable data set not included in PROC MI. This is not really a limitation in most cases; you should just know what you are getting. If this does become a problem, it is an easy matter to use KEEP or DROP statements prior to running PROC MI in order to keep the output data set of manageable size.

### Number of Variables to Be Imputed

In this regard, many of the statements I made in Chap. 3 for running Norm, also apply here. You cannot simply include all of your variables in your PROC MI variable list. Just as with Norm, it is advisable to keep your input data set to a maximum of around $k=100$ variables regardless of how many cases you might have. I have gone above this number over the years, but I begin feeling uneasy as the number of input variables exceeds 100, and with every added variable, that uneasiness increases exponentially, just as the number of parameters that must be estimated by the program increases exponentially with sample size (please see Table 7.6).

---

[1] Note that the variable *Program*, used in the Proc Mixed example near the end of the chapter, is a simulated program variable, and results based on that variable are somewhat different from true program effects observed for the AAPT project.

So be judicious in selecting the variables for analysis. Follow these general rules:

(a) Start with the analysis model of interest.
(b) Judiciously include a few auxiliary variables (please see Chaps. 1 and 11). If you have a longitudinal data set, the best auxiliary variables are variables that are the same as the variables in your analysis model, but that are not being used in this analysis. For example, if I were looking at a program effect at seventh grade on cigarette smoking at tenth grade, I might well include smoking at eighth and ninth grades as auxiliary variables, along with smoking at seventh grade (if it is not being used as a covariate in the analysis model). Similarly, for any mediating variable used in the model, good auxiliary variables would be that same mediating variables measured at other waves not otherwise included in the analysis. Especially important in this context is to include measures that were measured after the mediating variable to be used in the analysis. For example, suppose beliefs about the prevalence of cigarette smoking among peers, measured at the immediate posttest (late seventh grade) was the mediating variable. I might well include as auxiliary variables prevalence beliefs at eighth and ninth grades (along with prevalence beliefs at seventh grade if that variable is not part of the analysis model).

In general, the variables that are included in PROC MI should all be continuous (or reasonably assumed to be continuous, including "ordered-categorical" variables), or dichotomous categorical. Any categorical variables with more than two levels must be recast as dummy variables before the MI analysis ($p-1$ dummy variables must be used to represent the categorical variable with $p>2$ categories). For example, suppose you have a variable describing political party affiliation, with three levels: Democrat, Republican, Independent. This variable (e.g., Party), would be dummy coded as shown below, and the dummy variables, not Party, would be include in the PROC MI analysis.

```
data a;set in1.mydata;
    if party='Democrat'   then do;dummy1= 1  ;dummy2= 0;  end;
    if party='Republican' then do;dummy1= 0  ;dummy2= 1;  end;
    if party='Independent' then do;dummy1= 0 ;dummy2= 0;  end;
run;
```

Note that each group in the categorical variable has a "1" for a different dummy variable, and "0" for all others, except the last group, which has "0" for all dummy variables.

I would like to make one general point about naming SAS data sets. Many PROC steps in SAS automatically writes out a new SAS data set. If you do not explicitly name the data set, for example with an "OUT=" statement, then SAS gives it an automatic name (starts with "DATA1", "DATA2", and so on). The problem is that you may not remember what it is for that particular PROC. So I usually encourage people to provide an explicit name for every data set generated. I usually use letters "a", "b", "c", and so on, but many explicit naming conventions are possible. Use what works for you. The bottom line is that when you run PROC MI, you should explicitly name the output file.

**Reading the Sample Data into SAS**

Over the years, one of the biggest headaches I have had with SAS is in getting the data into SAS so I can do my work. If you are comfortable reading data into SAS, then just do this part in your usual way. However, if you just cannot get it to work any other way, try placing the SAS data file into the folder: "c:\NormUtil". Then, the SAS code I show below may be used to access the sample data set and perform the simplest of PROC MI runs.[2]

```
***=====================================================***;
*** Reading Sample data into SAS ***;
***=====================================================***;
libname in1 'c:\NormUtil';

data a;set in1.ex7;
     keep school alc7 riskreb71 likepar72 posatt72 alc9;
run;

proc mi data=a nimpute=2 out=b;
     var alc7 riskreb71 likepar72 posatt72 alc9;
run;

***=====================================================***;
```

## *Running PROC MI (Step 3): Variables*

As I said above, one of the best things about doing MI with SAS is that the data are all right there and available. Assuming that you are already a SAS user, and that you have read the data in (e.g., as I suggest above), there is relatively little else to do.

With NORM 2.03, performing data transformations is handled at this step. The same is true for SAS. If you want to perform any transformations (e.g., log transformations to help with skew), I recommend that you do this prior to running PROC MI.

With NORM 2.03, you must select variables to be included in the MI model. The same is true with PROC MI. With most SAS PROCs, you select variables with a VAR statement (see the statement in the brief example; the VAR statement appears

---
[2] Note that in most of these preliminary PROC MI runs, I am setting NIMPUTE=2. Please do not take from this that I ever think just two imputations is enough. I am using NIMPUTE=2 for these preliminary runs to save time. When it matters, NIMPUTE will be set to a reasonable number.

just below the PROC MI statement in the sample code). In the example shown just above, just five variables were included in the MI model. However, note that in that example, I have used the KEEP statement within the prior DATA STEP to keep the School variable as well. As the sample code indicates, the School variable is not included in the MI model, but it will be in the output data set (OUT=B).

**Rounding**

Rounding is an interesting issue. My view is that rounding should be kept to a minimum. Multiple imputation was designed to restore lost variability in the data set as a whole. However, rounding after imputation is the same as adding a small amount of additional random error variance to the imputed values. This is easiest to see when calculating coefficient alpha when scale items have been rounded and unrounded. The rounded versions always have scale alpha that is one or two points lower (indicating more random error in the scale score).

So my rule for rounding is this: If the variable will be used in an analysis where the unrounded values will be no problem (e.g., using a gender variable as a covariate in a regression model), then leave it in its unrounded form. Of course, if the variable is to be used in an analysis where only certain values make any sense (e.g., using gender as a blocking variable or using a dichotomous smoking variable as the dependent variable in a logistic regression analysis), then by all means, round to the legal values (e.g., 0 and 1).

**Rounding in SAS**

Fortunately, no rounding is the default in PROC MI. That is, unless you do something special, imputed values will be imputed with no rounding. Unfortunately, when you want rounding, the rounding feature in PROC MI is a little clunky. See the following code:

```
proc mi data=a out=b nimpute=10;
    var alc7 riskreb71 likepar72 posatt72 alc9;
run;
```

To round all five variables to integers, the code is:

```
proc mi data=a out=b nimpute=10 round=1;
    var alc7 riskreb71 likepar72 posatt72 alc9;
run;

proc freq;tables alc7 riskreb71 likepar72 posatt72 alc9;
run;
```

Add a PROC FREQ statement as shown above in order to check the effects of using this rounding statement. You will see in the output that any imputed values rounded to 0 are actually rounded to some very small number (e.g., 3.274291E-17). The fact that SAS PROC MI rounds to a value very near zero, but not exactly to zero, may be a problem in many applications. For example, a problem would arise if you tried to act on those values using an IF statement:

```
data c;set b;
    if alc9=0;
run;
```

Try the kind of IF statement shown above. SAS does not see the very small value as 0. This problem may have been resolved in SAS (version 9.2). However, I believe that using the ROUND function within the SAS DATA STEP is a better way to do any necessary rounding following MI.

```
proc mi data=a nimpute=2 out=b;
    var alc7 riskreb71 likepar72 posatt72 alc9 xalc9;
run;

data c;set b;
    array x alc7 riskreb71 likepar72 posatt72 alc9 xalc9;
    do over x;
    x=round(x,1);
    end;
run;

proc freq;tables alc7 riskreb71 likepar72 posatt72 alc9
xalc9;
run;

data d;set c;
    if posatt72=0;
run;

data d;set c;
    if posatt72=1;
run;
```

Looking at the PROC FREQ results, you will see that all values rounded to 0 appear as exactly 0 in the PROC FREQ output. Double check by adding the two data steps following the PROC FREQ. Checking the SAS LOG, you will see that the number of cases for these two data steps is the same as shown in the PROC FREQ output. This verifies that IF statements correctly operate on values rounded to 0 and to 1.

**Table 7.1** Model information output from SAS

| Model Information | |
|---|---|
| Data Set | WORK.A |
| Method | MCMC |
| Multiple Imputation Chain | Single Chain |
| Initial Estimates for MCMC | EM Posterior Mode |
| Start | Starting Value |
| Prior | Jeffreys |
| Number of Imputations | 2 |
| Number of Burn-in Iterations | 200 |
| Number of Iterations | 100 |
| Seed for random number generator | 752953001 |

## Running PROC MI (Step 4): Summarizing the Missing Data

The first part of the SAS output summarizes the missing data, and the analysis, in several ways. This is an important step in the imputation process. First, I find it useful to add the SIMPLE option in the PROC MI statement (see sample code below).

```
proc mi data=a nimpute=2 out=b simple;
   var alc7 riskreb71 likepar72 posatt72 alc9;
run;
```

The first section of the output is entitled, "Model Information." In my main run, I got the output shown in Table 7.1.

I find it useful to scan quickly down the list of model parameters. Seeing what was in the model might remind you that something different was needed. I will come back to many of these options later in the chapter; here I am just talking about the output itself.

All of these were defaults: Single chain MCMC for imputation (always use this); initial estimates coming from EM estimates; prior is "Jeffreys" (uninformative prior). I will talk more later in this chapter about the prior. For now, suffice it to say that this prior should be used if it works. As I noted above, number of imputations was set to 2 only for these preliminary models just to save time. The default for number of "burn-in" iterations is 200. It is customary in using MCMC procedures to allow the procedure to work a while (burn in) before one attempts to make use of the results. The random starting seed is always set automatically. However, if you would like control over the solution (always get the same results), then you may choose the random starting seed with the SEED=option within the PROC MI statement.

The next section of the preliminary output is "Missing Data Patterns." Table 7.2 presents these patterns for the small example used here. This section can be useful for a variety of reasons. In the output, as shown below, an "x" means the cases have data for that variable, and a "." means the variable is missing. First, as shown below,

Table 7.2 Patterns of missing and observed values

|  | Missing Data Patterns | | | | | | |
|---|---|---|---|---|---|---|---|
| Group | alc7 | riskreb71 | likepar72 | posatt72 | alc9 | Freq | Percent |
| 1 | X | X | X | X | X | 499 | 18.11 |
| 2 | X | X | X | X | . | 266 | 9.65 |
| 3 | X | X | X | . | X | 554 | 20.10 |
| 4 | X | X | X | . | . | 308 | 11.18 |
| 5 | X | X | . | X | X | 5 | 0.18 |
| 6 | X | X | . | . | X | 3 | 0.11 |
| 7 | X | X | . | . | . | 1 | 0.04 |
| 8 | X | . | X | X | X | 2 | 0.07 |
| 9 | X | . | X | X | . | 2 | 0.07 |
| 10 | X | . | X | . | X | 2 | 0.07 |
| 11 | X | . | . | X | X | 531 | 19.27 |
| 12 | X | . | . | X | . | 327 | 11.87 |
| 13 | X | . | . | . | X | 42 | 1.52 |
| 14 | X | . | . | . | . | 37 | 1.34 |
| 15 | . | X | X | X | X | 3 | 0.11 |
| 16 | . | X | X | X | . | 1 | 0.04 |
| 17 | . | X | X | . | X | 3 | 0.11 |
| 18 | . | X | X | . | . | 2 | 0.07 |
| 19 | . | . | . | X | X | 2 | 0.07 |
| 20 | . | . | . | . | X | 166 | 6.02 |

pattern, or "Group" 1, contains the complete cases, if there are any. The last pattern displayed (Group 20 in Table b8.2) shows the group with the least data. If there happen to be any cases with no data at all, it will show up here. If this should happen, "." shows up for all variables, and those cases are automatically omitted from the MI analysis. Still, when that happens, it is better to go back to the previous DATA STEP and eliminate any cases with data missing for all of the variable to be included in PROC MI.

▶ **Sample Data.** There are three key things to see here. First, for this small example, there were some (18.11 %) complete cases. I know this, because the top row, which will show the complete cases if there are any, have no "." values. Second, there were just 20 different patterns of missing and observed data in this small example. Third, because the bottom row of this matrix contains at least one "X" value, I know there no cases missing all the data.

## SAS Proc MI (v. 9) Is Not Perfect

Please understand that I believe SAS Proc MI to be an amazingly useful product. However, there are a few areas where it could be improved. For example, I find that the first few sections of output from PROC MI are a little disorganized, so beware.

One example of this is that when there are many missing data patterns, you will first see a few patterns, then you will see the means for the variables within those patterns. Then you will see more patterns and more means. For sake of clarity in Table 7.2, I combined two bits of output to create a somewhat cleaner version of the information. With larger models, this section of output is almost impossible to keep straight. So with larger models, keep in mind what you are looking for.

(a) Does Pattern (group) 1 indicate complete cases? (If there are any complete cases, they will show up in this group).
(b) How many complete cases are there?
(c) Does the last pattern indicate that cases with this pattern have at least some data?

If you focus on just these three bits of information, you will be able to find them, even with the largest problems. A partial solution to the problem of disjointed output is to ask for a very wide output line, for example, with, "Options LS=255".

## What Is Most Useful About Missing Data Patterns?

A key part of the EM algorithm is identifying all these patterns and operating on each of them separately. So because identifying all these patterns is being done anyway, it is an easy thing to provide a table of these patterns.

Software makers display all of the patterns of missing values more for completeness and because it is easier to present all of them. They do not present all the patterns because it is important for the end user to view all the patterns. As I have pointed out above, relatively few bits of information must be gleaned from these patterns.

In fact, in terms of conveying useful information to readers of an article I might be writing, I find it useful to generate missingness patterns from a set of variables that might be slightly different from, or possibly just a subset of, the variables that I am actually analyzing. For example, in a longitudinal study, I often find it useful to present a missingness patterns table that shows how many participants provided any data at each wave. For this kind of thing, I find it more useful to calculate the missingness patterns "by hand" in SAS. Using the sample data for this chapter, the relevant SAS code might look like this:

```
data a;set in1.ex7;
    if n(of alc7 riskreb71-riskreb74 likepar71-likepar75
        posatt71-posatt73)>0 then r7=1;else r7=0;
    if n(of alc8 riskreb81-riskreb84)>0 then r8=1;else r8=0;
    if n(of alc9)>0 then r9=1;else r9=0;
run;

proc freq;tables r7*r8*r9/list;
run;
```

**Table 7.3** Patterns of missing and observed values for wave participation

| r7 | r8 | r9 | Frequency | Percent | Cumulative Frequency | Cumulative Percent |
|----|----|----|-----------|---------|----------------------|--------------------|
| 0  | 1  | 1  | 166       | 6.02    | 166                  | 6.02               |
| 1  | 0  | 1  | 213       | 7.73    | 379                  | 13.75              |
| 1  | 1  | 0  | 944       | 34.25   | 1323                 | 48.00              |
| 1  | 1  | 1  | 1433      | 52.00   | 2756                 | 100.00             |

**Table 7.4** Partial PROC MI output

Univariate Statistics

| Variable | Missing Values Count | Percent |
|----------|----------------------|---------|
| alc7     | 177                  | 6.42    |
| riskreb71| 1111                 | 40.31   |
| likepar72| 1114                 | 40.42   |
| posatt72 | 1118                 | 40.57   |
| alc9     | 944                  | 34.25   |

In this case, if a participant provided any data for the seventh grade wave, the variable r7 takes on the value "1". Otherwise, r7 takes on the value "0". Similarly, if a participant provided any data for the eighth or ninth grade wave, then r8 or r9 would take on the value of "1". Otherwise, those variables would take on the value "0". The SAS output from this code appears in Table 7.3.

I might trim this table a little for presentation in my article (e.g., removing the two columns on the right), but otherwise, this is essentially the table I would present. I find the information in this table to be a lot more useful in understanding the data than is the information (taken as a whole) shown in Table 7.2 (this is especially true for models with more variables). As needed, I might consider including something like Table 7.3 in my article and present the information in Table 7.2 (and Table 7.1) on a website for ancillary information related to the article.

As noted above, I find it very useful to include the option, SIMPLE, in the PROC MI statement. If you do so, then at the end of the next section on univariate statistics, you will see the following output relating to the number and percent of missing data for each variable in the model. I find it useful to scan down the percent missing column and make sure that each percent missing makes sense based on what I already know about the data set. Be especially watchful when the percent missing is high. Does it make sense that some variables have 50 % (or more) missing data? This sometimes happens for the right reasons, for example, the data are missing due to a planned missing data design. But it is also possible that a high percent missing could be due to a simple coding error. It is important not to go forward until you have an adequate explanation.

▶ **Sample Data.** Table 7.4 shows the part of the SAS output that relates the number and percent missing for each variable in the model.

Note that a small percentage (6.42 %) of students had missing data for Alc7, alcohol use at seventh grade. Normally there is virtually no missing data in this cohort on this variable at seventh grade. The small amount of missingness seen here is due mainly to the fact that in this data set, I included new students who "dropped in" to the study beginning at eighth grade. Also note that about 40 % of students were missing each of the other variables measured at seventh grade. This amount of missingness is due to the planned missingness design used in this study (see Chap. 12 for a discussion of this type of design). In this case, approximately a third of the students were not given these questions. Add to that the approximately 6 % not present at all at the seventh grade measure, and the number is very close to the 40 % missingness observed. The 34.25 % missing on Alc9 reflects the somewhat greater attrition between eighth and ninth grades. This, too, makes sense given what I already know about these data.

## *Running PROC MI (Step 5): EM Algorithm*

Just as with NORM, PROC MI first runs EM and then runs MCMC using the EM parameter estimates as starting values. However, unlike NORM, PROC MI runs the whole thing at once, so it is not as obvious which part is EM and which part is MCMC.

However, it is important to see how EM is performing before going ahead with MCMC. For example, are the defaults for MCMC appropriate? As described in Chap. 2, having enough steps of MCMC (or DA) between imputed data sets is what allows normal-model MI to simulate random draws from the population. If too few steps are used, then the results of the MI inference will not be valid (because the between-imputation variance will be too small).

Thus, I strongly recommend running PROC MI in stages. First, examine the performance of EM without imputing anything. Sample PROC MI code for this is as follows:

```
proc mi data=a nimpute=0 simple;
   em itprint;
     var
       alc7 alc8 alc9
       riskreb71-riskreb74
       likepar71-likepar75
       posatt71-posatt73
       riskreb81-riskreb84;
run;
```

Adding the nimpute=0 option just saves the time of imputation during this step. In older versions (version 9.1), EM is run with PROC MI even without the "EM ITPRINT" statement. However, with SAS version 9.2, if the EM statement is omitted, EM is not run. If EM option is given (as shown), the output is given for

EM (MLE). If just the "MCMC" option is given (EM omitted), then output for EM (posterior mode) is given. If both EM and MCMC statements are present, then output is given for both EM (MLE) and EM (posterior mode).

Adding the "ITPRINT" option for EM produces the fit function value at each iteration (crucial information), along with means for each variable at each iteration (much less important information).

▶ **Sample Data.** If you run the SAS statements shown just above, look in the output for "EM (MLE) Iteration History". The first thing listed for each iteration uses the value of the fit function (-2 Log L). This value should change monotonically over the iterations. In this example, note that the value is 39,047 at iteration 0. At iteration 1, the value is 30,863. The values become smaller and smaller, until by iteration 24, the value is 28,813. Because only integers are shown in the output, you see no further changes in the function value through convergence at iteration 51.

As with the initial output, this part of the output is somewhat cluttered with information of secondary importance (e.g., means for all variables at each iteration). On my screen (using options LS=100), I first see all information for the first three iterations. It is five output pages before I see the function values for iterations 49–51. But persevere. It is important to verify that the function changes monotonically over the iterations.

The number of iterations to EM convergence can be seen in the output, but it also appears in the SAS LOG:

▶ **NOTE:** The EM algorithm (MLE) converges in 51 iterations.

The key information from the log is the number of iterations for EM (MLE) convergence.

## EM Convergence: Maximum Iterations

The default is 200 for EM (MLE) convergence in PROC MI. Verify (in the SAS LOG or in the output) that EM (MLE) has indeed converged. There will be warning in the SAS log if EM (MLE) fails to converge in the default 200 iterations:

▶ **WARNING:** The EM algorithm (MLE) fails to converge after 200 iterations. You can increase the number of iterations (MAXITER=option) or increase the value of the convergence criterion (CONVERGE=option).

If you see this message, it is important. Although EM taking more than 200 iterations to converge is not necessarily indicative of a problem, it is usually a good idea to take steps (e.g., modify or delete variables) if EM takes too long to converge. My rule of thumb is that if EM has not converged in 1,000 iterations, I can almost always make changes that will allow it to converge in fewer iterations. It is often a sign of a fundamental data problem when EM takes as many as 1,000 iterations to converge.

**Table 7.5** Converge rates for three EM programs

|  | Convergence Criterion | | | |
|---|---|---|---|---|
|  | 1E-3 | 1E-4 | 1E-5 | 1E-6 |
| Norm 2.03 | 54 | **72** | 91 |  |
| EMCOV | 52 | **70** | 94 |  |
| PROC MI |  | 51 | **70** | 89 |

If you see the warning that EM has not converged, it is important that you increase the maximum number of iterations (with the MAXITER=option), but you should NOT increase the value of the convergence criterion (see below) simply to get EM to converge within the 200 iteration limit.

**Convergence Criterion**

In Chap. 2, I noted that EM converges when the elements of the covariance matrix stop changing appreciably from one iteration to the next. Of course, what constitutes "appreciable" change can vary. The default convergence criterion for NORM is 1E-04 (.0001). It is important to know that with NORM, convergence is reached when the largest absolute change in any of the variance-covariance parameters, divided by that parameter's value, is less than the criterion. But other criteria are possible. For example, with EMCOV (Graham and Hofer 1992; Graham and Donaldson 1993), convergence is reached when the largest change in any of the variance-covariance parameters is smaller than the criterion (without dividing by the parameter's value). With SAS, the convergence criterion is partly what is used with NORM (for parameter values greater than .01), and partly what is used for EMCOV (values less than .01). The upshot is that what constitutes "appreciable" change is a little different for NORM and for PROC MI.

In any event, the convergence rates for the three programs were different for the sample data set used for this book. Table 7.5 presents the convergence rates for the three programs with different convergence criteria. It is important to realize that these convergence rates do not generalize perfectly to other input data sets. However, it does point up the fact that, for whatever reason, PROC MI converges in fewer iterations than does NORM. The figures in Table 7.5 suggest that in order to achieve comparable estimates of number of iterations to EM convergence, EM from PROC MI should specify CONVERGE=1E-5.

I am not saying that NORM is right and PROC MI is wrong. I am saying that I have extensive experience with the number of iterations for EM convergence with NORM, so that is the number I want to use. I will do whatever I need to within PROC MI EM to get a similar number. And that "whatever" appears to be to use CONVERGE=1E-5.

## Maximum-Likelihood Estimate or Posterior Mode

I describe the difference between these two modes of estimation here. SAS (v. 9) PROC MI does not have a separate PRIOR=statement for EM. But the PRIOR=option used under the MCMC statement also applies to the estimation of EM.

The decision to be made here is whether to ask for the standard maximum-likelihood estimate or to use the Bayesian posterior mode under ridge prior with hyperparameter. My view is that the ML solution is better if it works, so it is always best to try that first. But occasionally, the ML mode does not work well (e.g., EM takes more than 1,000 iterations to converge, or never converges). I have found that having few or no cases with complete data can often (but not always) produce this problem. The problem can also manifest itself when one or more variables have a very high percent missing data.

The posterior mode under ridge prior is like ridge regression (e.g., see Price 1977) in some respects. Ridge regression has been used when the predictors in multiple regression are so highly correlated as to produce unstable results. In ridge regression, one adds a small constant to all of the diagonal elements of the input correlation matrix (e.g., making them all 1.01 rather than 1.00). It is easy to see that all correlations in this new input matrix are slightly biased toward 0. The result is that the regression results will be slightly biased, but the solution will also be more stable because the predictors are less correlated.

A similar thing happens with multiple imputation. The idea is to introduce a little bias in order to make the MI solution more stable. Adding a ridge prior with hyperparameter is a little like adding some number of cases at the bottom of one's data set, such that all of the variables are uncorrelated. The number of cases added is similar to the value of the hyperparameter. So, if one sets the hyperparameter to 5 (with PRIOR=RIDGE=5), it is a little like adding five cases at the bottom of one's data set. It makes sense why this should work. If your data set has no complete cases, then adding these five cases means that your data set now has five complete cases. But the cost of doing this is that all correlations are biased slightly toward 0. This is why I say that I prefer using the ML mode if it works; I would like to avoid this bias if possible. Also, even if you must use the posterior mode, it is a good idea to use a hyperparameter as small as possible. My rule of thumb here is to use a hyperparameter no larger than 1 % of the overall sample size. In order to help keep that number as low as possible, think of the hyperparameter as adding "bogus" cases to the bottom of your data sets. What reviewer will respond favorably to your adding a large number of bogus cases to your data set?

## Informative Prior

The uninformative prior (Jeffreys prior) is a way to use the Bayesian posterior mode that is most similar to ML estimation. However, in addition to using the Ridge prior, it is also possible in SAS to use an informative prior. Let me talk briefly about a study that used a skip pattern (very common in survey research). That survey first asked adolescent participants if they had ever smoked in their life (yes or no). If the person responded "yes," then he or she received the follow-up question asking how much was smoked in the previous 30 days. But if the person answered "no," the follow-up 30-day smoking question was not presented.

With data like these, it makes sense that one could estimate the correlation between the lifetime smoking question and some other variable (e.g., grades in school), and between the 30-day smoking question and grades in school. But the correlation between lifetime smoking and 30-day smoking is not estimable in these data, because the only people with data for the 30-day question have a constant ("1") on the lifetime smoking question. Nevertheless, just because it is not estimable in these data, it makes sense that there is a correlation between one's lifetime smoking and one's smoking in the previous 30 days. And under some circumstances, it might be useful to have both of these variables in the same analysis model.

Suppose you had another data set based on a comparable population for which the dichotomous lifetime smoking and 30-day smoking questions were both observed. That data set would provide a reasonable basis for estimating the correlation between lifetime and 30-day smoking in the data with the skip pattern. Under these circumstances, you can make use of the *PRIOR=INPUT=[SAS data set]* option (under the MCMC statement) to provide enough information to allow the estimation of the correlations for the three variables, lifetime smoking, 30-day smoking, and grades in school. This data set is a TYPE=COV data set in SAS, where the N provided in the data set is like the hyperparameter given with the PRIOR=RIDGE option.

As I suggested above, using the ridge option with hyperparameter is a little like adding a certain number of bogus cases to the bottom of your data set, such that all of the variables are uncorrelated. Similarly, using this informative prior is a little like adding a certain number of bogus cases to the bottom of your data set such that the variables in question have the correlation specified in the TYPE=COV data set. And as with using the ridge prior, the N used with the PRIOR=INPUT=option should be kept as small as possible.

### Using an Informative Prior: Be Very Cautious

I very much like the fact that adding an informative prior is even possible with SAS PROC MI. But one of my basic philosophies of life is that just because something is possible, it does not mean one should do it. In this case, adding an informative prior to one's analysis requires rather strong assumptions. I would say that this approach should be attempted, first with great caution, and only then when the potential payoffs are substantial.

### EM Output: ML Estimates

Near the bottom of the EM output are EM (MLE) parameter estimates: means, standard deviations, and the correlation or covariance matrix. I believe these are the best

Table 7.6 Increase in parameters estimated in EM as number of variables increases

| Variables k | Parameters estimated $[(k(k+1)/2)+k]$ |
|---|---|
| 20 | 230 |
| 40 | 860 |
| 60 | 1,890 |
| 80 | 3,320 |
| 100 | 5,150 |
| 120 | 7,380 |
| 140 | 10,010 |
| 160 | 13,040 |
| 180 | 16,470 |
| 200 | 20,300 |

point estimates for these parameters. If you want to report these quantities in your article, I believe they should come from this output. Your table (or text) should, of course, be clear that these means and standard deviations (and correlation matrix) are EM parameter estimates. Remember that in order to get these EM estimates (MLE), you must have the EM statement in PROC MI.

## Speed of EM

How long it takes EM to converge depends on many factors. The two biggest factors are the number of variables ($k$) in the model and the amount of missing information (related to the amount of missing data). EM estimates $k(k+1)/2$ variances and covariances and $k$ means. Table 7.6 shows how the number of parameters to be estimated increases exponentially with the number of variables. Because the EM algorithm works primarily with the variance-covariance matrix, and other matrices of the same size, the number of variables is far more important to the time to EM convergence than is the number of cases.

The second major factor in EM convergence rate is the amount of missing data. The more missing data, the longer it takes EM to converge. Another factor is the correlation between other variables in the model and the variables with missing data (higher correlations mean faster convergence). The number of different missing data patterns also contributes to the convergence rate (more patterns take longer). I have also observed that EM with highly skewed variables can take longer to converge.

## Output the EM (MLE) Variance-Covariance Matrix

A very useful feature in SAS is the ability to produce TYPE=COV data sets. Of course, such data sets come most commonly from PROC CORR, and can be used as input to several other procedures, including PROC FACTOR and PROC REG. It is especially important that PROC MI also has the capability of producing an EM (MLE) variance-covariance matrix as a TYPE=COV data set. The code for writing out this data set is given below.

```
proc mi data=a nimpute=0;
    em outem=b;
        alc7 alc8 alc9
        riskreb71-riskreb74
        likepar71-likepar75
        posatt71-posatt73
        riskreb81-riskreb84;
run;
```

The description of using this output data set with PROC FACTOR and PROC REG is given later in this chapter.

## *Running PROC MI (Step 6): Impute From (EM) Parameters*

Imputing from EM parameters is with PROC MI is easy. The only major difference between the imputing from EM parameters with PROC MI and NORM is that with PROC MI, the EM estimates for imputation are the EM (posterior mode) estimates, whereas with NORM, the EM estimates for imputation are the ML estimates. These two sets of estimates do tend to be very similar, as long as the uninformative (Jeffreys) prior is used for posterior mode (this is the default in PROC MI).

The key here is that one does not want to iterate at all. This can be accomplished by suppressing all MCMC iteration. The sample code for generating this single data set imputed from EM parameters is given below.

```
proc mi data=a nimpute=1 out=b;
    mcmc nbiter=0 niter=0;
        alc7 alc8 alc9
        riskreb71-riskreb74
        likepar71-likepar75
        posatt71-posatt73
        riskreb81-riskreb84;
run;
```

The data set resulting from the OUT=B statement can then be used like any other regular SAS data set. As I suggest in later in this chapter, this data set is particularly useful for conducting data quality (coefficient alpha) analysis. However, this data set should not be used for hypothesis testing. Hypothesis testing should be carried out only with multiple imputations.

## Running PROC MI (Step 7): MCMC (and Imputation)

The MCMC (and imputation) part of this process should be run as a separate step after verifying that EM converges normally and knowing the number of iterations it took for EM convergence (using CONVERGE=1E-5). Note that I am now asking for 40 imputations with the NIMPUTE=40 option.

```
proc mi data=a nimpute=40 out=b;
   mcmc nbiter=200 niter=70;
      var
      alc7 alc8 alc9
      riskreb71-riskreb74
      likepar71-likepar75
      posatt71-posatt73
      riskreb81-riskreb84;
run;
```

Recall that EM (with CONVERGE=1E-5) converged in 70 iterations (see Table 7.5). So the number of MCMC iterations between imputed data sets should be 70. Accomplish this with the NITER=70 option within the MCMC statement. For the number of burn-in iterations (i.e., the number of MCMC iterations before imputing the first data set), my rule of thumb is to use the SAS default (NBITER=200) whenever EM converged in 200 or fewer iterations. After that, allow NBITER and NITER to increase to the same value (although it may be necessary to see the plots to judge whether a larger number of burn-in iterations is required). For example, if EM converged in 237 iterations, then the settings for MCMC would be NBITER=237 and NITER=237. I encourage you to use the NBITER= and NITER= statements even when the defaults are used. I find that this keeps me from omitting these statements mistakenly when they should be used.

Note that when you run MCMC without the EM statement, EM convergence will revert to the default convergence levels. This is reasonable; EM estimates are used only as starting values for MCMC iteration. As long as these estimates are reasonable, and they will be even with the default, CONVERGE=1E-4, the burn-in iterations for MCMC will produce a meaningful first imputed data set. However, if for some reason you would like to retain the more stringent convergent criteria for both the MLE and posterior mode EM estimates, do so with separate CONVERGE=statements within the EM and MCMC statements:

```
proc mi data=a nimpute=40 out=b;
   em converge=1e-5;
   mcmc nbiter=200 niter=70 initial=em(converge=1e-5);
```

The CONVERGE=option within the EM statement controls the convergence criterion for EM (MLE), and the CONVERGE=option within the MCMC statement controls the convergence criterion for EM (posterior mode).

At the same time you are doing the MCMC and imputation part of the process, I strongly encourage you to ask for the diagnostic plots. These plots must be specified explicitly in SAS:

```
proc mi data=a nimpute=40 out=b;
  mcmc nbiter=200 niter=70 acfplot(cov mean wlf)
  timeplot(cov mean wlf);
```

The ACFPLOT is a plot of the auto correlations of parameters over iterations of MCMC. The TIMEPLOT is the plot of the parameter estimates themselves over all iterations of MCMC. For the two plots, COV refers to the elements of the variance-covariance matrix, MEAN refers to the estimates of the means, and WLF refers to the "worst linear function." I suggest you typically ask for both kinds of plots with all three of kinds of estimates.

▶ **Sample Data**. This problem took just under 2.5 min with a Dell Latitude D620 laptop (2 GHz Core Duo processor with 1 GB RAM) and just under 28 s with a Dell Latitude E6320 laptop (Intel® Core(TM) i7-2620 M CPU @ 2.70 GHz, with 4 GB RAM).

▶ **Results of Imputation**. Once completed, there will be $m$ (e.g., 40) imputed data sets in the specified SAS output file.

## *Running PROC MI (Step 8): MCMC Diagnostics*

The final step in the imputation process is to check the diagnostic plots. The goals of checking these plots are to verify (a) that the number of MCMC steps between imputed data sets was sufficient, and (b) that the imputation solution was "acceptable," and not "pathological." Remember that we use the MCMC procedure to simulate random draws from the population. So it makes sense that each parameter estimate from each random draw from the population would come from legal parameter space. That is, each parameter value would fall in a reasonable range of values. If the time series (trace) plot is somewhat rectangular in appearance, that suggests that a parameter value drawn anywhere along the width of the plot would fall in the same range of values. I say this is an "acceptable" plot, because it means that imputed data sets from the DA run are a good representation of multiple random draws from the population. The trace plot displayed in Fig. 7.1 (panel a1) is an example of an acceptable plot. However, the 1,000 MCMC iterations in this plot is not a very large number; because of this, the plot does look a little ragged. The plot displayed in Fig. 7.1 (panel a2) was based on 5,000 MCMC iterations. This plot is more clearly an example of an acceptable MCMC run.

On the other hand, if the time series (trace) plot snakes slowly up or down over the width of the plot, then it is likely that parameter values drawn at one point will

**a1** Acceptable

**a2** More Clearly Acceptable with 5000 Iterations of MCMC

**b1** Possibly Unacceptable

**b2** Plot More Clearly Acceptable with More MCMC Iterations (note that a large number of burn-in iterations may be needed)

**b3** WLF Plot Shows Clear Need for Large Number of Burn-in Iterations

**C1** Clearly Pathological

**C2** 5000 MCMC Iterations

**C3** 5000 MCMC Iterations with Prior=Ridge=5

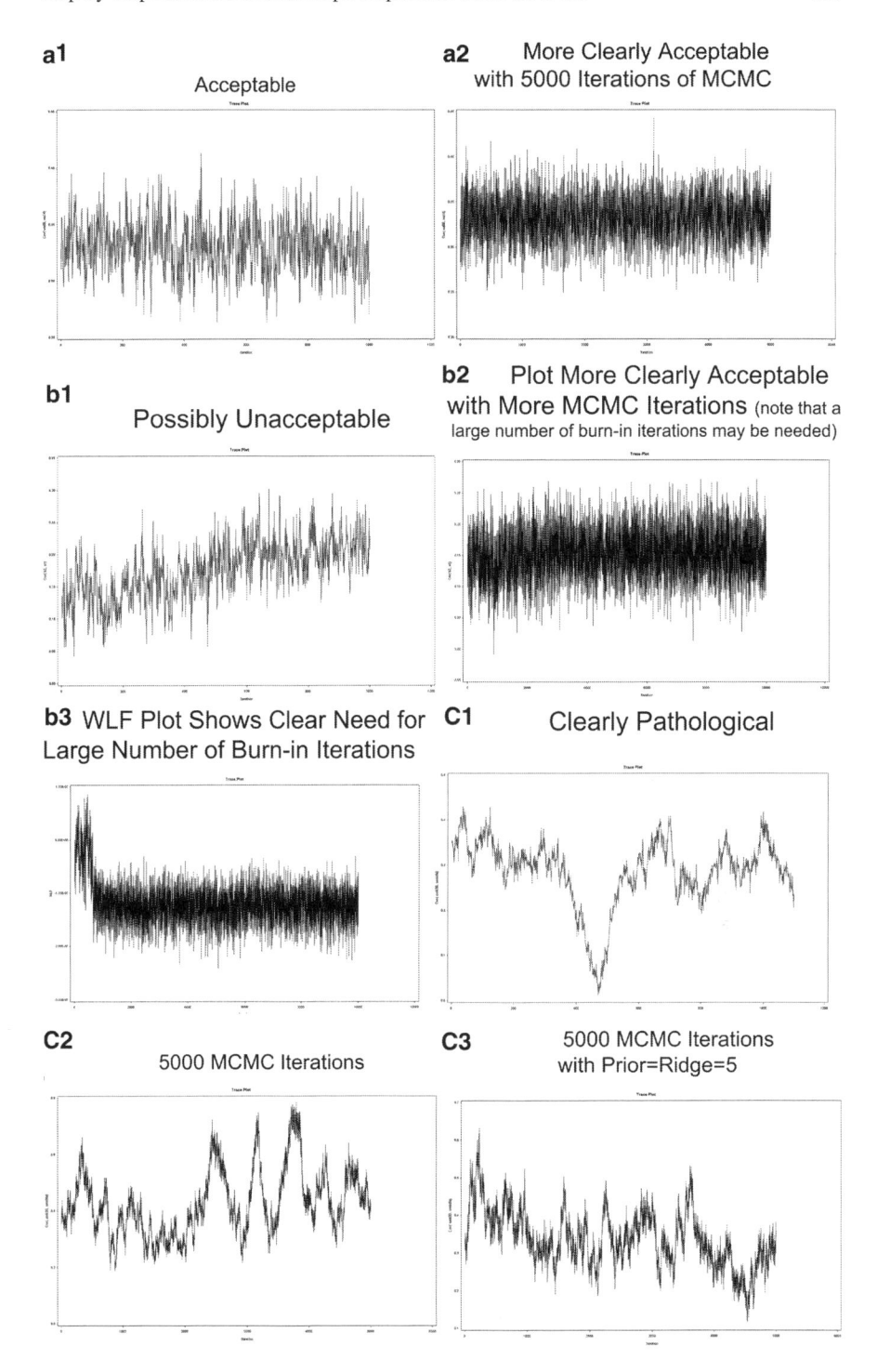

**Fig. 7.1** Diagnostic plots. Plots depict MI solutions that range from clearly acceptable to clearly pathological

be larger or smaller than parameter values drawn at other points along the width of the plot. I refer to this as a "pathological" plot, because it does not reflect a good simulation of random draws from the population. The plot displayed in Fig. 7.1 (panel b1) appears to have this problem. Parameter values early in the series are clearly lower than those later in the series. However, this may be an artifact of (a) a burn-in period that was too short, and (b) having too few overall MCMC iterations. Figure 7.1 (panel b2) displays the time series (trace) plot for the same data, but with 10,000 MCMC iterations. This plot is much more clearly acceptable; however, note that the first 1,000 or so iterations are still somewhat lower than the remainder of the plot. This is further evidence that the burn-in should have a larger number of MCMC iterations. Figure 7.1 (panel b3) displays the WLF plot for these same data. This plot much more clearly shows that at least 1,000 burn-in MCMC iterations are required (nbiter = 1,000), and that after about 1,000 iterations, the plot looks acceptable.

Figure 7.1 (panel c1) displays a time series (trace) plot that shows a clearly pathological MCMC run. However, one might question whether the shape of this plot is due to the relatively small number of MCMC iterations (1,100). Figure 7.1 (panel c2) displays the time series plot for the same data, but with 5,000 MCMC iterations. Clearly, the pathological nature of this plot was not due to the relatively small number of iterations. For these data, even with posterior mode and a small hyperparameter, the plot remains pathological (see Fig. 7.1, panel c3). These data came from two questions with a skip pattern. If the person responded with "0" to the first question ("never smoked"), then he or she did not see the second question (How many cigarettes smoked in past 30 days), that is, the second question was always missing. Because the first question had only two categories ("0" or "1"), the correlation between the two questions could not be estimated, even using posterior mode with a small hyperparameter.

## Options for the ACFPLOT

One option for the ACFPLOT is the number of lags for the autocorrelations. The value of examining these plots is to verify that the number of MCMC steps between imputed data sets was reasonable. Therefore, you need the number of lags to be larger than the number of MCMC steps between imputed data sets. In our example, EM converged with 70 iterations, so I set NITER = 70. In this case, then, the number of lags should be larger than 70; setting NLAG = 100 or NLAG = 150 would be a good idea in this case. The default for NLAG = 20, which is way too few to be useful in many instances. Be sure to set this value before you run PROC MI.

▶ **Sample Data.** I analyzed the 19 variable data set, asking for the Time Series (trace) and ACF plots, using the code shown below.

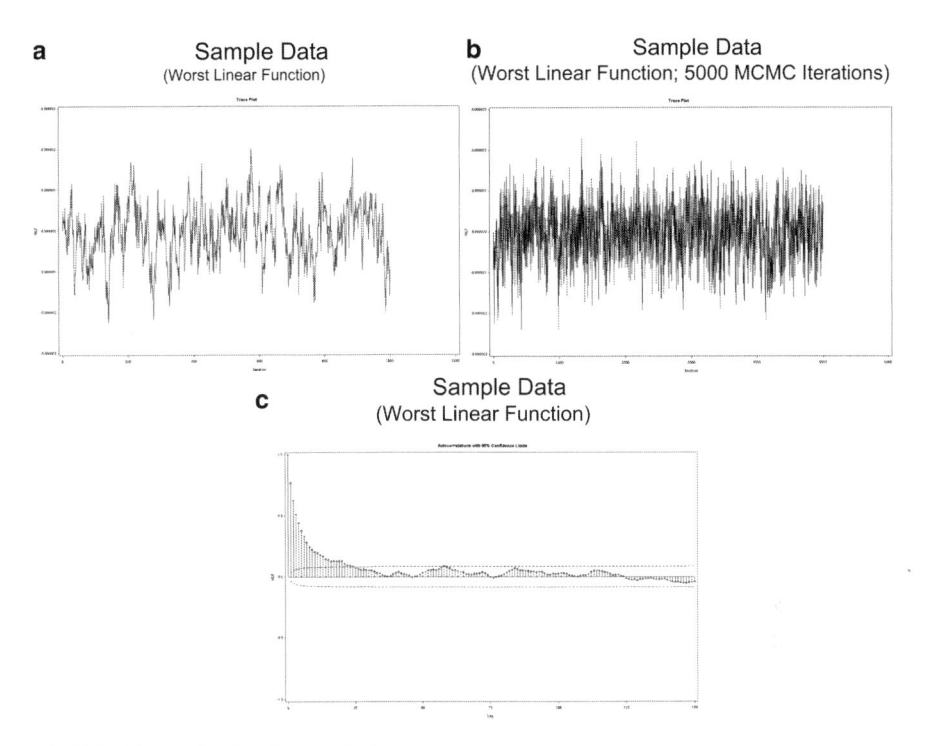

**Fig. 7.2** Diagnostic plots for sample data

```
proc mi data=a nimpute=1 out=b;
  em itprint converge=1e-5 maxiter=1000;
  mcmc nbiter=1000 niter=1000 acfplot(cov mean wlf/
  nlag=150) timeplot(cov mean wlf);

    var
    alc7 alc8 alc9
    riskreb71-riskreb74
    likepar71-likepar75
    posatt71-posatt73
    riskreb81-riskreb84;
```

The code given above illustrates how one might examine the diagnostic plots before performing the imputations. The time series (trace) plot for the worst linear function for these data appears in Fig. 7.2 (panel a). I would judge this plot to reflect an acceptable MCMC run. However, as with the plot shown in Fig. 7.1 (panel a1), this plot does look a little raged. Increasing the number of MCMC iterations (with nbiter=5,000) yielded the plot shown in Fig. 7.2 (panel b).

As with the plot shown in Fig. 7.1 (panel a2), increasing the number of MCMC iterations to 5,000 makes it clearer that this is an acceptable MCMC run. The plot shown in Fig. 7.2 (panel b) also shows that the burn-in should have a minimum of about 200 MCMC iterations.

ACF Plots. The ACF plot for the sample data appears in Fig. 7.2 (panel c). The plot shows that the autocorrelation for this parameter drops below the significance line at a lag of around 35. This plot verifies that writing out an imputed data set after every 70 MCMC iterations is reasonable for these data.

The diagnostic plots in PROC MI are a little less convenient to examine than are the plots produced by NORM. But they are good, readable plots. Wending your way through the plots may be a bit tedious (in PROC MI or NORM), but it is usually just a one-time job when you impute. Making use of the WLF does give you a sense of the worst it can get, but in my experience, it is better to take the time to examine the plots of individual parameters. Once you have gained experience with a particular set of variables, it is not necessary to keep examining the plots. And, you are often able to focus on the parameters that are likely to create the most problems. Also, in viewing the plots, it is not necessary to stare at each plot. You can move through them quickly and still comprehend all you need in a relatively short amount of time.

## Direct Analysis of EM (MLE) Covariance Matrix with PROC FACTOR, PROC REG

One of the beauties of working with SAS is that it is possible to estimate an EM (MLE) covariance matrix with PROC MI, and then analyze that matrix directly with other SAS PROCs such as PROC FACTOR, and to an extent PROC REG.

### *PROC FACTOR with an EM Covariance Matrix as Input*

I do not intend this to be a tutorial in performing exploratory factor analysis with PROC FACTOR. Mainly I want to familiarize you with the syntax for performing this very useful analysis. Here is the syntax:

```
proc mi data=a nimpute=0;
    em outem=b;
      var
      alc7 alc8 alc9
      riskreb71-riskreb74
      likepar71-likepar75
      posatt71-posatt73
      riskreb81-riskreb84;
run;
```

```
proc factor data=b(type=cov) method=prin rotate=promax
   round reorder;
   var
     riskreb71-riskreb74
     likepar71-likepar75
     posatt71-posatt73
     riskreb81-riskreb84;
run;
```

## PROC REG with an EM Covariance Matrix as Input

Before I present the material in this section, let me explain that I do NOT recommend that the EM covariance matrix be used directly for the regression analysis. In this book, I have said repeatedly that the EM covariance cannot be used for hypothesis testing. My use of PROC REG with an EM covariance matrix is a special case and does NOT involve hypothesis testing.

One of the most frequently asked questions I get is:
How do I estimate the $R^2$ in multiple regression with multiple imputation?

And the related question:
How do I get standardized regression coefficients with multiple imputation?

I have two answers to both of these questions. First, the $R^2$ and standardized regression coefficients are parameter estimates. So one can certainly use multiple imputation to estimate them. The biggest problem with that approach, however, is that these two parameter estimates typically do not have associated standard errors. Thus, one must fiddle with the multiple imputation solution in order to get it to work. Or one must use some other way to calculate the mean of these quantities over the $m$ imputed data sets.

But a much easier and completely acceptable alternative is available. Simply perform a single multiple regression analysis with the EM covariance matrix as input. Because researchers typically use the $R^2$ and standardized regression coefficients without significance tests, all one is really interested in here are the parameter estimates themselves. And, we know that EM produces excellent parameter estimates.

I do not intend this to be a tutorial on performing multiple regression analysis, so I am presenting this section mainly to familiarize you with the syntax necessary to carry out this analysis. So here is one, very simple, multiple regression analysis with the EM covariance matrix as input.

```
proc mi data=a nimpute=0;
   em outem=b;
     var
     alc7 alc8 alc9
     riskreb71-riskreb74
     likepar71-likepar75
     posatt71-posatt73
     riskreb81-riskreb84;
run;
proc reg data=b(type=cov);
   model alc9=alc7 riskreb71 likepar72 posatt72/stb;
run;
```

The standardized regression coefficients and $R^2$ from this analysis may be placed directly into your article. Usually this information would be used in conjunction with regular MI (see below) for the main hypothesis tests.

## Analysis of Single Data Set Imputed from EM Parameters with PROC CORR ALPHA

Again, in this section, my goal is not to provide a tutorial for performing coefficient alpha analysis. I simply wish to acquaint you with this strategy for performing these analyses with missing data, using the single data set imputed from EM parameters input for the analysis.

In the code that follows, by using NBITER = 0, and NITER = 0, and NIMPUTE = 1, I am asking that the one data set be imputed from the starting values provided to MCMC. Those starting values are the EM (posterior mode) estimates. Although they are not identical to the EM (MLE) estimates, they are very close. I believe this to be an excellent option for performing this analysis.

```
proc mi data=a nimpute=1 out=b;
   mcmc nbiter=0 niter=0;
       var
       alc7 alc8 alc9
       riskreb71-riskreb74
       likepar71-likepar75
       posatt71-posatt73
       riskreb81-riskreb84;
proc corr data=b alpha;var riskreb71-riskreb74;
proc corr data=b alpha;var likepar71-likepar75;
proc corr data=b alpha;var posatt71-posatt73;
proc corr data=b alpha;var riskreb81-riskreb84;
run;

proc corr data=b;var alc7 alc8 alc9;
run;
```

The last PROC CORR statement was included in the syntax above simply to illustrate that this approach may also be used to examine the test-retest correlation between two scales. Note that in all of these analyses, all correlations are conditioned on all 19 variables included in the PROC MI analysis, even though only a few of those variables are included in each PROC CORR analysis.

## Analysis of Multiple-Imputed Data with PROC REG, PROC LOGISTIC, PROC MIXED

One of the real joys of doing multiple imputation with PROC MI is that once the data have been imputed (successfully), it is an easy matter to perform analyses with procedures like PROC REG, PROC LOGISTIC, and PROC MIXED.

### Analysis of Multiple-Imputed Data with PROC REG

Analysis of multiple-imputed data sets with PROC REG is exceptionally easy. Below is the syntax for the PROC MI, PROC REG, and PROC MIANALYZE. Given that this is the first time PROC MIANALYZE has been discussed, let me say that this is the program with which the saved results from the PROC REG analysis are combined using Rubin's Rules for MI inference.

```
proc mi data=a nimpute=40 out=b;
    mcmc nbiter=200 niter=70 acfplot(cov mean wlf/nlag=150)
        timeplot(cov mean wlf);
    var
    alc7 alc8 alc9
    riskreb71-riskreb74
    likepar71-likepar75
    posatt71-posatt73
    riskreb81-riskreb84;

proc reg data=b outest=c covout noprint;
    model alc9=alc7 riskreb71 likepar72 posatt72;
    by _imputation_;
run;

proc mianalyze data=c;
    modeleffects intercept alc7 riskreb71 likepar72
    posatt72;
run;
```

Let me go through the syntax for the PROC REG statement. The DATA=B option specifies which data set will be read into PROC REG. DATA=B is the default in this case, but I find it useful to be explicit about this. With complicated or repetitive code, it is sometimes possible to read in the wrong data set.

OUTEST=C is the option that writes the parameter estimates from PROC REG out to a SAS file named "C". The "BY _IMPUTATION_" statement tells SAS to perform the PROC REG and the writing out of results separately for each of the $m=40$ imputed data sets. The COVOUT option specifies that the covariance matrix of the estimates be output along with the parameter estimates, for each of the $m=40$ imputations. The main diagonal of this matrix is the variance of the estimates. The square roots of these variances are the standard errors of the estimates.

As an exercise, specify PROC PRINT;RUN; immediately after the RUN; statement for PROC REG. This will help you see the organization of the SAS data set containing the results of PROC REG for each of the $m=40$ imputed data sets. It is:

1. Parameter estimates for imputation 1
2. Covariance matrix of estimates for imputation 1
3. Parameter estimates for imputation 2
4. Covariance matrix of estimates for imputation 2 and so on

The NOPRINT option with PROC REG suppresses the output for the individual PROC REG analyses. I find this useful because (a) there is typically too much output, and (b) examining that output almost always leads people to make incorrect inferences about their data. Remember, it is not the individual imputed values or the results from the individual imputed data sets that are important. It is the combined results. Thus, I encourage you to ignore the individual results and focus on the combined results.

The syntax for PROC MIANALYZE is also given above. I am generally explicit in specifying the input data set, but PROC MIANALYZE generally follows immediately after the relevant PROC statement, and the default data set will almost always be the correct one. The MODELEFFECTS statement replaces the VAR statement from the earlier versions of PROC MI. The "INTERCEPT" may be specified as one of the MODELEFFECTS. In this version of SAS, the variable "INTERCEPT" has all its letters (version 8.2 did not include the last "T" in order to keep the variable name to eight characters). If you forget what it is called, run the PROC PRINT I described just above.

## *PROC MIANALYZE Output for PROC REG*

Table 7.7 presents the results of PROC MIANALYZE produced from the code given just above. This output is based on the PROC REG analysis of 40 imputed data sets. The presentation of the results in MIANALYZE is a little unfortunate in that it does not bear much resemblance to the output from PROC REG or the other PROCs. Still, all the relevant information is there, and you will grow accustomed to reading it. Note that the output from PROC MIANALYZE is a little more readable if you specify a long output line length (e.g., OPTIONS LS=120, or OPTIONS LS=255).

**Table 7.7** PROC MIANALYZE: output from PROC REG

```
Formatted with OPTIONS LS=80
```

The MIANALYZE Procedure

Model Information

| Data Set | WORK.C |
|---|---|
| Number of Imputations | 40 |

Variance Information

| Parameter | Between | Within | Total | DF |
|---|---|---|---|---|
| intercept | 0.052060 | 0.028638 | 0.081999 | 92.093 |
| alc7 | 0.000290 | 0.000471 | 0.000768 | 260.77 |
| riskreb71 | 0.003102 | 0.002159 | 0.005338 | 109.94 |
| likepar72 | 0.001754 | 0.001198 | 0.002995 | 108.31 |
| posatt72 | 0.004029 | 0.002386 | 0.006516 | 97.069 |

Variance Information

| Parameter | Relative Increase in Variance | Fraction Missing Information | Relative Efficiency |
|---|---|---|---|
| Intercept | 1.863328 | 0.658101 | 0.983814 |
| alc7 | 0.630601 | 0.391379 | 0.990310 |
| riskreb71 | 1.472799 | 0.602761 | 0.985155 |
| likepar72 | 1.500476 | 0.607262 | 0.985045 |
| posatt72 | 1.731175 | 0.641175 | 0.984224 |

Parameter Estimates

| Parameter | Estimate | Std Error | 95% Confidence Limits | | DF |
|---|---|---|---|---|---|
| Intercept | 2.908503 | 0.286355 | 2.33979 | 3.47722 | 92.093 |
| alc7 | 0.607158 | 0.027707 | 0.55260 | 0.66172 | 260.77 |
| riskreb71 | 0.143061 | 0.073065 | -0.00174 | 0.28786 | 109.94 |
| likepar72 | -0.214834 | 0.054731 | -0.32332 | -0.10635 | 108.31 |
| posatt72 | 0.103754 | 0.080721 | -0.05645 | 0.26396 | 97.069 |

Parameter Estimates

| Parameter | Minimum | Maximum |
|---|---|---|
| Intercept | 2.419720 | 3.310048 |
| alc7 | 0.556408 | 0.633649 |
| riskreb71 | 0.030990 | 0.243192 |
| likepar72 | -0.285737 | -0.117881 |
| posatt72 | -0.032115 | 0.260663 |

Parameter Estimates

| Parameter | Theta0 | t for H0: Parameter = Theta0 | Pr > \|t\| |
|---|---|---|---|
| Intercept | 0 | 10.16 | <.0001 |
| alc7 | 0 | 21.91 | <.0001 |
| riskreb71 | 0 | 1.96 | 0.0528 |
| likepar72 | 0 | -3.93 | 0.0002 |
| posatt72 | 0 | 1.29 | 0.2017 |

**Table 7.8** Reformatted MI output

| Parameter | EST | SE | t | df | % mis inf | p |
|---|---|---|---|---|---|---|
| intercept | 2.909 | 0.2864 | 10.16 | 92 | 65.8 | .0000 |
| alc7 | 0.607 | 0.0277 | 21.91 | 260 | 39.1 | .0000 |
| rebel71 | 0.143 | 0.0731 | 1.96 | 109 | 60.3 | .0528 |
| likpar72 | -0.215 | 0.0547 | -3.93 | 108 | 60.7 | .0002 |
| posatt72 | 0.104 | 0.0807 | 1.29 | 97 | 64.1 | .2017 |

All of the relevant information is there in the output. When I do PROC REG with MI, however, I tend to focus on a few bits of information. And, to help me focus on the key results, I prefer to reformat the results every time I do this analysis. For example, I would reformat these results to what is shown in Table 7.8.

For me, the key information is the parameter estimate, its standard error (based on Rubin's rules), and the *t*-value (estimate divided by its standard error). And at the far right, the *p*-value. The DF and %MisInf, or fraction of missing information (FMI), are two quantities that are peculiar to multiple imputation.

## Fraction of Missing Information

The FMI, as discussed in Chap. 2, is related to the simple percent of missing data. But it is adjusted (downward) by the presence of other variables that are highly correlated with the variables with missing data. Remember that what appears in the output is just an estimate of the FMI; the estimate becomes stable only with a large number of imputations. Even with $m=40$ imputations, there can still be considerable "wobble" in the FMI estimate.

## Multiple Imputation Degrees of Freedom

As described in Chap. 2, DF has unique meaning in multiple imputation. It is not related to the sample size, as in the common complete cases analysis. I like to think of it as an indicator of the stability of the estimates. When DF is low (the minimum is $m-1$), it indicates that $m$ was too low, and that the parameter estimates remain unstable. When DF is high (substantially higher than $m$), it is an indicator that the estimation has stabilized. The bottom line is that whenever the DF is only marginally higher than $m$, it is an indicator that more imputations are needed.

## Proc Reg with Multiple Dependent Variables

The code described above for using PROC REG with multiple implementation works only with one dependent variable at a time, even though PROC REG itself works well with multiple dependent variables. A simple trick allows you to use PROC REG with two or more dependent variables at the same time. The trick is to sort the output data set by the dependent variable and to use BY processing with PROC MIANALYZE. The code assumes that you have already run PROC MI and that you have specified the output stacked data set with OUT=B. These differences between this code and the previous code for one dependent variable are highlighted in bold print.

```
proc reg data=b outest=c covout noprint;
     model alc8 alc9=alc7 riskreb71 likepar72 posatt72;
     by _imputation_;
run;
```

**proc sort;by _depvar_;run;**

```
proc mianalyze data=c;
     modeleffects intercept alc7 riskreb71 likepar72
     posatt72;
```
**by _depvar_;**
```
run;
```

The output for this analysis appear in Table 7.9 (for Dependent Variable=Alc8 only). In this analysis, I examined the effects alc7, riskreb71, likepar72, and posatt72 on alcohol use at eighth (alc8) and ninth (alc9) grades. A nice by-product of inserting the PROC SORT statement between the PROC REG and PROC MIANALYZE statements is that the dependent variable is listed at the top of each output page (something that does not happen normally). So I usually like to make use of this "trick" even when dealing with just one dependent variable at a time.

Note that this analysis shows that all three seventh grade predictors (risk-taking/rebelliousness, liking for parents, and beliefs about the positive consequences of alcohol use) were significant predictors of eighth grade alcohol use (alc8) after controlling for seventh grade alcohol use (alc7).

**Table 7.9** PROC MIANALYZE output sorted by _depvar_

**Dependent variable=alc8**

The MIANALYZE Procedure

Model Information

| Data Set | WORK.C |
|---|---|
| Number of Imputations | 40 |

### Variance Information

| Parameter | Between | Within | Total | DF |
|---|---|---|---|---|
| Intercept | 0.014139 | 0.021589 | 0.036082 | 241.73 |
| alc7 | 0.000110 | 0.000351 | 0.000464 | 664.88 |
| riskreb71 | 0.001101 | 0.001622 | 0.002751 | 231.53 |
| likepar72 | 0.000616 | 0.000897 | 0.001528 | 228.39 |
| posatt72 | 0.002107 | 0.001788 | 0.003948 | 130.27 |

### Variance Information

| Parameter | Relative Increase in Variance | Fraction Missing Information | Relative Efficiency |
|---|---|---|---|
| Intercept | 0.671317 | 0.406559 | 0.989938 |
| alc7 | 0.319595 | 0.244461 | 0.993926 |
| riskreb71 | 0.696125 | 0.415449 | 0.989721 |
| likepar72 | 0.704246 | 0.418302 | 0.989651 |
| posatt72 | 1.208283 | 0.553955 | 0.986340 |

### Parameter Estimates

| Parameter | Estimate | Std Error | 95% Confidence Limits | | DF |
|---|---|---|---|---|---|
| Intercept | 1.371896 | 0.189952 | 0.99772 | 1.74607 | 241.73 |
| alc7 | 0.676670 | 0.021534 | 0.63439 | 0.71895 | 664.88 |
| riskreb71 | 0.193980 | 0.052447 | 0.09064 | 0.29731 | 231.53 |
| likepar72 | -0.108091 | 0.039093 | -0.18512 | -0.03106 | 228.39 |
| posatt72 | 0.227718 | 0.062832 | 0.10342 | 0.35202 | 130.27 |

### Parameter Estimates

| Parameter | Minimum | Maximum |
|---|---|---|
| Intercept | 1.106418 | 1.565042 |
| alc7 | 0.655318 | 0.698939 |
| riskreb71 | 0.123783 | 0.245823 |

**Dependent variable=alc8**

The MIANALYZE Procedure

### Parameter Estimates

| Parameter | Minimum | Maximum |
|---|---|---|
| likepar72 | -0.159370 | -0.055149 |
| posatt72 | 0.116454 | 0.308355 |

### Parameter Estimates

| Parameter | Theta 0 | t for H0: Parameter = Theta 0 | Pr > \|t\| |
|---|---|---|---|
| Intercept | 0 | 7.22 | <.0001 |
| alc7 | 0 | 31.42 | <.0001 |
| riskreb71 | 0 | 3.70 | 0.0003 |
| likepar72 | 0 | -2.76 | 0.0062 |
| posatt72 | 0 | 3.62 | 0.0004 |

## Analysis of Multiple-Imputed Data with PROC LOGISTIC

The syntax for performing logistic regression with PROC LOGISTIC is virtually the same as that used for PROC REG.

```
proc mi data=a nimpute=40 simple out=b;
   mcmc nbiter=200 niter=70 ;
     var
       alc7 alc8 alc9
       riskreb71-riskreb74
       likepar71-likepar75
       posatt71-posatt73
       riskreb81-riskreb84;
run;

data b2;set b;
*** ====================================================== ***;
*** create a meaningful dichotomous version of alc9 variable
*** for use with logistic regression ***
*** I am not recommending this dichotomizing procedure in
    general.
*** I am simply using it for this example.;
*** ====================================================== ***;
   if -100<alc9<=2 then xalc9=0;
     else if alc9>2 then xalc9=1;
run;

proc logistic data=b2 outest=c covout;
   model xalc9 (event='1')=alc7 riskreb71 likepar72 posatt72;
   by _imputation_;
run;

proc print;run;

proc mianalyze data=c;
   modeleffects intercept alc7 riskreb71 likepar72 posatt72;
run;
```

The PROC MIANALYZE output from these statements, which appears in Table 7.10, is laid out exactly as it was for PROC REG.

Differences in these results from the PROC REG analysis shown with the same data could stem from two sources. First, of course, the two analyses are different, and the dependent variable itself was dichotomized for PROC LOGISTIC for illustrative purposes. Second, because I imputed $m=40$ data sets twice, there would naturally be a little imputation wobble (slightly different results even if the same analysis were used, e.g., see the differences in results displayed in Tables 4.2 and 4.3).

**Table 7.10** PROC MIANALYZE: output from PROC LOGISTIC

```
The MIANALYZE Procedure
          Model Information
Data Set           WORK.C
Number of          40
  Imputations
```

Multiple Imputation Variance Information

| Parameter | Between | Within | Total | DF |
|---|---|---|---|---|
| Intercept | 0.052228 | 0.055363 | 0.108896 | 161.38 |
| alc7 | 0.001136 | 0.002236 | 0.003400 | 332.48 |
| riskreb71 | 0.003106 | 0.004301 | 0.007485 | 215.53 |
| likepar72 | 0.002190 | 0.002184 | 0.004428 | 151.82 |
| posatt72 | 0.005125 | 0.005153 | 0.010407 | 153.03 |

Multiple Imputation Variance Information

| Parameter | Relative Increase in Variance | Fraction Missing Information | Relative Efficiency |
|---|---|---|---|
| Intercept | 0.966958 | 0.497787 | 0.987708 |
| alc7 | 0.520896 | 0.346413 | 0.991414 |
| riskreb71 | 0.740273 | 0.430636 | 0.989349 |
| likepar72 | 1.027715 | 0.513205 | 0.987332 |
| posatt72 | 1.019494 | 0.511174 | 0.987382 |

Multiple Imputation Parameter Estimates

| Parameter | Estimate | Std Error | 95% Confidence Limits | | DF |
|---|---|---|---|---|---|
| Intercept | 0.298351 | 0.329994 | -0.35331 | 0.95001 | 161.38 |
| alc7 | 0.689592 | 0.058313 | 0.57488 | 0.80430 | 332.48 |
| riskreb71 | 0.087063 | 0.086518 | -0.08347 | 0.25759 | 215.53 |
| likepar72 | -0.191643 | 0.066547 | -0.32312 | -0.06017 | 151.82 |
| posatt72 | 0.025475 | 0.102013 | -0.17606 | 0.22701 | 153.03 |

Multiple Imputation Parameter Estimates

| Parameter | Minimum | Maximum |
|---|---|---|
| Intercept | -0.121228 | 0.668341 |
| alc7 | 0.615055 | 0.758255 |
| riskreb71 | -0.060911 | 0.194486 |
| likepar72 | -0.264078 | -0.085495 |
| posatt72 | -0.161954 | 0.196999 |

Multiple Imputation Parameter Estimates

| Parameter | Theta 0 | t for H0: Parameter = Theta 0 | Pr > \|t\| |
|---|---|---|---|
| Intercept | 0 | 0.90 | 0.3673 |
| alc7 | 0 | 11.83 | <.0001 |
| riskreb71 | 0 | 1.01 | 0.3154 |
| likepar72 | 0 | -2.88 | 0.0046 |
| posatt72 | 0 | 0.25 | 0.8031 |

## Analysis of Multiple-Imputed Data with PROC MIXED

Before tackling analysis with PROC MIXED, I want to talk about some special challenges that arise for MI with cluster data (please see my discussion of this issue in Chap. 6). In previous written work, I have suggested that multilevel data could be handled with normal-model MI simply by dummy-coding cluster membership, as illustrated below, and including the dummy variables in the MI analysis. I have argued that including these dummy variables in the MI model allows the cluster means to be different during imputation, thus yielding unbiased estimates of the cluster means. I have argued that this model is equivalent to the random intercepts model. Indeed, ignoring cluster membership during MI is the same as imputing under the model that the means are all the same across clusters, and this is known to produce an intraclass correlation (ICC) that is too small.

Very recent work by Andridge (2011), however, has shown that this dummy-coding strategy overcompensates for cluster structure. Although she verified that ignoring cluster structure produces ICCs that are too small, Andridge also showed that including cluster membership dummy variables in the normal-model MI analysis produces an artificially high ICC. The explanation for this latter effect is that including the dummy variable represents a fixed effect for cluster in the multilevel imputation model. However, in the corresponding multilevel analysis model, the effect for cluster is a *random* effect. In short, including the dummy variables in the normal-model MI analysis has the effect of increasing the between-cluster variance, thereby producing an inflated ICC.

The best solution to this problem is to use the PAN program (Schafer 2001; Schafer and Yucel 2002) for performing the MI analysis (Andridge 2011; also see my discussion in Chap. 6). The PAN program allows the cluster to be included in the model as a random effect, thereby providing better estimates of the ICC. A potentially excellent new option in this context for SAS users is a PAN-like SAS macro being developed by Enders and colleagues (e.g., Mistler and Enders 2011). The early versions of this macro suggest that this is an excellent product that will be of enormous benefit to SAS users.

For the time being, PAN remains the best option. However, PAN, which is a program that must be executed from within the R package is not nearly as accessible as normal-model MI. In Chap. 6, I suggested that there is a compromise that can be used with normal-model MI. Ignoring cluster structure is known to produce ICCs that are too small, and including the dummy variables to represent cluster membership is now known to produce ICCs that are too large. So my compromise is to impute half the time under each model, thereby producing ICCs that are between these two extremes. Although this hybrid dummy variable strategy not as good as using PAN or other PAN-like programs, it will provide ICCs that are much closer to true ICCs than using the dummy-coding strategy alone. Also, my preliminary simulation work suggests that this hybrid dummy-coding strategy still produces ICCs that are a little too large. Thus with cluster randomized trials, program effects analyses will yield results that are somewhat too conservative. I illustrate the use of this hybrid dummy-coding strategy below with an empirical example.

▶ **Sample Data.** In the sample data, ex7.sas7bdat, the variable School, takes on 12 values (1–12). This sample data set is taken from the AAPT study (Hansen and Graham 1991). The participants were seventh graders at the first wave (when they received the program). These sample data involve seventh, eighth, and ninth grade data from this cohort. Listed below are the variables on the data set, along with brief descriptions.

| | |
|---|---|
| school | school membership (schools 1–12) |
| program | received program=1; control=0 |
| alc7 | alcohol use in seventh grade |
| riskreb7 | risk-taking/rebelliousness in seventh grade |
| likepar7 | relationship with parents in seventh grade |
| posatt7 | positive alcohol expectancies in seventh grade |
| alc8 | alcohol use in eighth grade |
| riskreb8 | risk-taking/rebelliousness in eighth grade |
| alc9 | alcohol use in ninth grade |

In order to generate the 11 dummy variables for inclusion into PROC MI, I did the following:

```
Data a;set in.ex7;
    if school=1 then do;s1=1;s2=0;s3=0;s4=0;s5=0;s6=0;s7=0;s
    8=0;s9=0;s10=0;s11=0;end;
    if school=2 then do;s1=0;s2=1;s3=0;s4=0;s5=0;s6=0;s7=0;s
    8=0;s9=0;s10=0;s11=0;end;
    if school=3 then do;s1=0;s2=0;s3=1;s4=0;s5=0;s6=0;s7=0;s
    8=0;s9=0;s10=0;s11=0;end;
    if school=4 then do;s1=0;s2=0;s3=0;s4=1;s5=0;s6=0;s7=0;s
    8=0;s9=0;s10=0;s11=0;end;
    if school=5 then do;s1=0;s2=0;s3=0;s4=0;s5=1;s6=0;s7=0;s
    8=0;s9=0;s10=0;s11=0;end;
    if school=6 then do;s1=0;s2=0;s3=0;s4=0;s5=0;s6=1;s7=0;s
    8=0;s9=0;s10=0;s11=0;end;
    if school=7 then do;s1=0;s2=0;s3=0;s4=0;s5=0;s6=0;s7=1;s
    8=0;s9=0;s10=0;s11=0;end;
    if school=8 then do;s1=0;s2=0;s3=0;s4=0;s5=0;s6=0;s7=0;s
    8=1;s9=0;s10=0;s11=0;end;
    if school=9 then do;s1=0;s2=0;s3=0;s4=0;s5=0;s6=0;s7=0;s
    8=0;s9=1;s10=0;s11=0;end;
    if school=10 then do;s1=0;s2=0;s3=0;s4=0;s5=0;s6=0;s7=0;
    s8=0;s9=0;s10=1;s11=0;end;
    if school=11 then do;s1=0;s2=0;s3=0;s4=0;s5=0;s6=0;s7=0;
    s8=0;s9=0;s10=0;s11=1;end;
    if school=12 then do;s1=0;s2=0;s3=0;s4=0;s5=0;s6=0;s7=0;
    s8=0;s9=0;s10=0;s11=0;end;
run;
```

To produce 40 imputed data sets using the hybrid dummy-coding strategy, I first generated 20 imputed data sets using each model (with and without dummy variables). I then added 20 to the variable _imputation_ in the second imputed data set and stacked the two sets of imputed data sets together using the SET command:

```
proc mi data=a nimpute=20 out=b1;
    em itprint converge=1e-5;
    mcmc nbiter=200 niter=50 initial=em(converge=1e-5);
    var alc7 riskreb7 likepar7 posatt7 alc8 riskreb8 alc9
    s1-s11;
run;
proc mi data=a nimpute=20 out=b2;
    em itprint converge=1e-5;
    mcmc nbiter=200 niter=50 initial=em(converge=1e-5);
    var program alc7 riskreb7 likepar7 posatt7 alc8
    riskreb8 alc9;
run;
data b2x;set b2;
    _imputation_=_imputation_+20;
run;
data b;set b1 b2x;
run;
```

**Notes**

With the EM convergence criterion set to 1E-5, EM converged in 39 iterations for the first analysis and in 37 iterations for the second analysis. Thus, setting mcmc niter=50 in both analyses was a conservative number. Note that the variable "program" was omitted from the first analysis (which contained the dummy variables representing school), and that "program" was included in the second analysis that omitted the dummy variables.

The syntax with PROC MIXED is a little different from the previous analyses. I do not pretend to be an expert with MIXED models, but I have had good luck with this one for taking the multilevel (cluster) structure of my data (e.g., students within schools) into account. The model I have used for this is a random intercepts model (i.e., allowing intercepts, but not slopes to vary across schools).

```
proc mixed noclprint covtest;
   class school;
   model alc9=program alc7 riskreb71 likepar71 posatt71 /
   solution ddfm=bw;
   random intercept /sub=school;
   by _imputation_;
   ods output SolutionF=mixparms CovParms=mixparmsR;
run;

proc mianalyze parms=mixparms;
   modeleffects intercept program alc7 riskreb71 likepar71
   posatt71;
run;
```

The output for this analysis is presented in Table 7.11.

Not surprisingly, the MIANALYZE output based on PROC MIXED is the same as with the other two programs. Note that the final results are very similar to the results obtained from PROC REG. The differences that did appear between PROC MIXED and PROC REG could be due to the differences in the analysis; but they could also be due simply to imputation wobble, that is, to minor differences in results that are found between two sets of imputed data sets. As I have point out previously (e.g., please see the discussion of this topic in Chap. 4), those differences tend to be small, especially when the number of imputations is reasonably large. I used $m=40$ imputations in these examples, so I expect the differences in results based on different sets of imputed data sets to be tolerably small.

**Table 7.11** PROC MIANALYZE: output from PROC MIXED

The MIANALYZE Procedure

Model Information

PARMS Data Set   WORK.MIXPARMS
Number of        40
  Imputations

Variance Information

| Parameter | Between | Within | Total | DF |
|---|---|---|---|---|
| intercept | 0.064584 | 0.043222 | 0.109420 | 106.55 |
| program | 0.003076 | 0.013270 | 0.016423 | 1058.3 |
| alc7 | 0.000303 | 0.000415 | 0.000725 | 212.64 |
| riskreb7 | 0.003619 | 0.002084 | 0.005794 | 95.124 |
| likepar7 | 0.004439 | 0.002310 | 0.006860 | 88.647 |
| posatt7 | 0.002145 | 0.001675 | 0.003874 | 121.06 |

(continued)

### Analysis of Multiple-Imputed Data with PROC REG, PROC LOGISTIC, PROC MIXED    189

**Table 7.11** (continued)

The MIANALYZE Procedure

Variance Information

| Parameter | Relative Increase in Variance | Fraction Missing Information | Relative Efficiency |
|---|---|---|---|
| intercept | 1.531589 | 0.612202 | 0.984926 |
| program | 0.237574 | 0.193490 | 0.995186 |
| alc7 | 0.749066 | 0.433569 | 0.989277 |
| riskreb7 | 1.780149 | 0.647638 | 0.984067 |
| likepar7 | 1.969869 | 0.670633 | 0.983511 |
| posatt7 | 1.312545 | 0.574547 | 0.985840 |

Parameter Estimates

| Parameter | Estimate | Std Error | 95% Confidence Limits | | DF |
|---|---|---|---|---|---|
| intercept | 3.241134 | 0.330787 | 2.58536 | 3.89691 | 106.55 |
| program | -0.443729 | 0.128151 | -0.69519 | -0.19227 | 1058.3 |
| alc7 | 0.626909 | 0.026927 | 0.57383 | 0.67999 | 212.64 |
| riskreb7 | 0.188625 | 0.076115 | 0.03752 | 0.33973 | 95.124 |
| likepar7 | -0.286244 | 0.082826 | -0.45083 | -0.12166 | 88.647 |
| posatt7 | 0.010754 | 0.062241 | -0.11247 | 0.13398 | 121.06 |

Parameter Estimates

| Parameter | Minimum | Maximum |
|---|---|---|
| intercept | 2.718170 | 3.825570 |
| program | -0.574173 | -0.353057 |
| alc7 | 0.596191 | 0.668577 |
| riskreb7 | 0.066776 | 0.332532 |
| likepar7 | -0.433510 | -0.143740 |
| posatt7 | -0.094267 | 0.087881 |

Parameter Estimates

| Parameter | Theta 0 | t for H0: Parameter = Theta 0 | Pr > \|t\| |
|---|---|---|---|
| Intercept | 0 | 9.80 | <.0001 |
| Program | 0 | -3.46 | 0.0006 |
| alc7 | 0 | 23.28 | <.0001 |
| riskreb7 | 0 | 2.48 | 0.0150 |
| likepar7 | 0 | -3.46 | 0.0008 |
| posatt7 | 0 | 0.17 | 0.8631 |

It is not clear that this is the correct DF for the level-2 predictor, Program. It could be that the appropriate DF = 10 for this predictor (e.g., Barnard and Rubin 1999)

# References

Andridge, R. R. (2011). Quantifying the impact of fixed effects modeling of clusters in multiple imputation for cluster randomized trials. *Biometrical Journal, 53*, 57–74.

Barnard, J., and Rubin, D. B. (1999). Small-sample degrees of freedom with multiple imputation. *Biometrika, 86*, 948–955.

Hansen, W. B., & Graham, J. W. (1991). Preventing alcohol, marijuana, and cigarette use among adolescents: Peer pressure resistance training versus establishing conservative norms. *Preventive Medicine, 20*, 414–430.

Graham, J. W., & Donaldson, S. I. (1993). Evaluating interventions with differential attrition: The importance of nonresponse mechanisms and use of followup data. *Journal of Applied Psychology, 78*, 119–128.

Graham, J. W., & Hofer, S. M. (1992). *EMCOV Users Guide*. Unpublished Manuscript, University of Southern California.

Mistler, S. A., and Enders, C. K. (2011). Applying multiple imputation to multilevel data sets: A practical guide. Paper presented at the Annual Convention of the American Psychological Association, Washington, DC, August 6, 2011.

Price, B. (1977). Ridge regression: Application to nonexperimental data. *Psychological Bulletin, 84*, 759–766.

Schafer, J. L. (1997). *Analysis of Incomplete Multivariate Data*. New York: Chapman and Hall.

Schafer, J. L. (2001). Multiple imputation with PAN. In L. M. Collins & A. G. Sayer (Eds.), *New methods for the analysis of change* (pp. 357–377). Washington, DC: American Psychological Association.

Schafer, J. L., & Yucel, R. M. (2002). Computational strategies for multivariate linear mixed-effects models with missing values. *Journal of Computational and Graphical Statistics, 11*, 437–457.

# Section 3
# Practical Issues in Missing Data Analysis

# Chapter 8
# Practical Issues Relating to Analysis with Missing Data: Avoiding and Troubleshooting Problems

If you follow the advice I have given in previous chapters, the chances are good that the results of your multiple imputation and analysis will be good. However, unforeseen things happen. Also, if you happen to be helping another person with these analyses, the material in this chapter will give some strategies for working through the problems.

When you have problems with the missing data analysis, the root problem is most likely in your data. In this chapter, I talk about several kinds of problems that you may face, and I talk about some strategies you can employ, at different stages of the research, to help with the problem. I cannot guarantee that my strategies will always work, but I have found them to be useful in solving a wide variety of problems in MI analysis.

One idea that came out in the early days of missing data analysis was the "impute once, analyze many times" strategy. The idea was that if the analyst could get, say, 50 different analyses out of one multiple imputation analysis, then any tedium involved could be spread over the "life" of the imputed data set, and would therefore be lessened. Unfortunately, this thinking can lead analysts to believe that throwing everything into the MI model is an acceptable thing to do. I sometimes refer to this as the "kitchen sink" approach to MI.

Although this approach might work in theory, the practicalities of such an analysis virtually always make it infeasible (for reasons I describe below in this chapter and in the next chapter). It is for this reason that I have taken the opposite stance in my own work and in this book. I take the "impute once, analyze once" approach (although it does often work out that one can perform several analyses based on a single imputation). As the software options (as with the current version of Proc MI in SAS) become more automated, the "impute once, analyze once" approach will be an obvious solution to one's missing data problems.

## Strategies for Making It Work: Know Your Analysis

Often one of the first questions I ask of people wanting to do missing data analysis is: What analysis are you planning? What would you be doing if you had no missing data? I often find that a big problem with missing data analysis stems from the fact that the people do not have ready answers to these questions.

So an important point about understanding missing data analysis is to know your analysis. Think through what hypothesis you want to test. Maybe even try it out first with complete cases analysis. Although this is not always a good strategy (e.g., when the complete cases N is small compared to the total N), I often find that doing an analysis helps me think through the wisdom of the analysis. Once you are very clear about the analysis you want and need, solving the missing data part of the problem becomes much more straightforward.

## Strategies for Making It Work: Know Your Data

Once you know what analysis you want, the next thing to be clear about is your data. First, rule out simple problems. For example, verify that no variable you are using is a constant in the sample you are using. Also, take care of mundane issues. For example, be sure that the missing data indicator you are using is appropriate for your analysis. If you are using PROC MI, missing values should be represented by the system missing indicator in SAS, that is, by a period, ".". On the other hand, if you will be imputing with an outside program such as NORM, then the missing value indicator needs to be something numeric (e.g., −9), and the system missing indicator will be improper. Finally, along these same lines, sometimes missing values appear as a blank space. That can create all kinds of problems for MI programs.

Once the more mundane issues have been dealt with, determine what variables are relevant – from the *analysis* perspective? For example, if you were planning a multiple regression analysis, you may need to form scales out of individual items prior to the analysis. Should scales be formed before or after imputation? What background or demographic variables will be included in the analysis, for example, as covariates? Do any of these variables, which are often categorical, need to be transformed into dummy variables prior to the analysis?

When you have identified and dealt with (e.g., transformed) all of the variables that will be in your analysis model, why would you need any additional variables in the imputation model? That is, what variables are relevant from a ***missing data*** perspective?

## *Causes of Missingness*

The first answer is that you may want to include the cause(s) of missingness in the missing data model. In the early days following the missing data revolution, there was a lot of confusion about the necessity of including these variables in the model. Many people (including me) did simulations to show that omitting the cause of missingness produced estimation bias. These people (including me) concluded that it was therefore critical to include the cause(s) of missingness in the missing data model. My early writings were replete with statements such as these:

> When data are missing, work hard to find the cause of missingness and include the cause in the analysis model. When planning a study, think about what the causes of missingness are likely to be and obtain measures for as many causes as possible (Graham et al. 1994).

Although I believe it is still good advice to think about the causes of missingness and to include measures of such variables where possible, our implying that there was a dire need to do so rather substantially overstated the case, and said more about our misunderstanding of the processes involved than about the true need.

Recent work, most notably Collins et al. (2001; also see my discussion in Chaps. 1 and 10), has shown rather clearly that for many important parameter estimates (e.g., the regression coefficient for X predicting Y when Y has MNAR missingness) the biases are tolerably small when the cause of missingness is omitted from the model.

The key here is that failing to include a cause of missingness will, to be sure, introduce estimation bias into the analysis. With very few exceptions, it is safe to say this is always true. However, what is seldom said in this context is that the amount of bias can be anywhere from trivial to substantial. In those early days, most of us acted as though any bias was important. But the recent work has shown that the magnitude of the bias is dependent on several factors, and that bias that has an appreciable effect on statistical conclusions requires circumstances are that are relatively rare in many types of research (see Chapts. 1 and 10).

The bottom line is that you should definitely make an attempt to identify the causes of missingness, to measure them, and to include them in the missing data model to the extent that is possible. But it is important to select variables that you know are causes of missingness, and to ignore variables for which you have no clear expectations about them being causes of missingness.

So, for example, when designing your measurement procedures, try to include as many causes of missingness as is feasible, but do not go overboard. Graham et al. (1994) suggested several possibilities (also see Chap. 1). For example, research participants may fail to complete a self-administered survey because they are slow readers. Thus, we often include measures of reading speed early in the survey. They may fail to complete the survey because they lack the motivation. So we often include measure of general motivation to comply, for example, by measuring the personality trait, conscientiousness. Or they may fail to complete the survey because they are motivated to behave contrary to what is asked of them. Thus, we often include measures of rebelliousness or related concepts.

Another cause of missingness relates to attrition from longitudinal studies. For example, schoolchildren may be drop out of a longitudinal study because their parents move away. Thus, a measure of family transiency would be a predictor of later attrition (e.g., something like, "How many different schools have you attended since first grade?"). It might even work in this context simply to ask respondents how likely it is that they will still be in the present school system next year.

All of this will help, but to be honest, it may not help all that much (e.g., see Collins et al. 2001). So it is important to balance your attempts to measure causes of missingness against other needs of the project. What I described above could be handled with seven questions (five for predicting survey completion and two for predicting attrition). In short, keep relatively small the number of variables measuring causes of missingness.

## Auxiliary Variables

A second answer to the question of what variables are relevant from a *missing data* perspective is auxiliary variables (see Chap. 11). In the early days after the missing data revolution, people would often say that such variables were included "to help with the imputation." I probably made statements like that in my early writing. The problem was that in those early days we did not have a clear idea of how, and to what extent, adding auxiliary variables would help with the imputation. Because of the fuzziness surrounding the value of auxiliary variables, researchers often got the idea that they should include all variables in the imputation model.

Now, however, we know a lot more about the value of auxiliary variables. From the work in Chap. 11, for example, we know that a key factor is the correlation between the potential auxiliary variable and the variable with missing data. From what we said in Chap. 11, it is clear that auxiliary variables have significant impact when they correlate $r=.50$ or more with the model variables that are sometimes missing. It is true that there is some benefit with auxiliary variables with smaller correlations, but I would argue that the point of diminishing returns is around $r=.50$. You are, of course, free to draw the line wherever you like, but the benefits of auxiliary variable correlations below $r=.50$ drop off rather substantially. For example, from the work described in Chap. 11, ($N_{TOT}=1,000$; $N_{CC}=500$; $\%Z=100\%$), $r=.50$ returns a 14 % increase in the $N_{EFF}$; $r=.40$ returns an 8.4 % increase; and $r=.30$ returns a 4.4 % increase.

My main point here is that correlations in the neighborhood of $r=.50$ are possible for variables measured at the same wave, but they are not common. Thus, in cross-sectional studies, good auxiliary variables are rare. In longitudinal studies in which a person left blank one or more items at the wave 2 measure, the best auxiliary variable may come from the wave 1 measure, and not from other variables measured at wave 2. That is, the wave 1 measure of construct X is likely to be a better auxiliary variable for the missing wave 2 measure of construct X than is any other variable measured at wave 2.

Also, as we pointed out in Chap. 11, the incremental benefit of adding a second auxiliary variable is often quite small, assuming a realistic correlation between the two auxiliary variables. So, for example, if the main dependent variable were alcohol use at tenth grade (alc10; see Table 11.9), and the auxiliary variables were alc9 ($r=.57$ with alc10) and alc8 ($r=.48$ with alc10; $r=.56$ between alc8 and alc9), the incremental benefit of adding alc8 as a second auxiliary variable would only be $N=13$. The reason for this is that the partial correlation between alc8 and alc10, partialling alc9, is only $r=.24$. Adding a second auxiliary variable that is a different variable almost always has an even smaller benefit (see Table 11.9).

## *Bottom Line: Think FIML*

My strategy for selecting variables for MI reduces to the following. Start by thinking only of the variables that would be included in the analysis if there were no missing data. Then, judiciously, add variables that are the causes of missingness or auxiliary variables. I say "think FIML" here because if you were using a FIML model, this would be the basic strategy you would use (although adding auxiliary variables to FIML models is certainly desirable and feasible; e.g., see Graham 2003; Muthen and Muthen 2010).

For causes of missingness, a rule of thumb is to include such variables only if (a) $r>.40$ between the variable and your main DV, AND (b) $r>.40$ between the variable and missingness itself. For auxiliary variables, a good rule of thumb is to include variables only if $r>.50$ between the variable and the main DV. Of course, if the number of variables in your analysis is relatively small, you can move these values down to include more variables.

## Troubleshooting Problems

I have organized this section according to the symptoms one might observe in the process of doing MI. The symptoms fall into three basic categories revolving around three diagnostic elements: (1) speed of EM convergence; (2) monotonicity of EM function values over iterations; (3) data augmentation (or MCMC) diagnostic plots.

## *Disclaimer*

Note that I have selected the examples in this chapter to be rather straightforward examples of each problem. Although these examples are representative of the kinds of problems you will encounter in real data (all these examples do come from real data), you need to know that the solutions you will encounter will not always be as clean as those shown. For example, in the first example shown, the EM convergence numbers shown change monotonically over the examples, and the effect of adding the small hyperparameter also changes monotonically over the examples shown. Although the general patterns should nearly always hold as I have shown them, you may find inconsistencies in your own data.

*Symptom: EM Doesn't Converge (or Very Slow Convergence)*
*Function Value Changes Monotonically*

With this problem, EM seems to be converging, in the sense that the function value is changing monotonically, but EM just goes on and on without converging. It goes past 1,000, 2,000, and 3,000 iterations without converging. With this pattern, EM probably will converge eventually, but the number of iterations is so high that it is infeasible, or only marginally feasible to perform the corresponding multiple imputation (realizing that 40 or more imputations may be necessary).

## *Underlying Problem 1*

One of the most common reasons for this symptom is that one simply has too many variables in the model.

## *Solution 1*

The solution to this problem is to reduce the number of variables (please see Chap. 9; also read carefully the earlier sections in this chapter).

## *Underlying Problem 2*

Another common reason for this symptom is that some variables have a very large amount of missing data.

## *Solution 2a*

One solution in this situation is to remove at least some of the variables with the most missing data. This may seem like an undesirable option, but remember that you cannot address a particular hypothesis unless you have data. Having too much missing data is tantamount to having no data in this instance. On the bright side, it is sometimes necessary to remove just one or two variables with the most missing data.

## *Solution 2b*

In this situation, it is sometimes possible to switch from ML mode (for EM), and use posterior mode with a small hyperparameter. As I have noted previously, using a

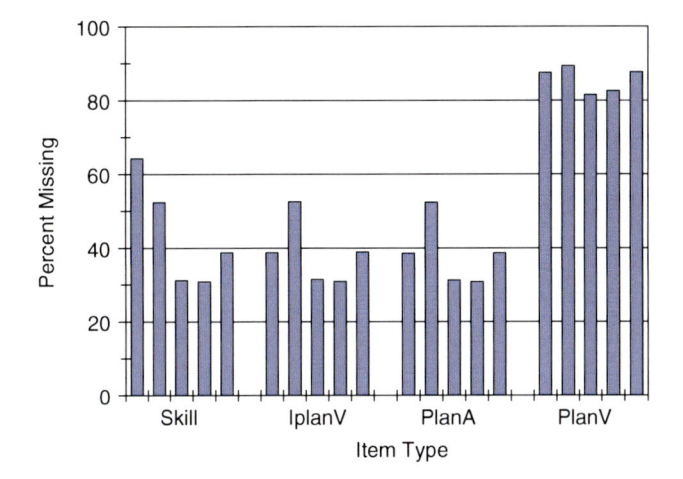

**Fig. 8.1** Percent Missing by Item Type, Skill = Planning Skill, IplanV = Intentions to make vehicle-related plans, PlanV = Actually made vehicle-related plans, PlanA = Actually made other kinds of harm-prevention plans

hyperparameter of, say, 5, is like adding 5 complete cases to the bottom of the data set, such that all variables are correlated $r=0$. Using a hyperparameter introduces a small amount of bias (all correlations are suppressed slightly toward 0), but in the process, the solution is often much more stable. Remember, however, to keep the hyperparameter small in comparison to the full sample size. My rule of thumb is to select a hyperparameter that is no more than 1 % of the nominal sample size. Smaller values are desirable.

▶ **Sample Data.** In a recent study, I asked college students about their skills for making plans to avoid alcohol-related harm, about their intentions for making such plans, and about actually making such plans. The first two kinds of questions were relevant for all participants, and with four relatively minor exceptions (see Fig. 8.1), missingness on these variables was in the 31–39 % range. However, for the five variables measuring actual vehicle-related plans, which required that the student participants found themselves in the situation requiring such plans, the missingness rate ranged from 82 % to 89 %.

Dataset: ex8a.dat
$N = 1,023$
Variables ($k = 20$)
    Variable names file: ex8a.nam
    skill1-5 = skill for making plans at waves 1-5
    iplanv1-5 = intention to make vehicle-related plans at waves 1-5
    planA1-5 = made actual plans for preventing alcohol-related harm
    planV1-5 = made actual vehicle-related plans
Missingness rates for the 20 variables are presented in Fig. 8.1.

**Table 8.1** EM convergence with high percent missing for some variables

| Variables | Number of iterations for EM convergence | |
|---|---|---|
| | ML mode | Posterior mode with hyperparameter = 5 (% improvement) |
| All 20 variables | 1,373 | 293 (79 %) |
| Drop PlanV2 (89 %) | 647 | 240 (63 %) |
| Drop PlanV5 (88 %) | 492 | 193 (61 %) |
| Drop PlanV1 (87 %) | 172 | 137 (20 %) |
| Drop all 5 PlanV variables | 67 | 61 (9 %) |

Next, with the Norm program, run EM on with all 20 variables. Then delete the variable with highest missingness (PlanV2, 89 %) and rerun EM. Then delete the variable with the next highest missingness (PlanV5, 88 %) and rerun EM. Then omit the variable with the next highest missingness (PlanV1, 87 %) and rerun EM. Finally, omit all five PlanV variables and rerun EM. The results of these EM runs appear in Table 8.1.

The numbers for EM convergence shown in Table 8.1 illustrate these points nicely. Under these circumstances, dropping even one variable with the most missing data cut the number of EM iterations in half. As it happens, dropping this wave 2 variable has limited substantive implications and is therefore a reasonable option in this case. Dropping the variable, PlanV5, however, might have more serious substantive implications; thus, dropping this variable might not be a good option. Also, in this case, switching to posterior mode with hyperparameter = 5 produced an even more striking improvement in EM convergence. In this case, it would seem that either of these options (dropping an item or switching to posterior model) would produce a viable solution.

*Symptom:* *EM May or May Not Converge*
*Function Value Changes Non-monotonically*

With this problem, EM sometimes does not converge, and sometimes EM does converge, but in a weird way. The key here is that the function values bounce back and forth between getting smaller and getting larger. When EM does converge in this context, it is "weird" because the function value seems to be changing in rather large chunks just before apparent convergence.[1]

## *Underlying Problem: Redundancies in Variable List (Matrix Not Positive Definite)*

The easiest, most common version of this problem is that the analyst inadvertently includes the individual items making up an additive scale and the scale score itself.

---

[1] But do recall that convergence is a function of the parameter values, and is not a direct function of the function value. Still, it is more common with "normal" EM convergence that the function value makes very small (monotonic) changes just prior to convergence.

# Troubleshooting Problems

**Table 8.2** Output from EM.OUT: input matrix not positive definite

| iteration # | Observed-data Loglikelihood |
|---|---|
| 990 | 21036.11128 |
| 991 | 20886.85934 |
| 992 | 22142.71381 |
| 993 | 21000.63380 |
| 994 | 21356.37234 |
| 995 | 21540.07565 |
| 996 | 21356.43041 |
| 997 | 20624.48552 |
| 998 | 20853.13673 |
| 999 | 21297.81517 |
| 1000 | 20976.37888 |

WARNING!!!!!
EM DID NOT CONVERGE BY ITERATION 1000

A more insidious version of the problem is usually referred to as multicollinearity, that is, there are redundancies in the data, but it just happens that a particular variable is perfectly predicted (linearly) by a rather large set of other variables. Whatever the source of the problem, in this situation, you have less information than is implied by the number of variables in the model. Virtually no multivariate procedures, including EM and multiple imputation, work under these circumstances.

▶ **Sample Data**.

Dataset: ex8b.dat
$N = 2,570$
Variables ($k = 6$)
  Variable names file: ex8b.nam
  riskreb1 = risk-taking/rebelliousness (item 1)
  riskreb2 = risk-taking/rebelliousness (item 2)
  posatt1 = beliefs about positive consequences of alcohol use (item 1)
  posatt2 = beliefs about positive consequences of alcohol use (item 2)
  posatt3 = beliefs about positive consequences of alcohol use (item 3)
  posatt = beliefs about positive consequences of alcohol use (scale score – average of other 3).

This data set was constructed to illustrate what happens when the individual items making up a summary scale, and the scale score itself, are included in the EM analysis. Start by running EM in Norm on all six variables in the data set. Note that the function value (Observed-data loglikelihood) is not monotonic over iterations. I show the last few iterations from the Norm output in Table 8.2.

Now repeat the EM analysis omitting the variable, posatt (the scale score). I show the iterations of EM in Table 8.3.

**Table 8.3** Output from EM.OUT: with problem variable omitted

| iteration # | Observed-data Loglikelihood |
|---|---|
| 1 | −4097.000000 |
| 2 | −3573.606946 |
| 3 | −3461.251865 |
| 4 | −3432.067301 |
| 5 | −3423.604506 |
| 6 | −3420.837124 |
| 7 | −3419.845559 |
| 8 | −3419.461072 |
| 9 | −3419.298466 |
| 10 | −3419.222811 |
| 11 | −3419.184264 |
| 12 | −3419.163138 |
| 13 | −3419.150954 |
| 14 | −3419.143699 |
| 15 | −3419.139294 |
| 16 | −3419.136589 |
| 17 | −3419.134917 |
| 18 | −3419.133879 |
| 19 | −3419.133233 |
| 20 | −3419.132831 |
| 21 | −3419.132580 |
| 22 | −3419.132423 |
| 23 | −3419.132325 |
| 24 | −3419.132264 |
| 25 | −3419.132226 |
| 26 | −3419.132202 |
| 27 | −3419.132187 |
| 28 | −3419.132178 |
| 29 | −3419.132172 |
| 30 | −3419.132168 |
| 31 | −3419.132166 |
| 32 | −3419.132164 |
| 33 | −3419.132163 |
| 34 | −3419.132163 |
| 35 | −3419.132162 |
| 36 | −3419.132162 |
| 37 | −3419.132162 |
| 38 | −3419.132162 |
| EM CONVERGED AT ITERATION 38 | |

Note that when the scale score was included in the analysis (Table 8.2), not only did the function values bounce around (getting larger, smaller, larger, etc.), but the changes were relatively large. Compare that to normal EM convergence shown in Table 8.3. With normal convergence, there may be large changes in the function

# Troubleshooting Problems

**Table 8.4** Output from EM.OUT: another pathological pattern

| iteration # | Observed-data Loglikelihood |
|---|---|
| 1 | −3237.500000 |
| 2 | −1587.081959 |
| 3 | −737.7915525 |
| 4 | 32.43368198 |
| 5 | 789.6940132 |
| 6 | 1544.946098 |
| 7 | 2299.900033 |
| 8 | 3054.809647 |
| 9 | 3809.712383 |
| 10 | 4564.613954 |
| 11 | 5319.515303 |
| 12 | 6074.416605 |
| 13 | 6829.317899 |
| EM CONVERGED AT ITERATION 13 | |

value early in the iterations, but it is not at all uncommon for the changes just before convergence to be very tiny.

Note, too, that the problem shown here may manifest itself in different ways. But in each case, the pattern of function values over iterations will deviate rather substantially from that shown for "normal EM convergence" in Table 8.3. One example comes from this same data set. Rerun EM in Norm, but this time select only the four Posatt variables (including the scale score; ignore for now the fact that many of the cases have no data at all for these four variables). EM did appear to converge in this case (as shown in Table 8.4). But note the highly unusual pattern of function values over iterations. Although the values did change monotonically over iterations, the values went from negative to positive, and the changes from iteration to iteration near "convergence" were very large – nothing at all like the normal convergence shown in Table 8.3.

## *Solution1*

This is not so much a solution as a method for discovering the solution. The ultimate solution in this case is to find the variables that render the matrix nonpositive definite and remove them from the analysis. The first step in this solution is to verify that the matrix is, indeed, not positive definite. To do this, analyze the *same* data using principal components analysis. Use pairwise deletion for this task.

**Table 8.5** Principal components eigenvalues and final communality estimates (based on pairwise deletion), including bad variable

```
The FACTOR Procedure
Initial Factor Method: Principal Components
Prior Communality Estimates: ONE
Eigenvalues of the Correlation Matrix: Total = 6 Average = 1
          Eigenvalue  Difference  Proportion  Cumulative
1         3.25069837  2.18208280  0.5418      0.5418
2         1.06861557  0.37637959  0.1781      0.7199
3         0.69223598  0.12380224  0.1154      0.8353
4         0.56843374  0.14640731  0.0947      0.9300
5         0.42202643  0.42403651  0.0703      1.0003
6         -.00201008              -0.0003     1.0000
The FACTOR Procedure
Rotation Method: Promax (power = 3)
          Final Communality Estimates: Total = 4.319314
rskreb71    rskreb72    posatt71    posatt72    posatt73    posatt
0.60765066  0.69463724  0.65657938  0.70695389  0.65462493  0.99886784
```

I did this analysis in SAS (I asked for promax rotation for this analysis).[2] The key results appear in Table 8.5. The first thing to notice from this analysis is that the last eigenvalue is negative. That demonstrates that the matrix for these six variables was not positive definite. Second, look the final communality estimates. Although this may not be so telling in all cases, note that in this case, the communality estimate for posatt was .999.

## Solution 1b

The follow-up to running principal components is to perform a multiple regression analysis on the same data (with pairwise deletion). I typically just pick the first variable in the variable list as the dependent variable and specify all other variables as predictors. You may sometimes need to test additional models, but that will often show the bad variable. For example, with the six variables from our sample data set, the key output from the SAS Proc Reg analysis is shown in Table 8.6.

Of course, had one of the other posatt variables been listed last in the analysis, that one would have been shown to be the problem variable. But at least this analysis

---

[2] I also performed the same analysis with SPSS 19. Strategies and code for performing these analyses in SAS and SPSS are provided on our website, http://methodology.psu.edu.

**Table 8.6** Multiple regression results (with pairwise deletion), including bad variable

```
The REG Procedure
Model: MODEL1
Dependent Variable: rskreb71
```

| Variable | DF | Parameter Estimate | Standard Error | t Value | Pr > \|t\| |
|---|---|---|---|---|---|
| Intercept | B | 0.78778 | 0.06079 | 12.96 | <.0001 |
| rskreb72 | B | 0.23227 | 0.02366 | 9.82 | <.0001 |
| posatt71 | B | 0.07998 | 0.02496 | 3.20 | 0.0014 |
| posatt72 | B | 0.22451 | 0.02969 | 7.56 | <.0001 |
| posatt73 | B | 0.01734 | 0.03755 | 0.46 | 0.6443 |
| posatt | 0 | 0 | . | . | . |

shows that the problem is in that set of variables. Once you see that, it should be a relatively straightforward to see the solution to the problem.[3]

*Symptom:* *EM Converges Quickly*
*Function is Monotonic over Iterations*
*MI Diagnostic Plots Are Pathological*

This problem is more difficult to see in the first place. But it points to the need to examine all of the diagnostics before proceeding with interpretation of the analysis results.

## *Underlying Problem*

Suppose that our data set has data from 12 schools. Normally, within each school, each variable would have some cases with data, and some cases with missing values, as depicted in Table 8.7 (in this case, "1" for variable S11 means that the case comes from school 11; "0" indicates the cases come from another school).

In this example (normal scenario), there are missing and nonmissing values both within school 11 and in other schools.

However, suppose that for whatever reason, all students in school 11 did not provide data for the alcohol use measure in seventh grade. Under these circumstances, the numbers would look as shown in Table 8.8.

Note that in this scenario, data coming from all other schools appear normal, in that some values are "1" (no alcohol use), some are "2" (some alcohol use), and some are "." (missing). However, in this case, all values from school 11 (S11 = 1) are missing.

---

[3] In SPSS, I found the principal components analysis to be as described above. However, I was somewhat less able to make use of the regression analysis to point further to the variable that should be removed, because SPSS does not have the option of including variables in the order presented. Thus, posatt1 was omitted from the analysis based on the F-to-enter criterion. On the other hand, the variable that was removed automatically (posatt1) did show that the problem was probably in that set of variables.

**Table 8.7** Normal data pattern within school 11 (S11)

| s11 | alc7 | Frequency | Percent |
|---|---|---|---|
| 0 | . | 174 | 6.31 |
| 0 | 1 | 831 | 30.15 |
| 0 | 2 | 1603 | 58.16 |
| 1 | . | 3 | 0.11 |
| 1 | 1 | 45 | 1.63 |
| 1 | 2 | 100 | 3.63 |

S11 = 1 indicates data come from School 11; S11 = 0 indicates data come from another school. Alc7 = Alcohol use at seventh grade. Alc7 = 1 indicates no use; Alc7 = 2 indicates at least some alcohol use

**Table 8.8** All missing data within school 11 (S11)

| s11 | xalc7 | Frequency | Percent |
|---|---|---|---|
| 0 | . | 174 | 6.31 |
| 0 | 1 | 831 | 30.15 |
| 0 | 2 | 1603 | 58.16 |
| 1 | . | 148 | 5.37 |

S11 = 1 indicates data come from School 11; S11 = 0 indicates data come from another school. Alc7 = Alcohol use at seventh grade. Alc7 = 1 indicates no use; Alc7 = 2 indicates at least some alcohol use.

Analyses of these data that do not take school membership into account will be fine, because data from school 11 will be grouped with data from other schools.

▶ **Sample Data**

Dataset: ex8c.dat
$N = 2,756$
Variables ($k = 16$)
  Variable names file: ex8c.nam
  S1–S11 = school membership dummy variables; 1 = member of the school; 0 = not a member of that school. Data with all "0" values for these 11 dummy variables come from School 12.
  xalc7 = alcohol use in seventh grade
  riskreb1 = risk-taking/rebelliousness (item 2)
  likepar1 = liking for parents (item 1)
  posatt1 = beliefs about positive consequences of alcohol use (item 1)
  alc8 = alcohol use in eighth grade

*When the school membership dummy variables were omitted* from the analysis, EM converged normally in 34 iterations.

Further, all diagnostic plots from data augmentation (MCMC) looked reasonable (see Chaps. 3 or 7).

*When the school membership dummy variables were included* in the model, EM converged normally in 52 iterations.

# Troubleshooting Problems

**a** Probably Pathological Diagnostic Plots for Covariance of xalc7 with S1

**b** Pathological Diagnostic Plots for Mean of xalc7

**c** Cleary Pathlogical Diagnostic Plot for covariance of xalc7 with s11

**d** Cleary Pathlogical Diagnostic Plot for Variance of xalc7

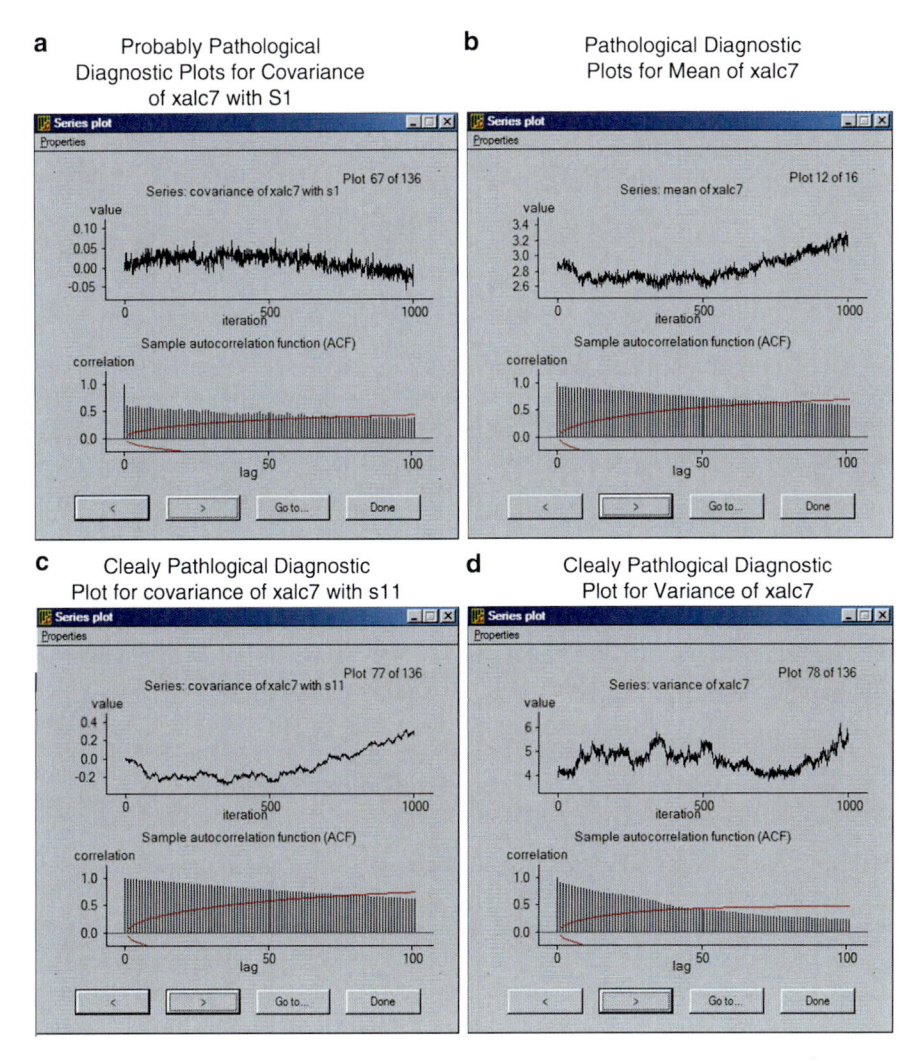

**Fig. 8.2** Diagnostic Plots. Plots depict MI solutions that range from probably pathological to clearly pathological

Diagnostic plots from data augmentation showed some pathological patterns. The plots for several parameter estimates involving the variable xalc7 looked questionable (e.g., see Fig. 8.2, panel a). But others were clearly pathological (see Fig. 8.2, panels b, c, and d).

Note that with this problem, adding a hyperparameter does not help. Even with a hyperparameter = 10, EM converged (apparently normally) in 912 iterations. Further, diagnostic plots were clearly pathological for the same parameters (mean of xalc7, variance of xalc7, and covariance of s11 with xalc7 were again the worst offenders).

## First Conceptual Basis for This Missingness Pattern

I have seen this pattern manifests itself in two contexts. First, in a large study in several communities, one whole community did not want its children responding do certain questions that were on the survey. The following solution applies in this context.

## Solution

The problem in this instance is that one cannot test hypotheses involving all of the dummy variables and the substantive variable (xalc in my example) that has the problem. So the solution is that one of the problem variables must be removed. If the substantive variable is key for testing study hypotheses, then one must drop the problem dummy variable. In this instance, I feel that relatively little is given up if you combine the problem school with another school. If you simply drop the problem dummy variable (s11), it means that school 11 is combined with school 12 (the school with 0 for all dummy variables). If you must do this combining, it is probably best to combine school 11 with another school that has the most similar school characteristics. At the very least, be sure to combine the school in question with another school that is in the same condition (e.g., program or control).

## Second Conceptual Basis for This Missingness Pattern

Another context for this missingness pattern is with certain skip patterns in questionnaire research. Skip patterns typically take this form: The participants are first shown a lead question, for example, "Have you ever smoked even one cigarette in your whole life?" (1 = "no", 2 = "yes"). If the answer is "yes," the person receives the follow-up questions, such as "How many cigarettes have you smoked in the past 30 days?" However, if the person answers "no" to the lead question, then he or she is not shown the follow-up questions. When the lead question is dichotomous, this situation creates exactly the missingness pattern we have been talking about in this section. Ignoring other forms of missingness, the missingness on the two questions (lead and follow-up questions) look as shown in Table 8.9.

As expected, everyone with a "1" on wa14 is missing on xa15. In this case, a correlation cannot be calculated between wa14 and xa15, and the missing values on xa15 cannot be imputed (with wa14 in the model).

## Solutions

There are solutions to this problem. However, none of them are particularly satisfying. One solution is to be sure that the lead question is not a categorical question.

# Troubleshooting Problems

**Table 8.9** Missingness on follow-up question based on response to lead question

| wa14 | xa15 | Frequency | Percent |
|---|---|---|---|
| 1 | . | 1875 | 61.94 |
| 2 | 1 | 933 | 30.82 |
| 2 | 2 | 39 | 1.29 |
| 2 | 3 | 66 | 2.18 |
| 2 | 4 | 59 | 1.95 |
| 2 | 5 | 29 | 0.96 |
| 2 | 6 | 20 | 0.66 |

wa14 = lead question: Have you ever smoked even one cigarette in your whole life (1 = no; 2 = yes). xa15 = follow-up question: How many cigarettes have you smoked in the past 30 days (1 = none; 2–6 = some)

The problem occurs when everyone with one level of a categorical variable has a missing value for some other question. So if the lead question has even three ordered categories, it is possible to estimate a correlation between the lead and follow-up questions. For example, suppose the lead question (wa14) was, "How many cigarettes have you smoked in your whole life?" 1 = none; 2 = part or all of one cigarette; 3 = more than one cigarette. In this case, the follow-up question (xa15; e.g., "How many cigarettes have you smoked in the past 30 days?") is missing whenever wa14 = 1. In this case, the correlation between wa14 and xa15 can be estimated using values of wa14 that are greater than 1. Unfortunately, when the lead question has only three levels, the correlation with the follow-up question can be substantially biased. That is, the correlation based on the last two values of wa14 is not representative of the correlation based on all three values of wa14.

A better solution is to have a lead question with several response options. For example, suppose the lead question (wa14) was, "How many cigarettes have you smoked in your whole life?", and the responses were 1 = none; 2 = only one puff; 3 = part or all of one cigarette; 4 = 2–4 cigarettes; 5 = 5–20 cigarettes; 6 = 1–5 packs; and 7 = more than 5 packs. Further suppose that the follow-up question (xa15) is, as before, "How many cigarettes have you smoked in the past 30 days?" (with six response categories). In this case, all values of xa15 are still missing if wa14 = 1. But in this case, the correlation between wa14 and xa15 can be estimated using values 2–7 for wa14. Thus, in this case, the correlation has a better chance of being representative of the correlation based on all the data. In this case, it is also possible to impute the missing values of xa15 with wa14 in the imputation model.

This solution will perform reasonably well when the observed correlation (omitting cases where wa14 = 1) is similar to the overall correlation. Table 8.10 shows the correlations with the key variables with and without the skip pattern using data from the Adolescent Alcohol Prevention Trial (AAPT; Hansen and Graham 1991). We did not actually use skip patterns in the AAPT questionnaire. However, it is possible to simulate a skip pattern in these data simply by setting all values of the follow-up questions (xa15 and xa16) to missing whenever the lead question (wa14) takes on the value 1 (in this example, xa15 = How many cigarettes have you smoked in the past 30 days?;

**Table 8.10** Correlations with and without skip pattern

| With skip pattern (simulated) | | | | | Without skip pattern | | |
|---|---|---|---|---|---|---|---|
| | wa14 | xa15 | xa16 | | wa14 | wa15 | wa16 |
| wa14 | 1.000 | | | wa14 | 1.000 | | |
| | 3023 | | | | 3023 | | |
| xa15 | .590 | 1.000 | | wa15 | .590 | 1.000 | |
| | <.0001 | | | | <.0001 | | |
| | 1146 | 1149 | | | 3020 | 3023 | |
| xa16 | .463 | .747 | 1.000 | wa16 | .455 | .754 | 1.000 |
| | <.0001 | <.0001 | | | <.0001 | <.0001 | <.0001 |
| | 1145 | 1148 | 1148 | | 3018 | 3021 | 3021 |

Below each correlation is the *p*-value for the correlation, and below that, the sample size on which the pairwise correlation was calculated. wa14 = lifetime smoking; wa15 = smoking in past 30 days; wa16 = smoking in past 7 days; xa15 = smoking in past 30 days with skip pattern (xa15 missing if wa14 = 1); xa16 = smoking in past 7 days with skip pattern (xa16 missing if wa14 = 1)

xa16 = How many cigarettes have you smoked in the past 7 days?). The variables xa15 and xa16 simulated data that would be observed with the skip pattern; the variables wa14, wa15, and wa16 were the actual data (i.e., without the skip pattern).

In this instance, it is pretty easy to see that the correlations based only on the reduced sample with data for both questions were good representations of the correlations based on the total sample. In general, however, this will occur only when the two variables are linearly related through the entire range of responses.

Another solution involves simply inserting "no use" values ("1" in this case) in the follow-up questions when "no use" ("1") was indicated on the lead question. Although this solution is admittedly ad hoc, it often performs well in practice. It works because the probability is very low that a person who indicates "no use" on the lead question will in fact indicate something other than "no use" on the follow-up questions, if given the chance. In the AAPT study, for example, 1,875 students indicated "no use" on the lead, lifetime smoking question. Of those, one was missing on the follow-up question about smoking in the past 30 days, and three (0.16 %) gave responses other than "no use" on the follow-up question. For the lead, lifetime alcohol use question in the AAPT study, 1,002 students gave the "no use" response. Of these, four students (0.4 %) gave responses other than "no use" to the 30-day alcohol use question. In short, given that the other solution described above (having a lead question with multiple response categories) may not always work well, this ad hoc solution could be the best option available.

## Summary of Troubleshooting Symptoms, Causes, and Solutions

Table 8.11 presents a convenient summary of the troubleshooting tips described in this chapter.

Summary of Troubleshooting Symptoms, Causes, and Solutions 211

**Table 8.11** Summary of troubleshooting symptoms, causes, and solutions

| Symptom | Function values | Diagnostic plots | Root cause | Fix* |
|---|---|---|---|---|
| EM fails to converge after 1,000 iterations | Change monotonically over iterations | | Large number of variables | Reduce the number of variables; see Chap. 9 |
| | | | Large amount of missing data on one or more variables | Consider dropping one or more variables with high missingness |
| | | | | Or try adding a small hyperparameter |
| EM fails to converge after 1,000 iterations (or EM seems to converges, but after large change in function value) | Large changes between iterations; change nonmonotonically over iterations | | Often means that matrix is not positive definite | Perform principal components on same variables to verify the problem; regression analysis to identify the problem variable |
| EM converges in relatively few iterations | Change monotonically over iterations | Pathological | EM converged to "ridge" (rather than point) solution; all cases on level p of categorical variable X are missing on variable Y | If categorical variable is dummy variable indicating cluster (e.g., school) membership, combine problem cluster with another, similar cluster |
| | | | | If categorical variable is lead question in a skip pattern, use a lead question with several, ordered, response categories; simply insert value in follow-up question (if possible) |

# References

Collins, L. M., Schafer, J. L., & Kam, C. M. (2001). A comparison of inclusive and restrictive strategies in modern missing data procedures. *Psychological Methods, 6*, 330–351.

Graham, J. W. (2003). Adding missing-data relevant variables to FIML-based structural equation models. *Structural Equation Modeling, 10*, 80–100.

Graham, J. W., Hofer, S. M., & Piccinin, A. M. (1994). Analysis with missing data in drug prevention research. In L. M. Collins and L. Seitz (eds.), *Advances in data analysis for prevention intervention research*. National Institute on Drug Abuse Research Monograph Series #142, pp. 13–63, Washington DC: National Institute on Drug Abuse.

Hansen, W. B., & Graham, J. W. (1991). Preventing alcohol, marijuana, and cigarette use among adolescents: Peer pressure resistance training versus establishing conservative norms. *Preventive Medicine, 20*, 414–430.

Muthén, L. K., & Muthén, B. O. (2010). *Mplus User's Guide. (6th ed.)*. Los Angeles: Author.

# Chapter 9
# Dealing with the Problem of Having Too Many Variables in the Imputation Model

John W. Graham, M. Lee Van Horn, and Bonnie J. Taylor

One of the most difficult problems with performing multiple imputation relates to having too many variables in the imputation model. In many instances, the problems associated with having too many variables in the model can be avoided by using the strategies suggested in the previous chapter. Still, situations arise in which more variables need to be included in the model than can feasibly be handled by the current software. In this chapter, we reiterate the "Think FIML" approach to multiple imputation, which will help you avoid many pitfalls in this regard. Also, for situations in which the Think FIML approach is not enough, we describe two other strategies for dealing with this problem. The first strategy involves reducing the number of variables by imputing whole scales rather than the individual items making up the scales. The second strategy involves dividing up the variables into two or more sets that can be imputed separately with minimal bias.

## Think FIML

As outlined in the previous chapter, the Think FIML strategy starts with the variables that are in the analysis model. Then add the few variables you know to be related to missingness on your model variables. Finally, add the few auxiliary variables that are most highly correlated with the analysis model variables that are sometimes missing. This strategy works very well to reduce any biases related to missing data, and to restore lost power due to attrition and other forms of missingness. Also, because these models tend to be relatively small, and with the kind of automation that is currently available (including the automation utilities described in this book), it is often quite practical to perform missing data analyses tailored to each analysis.

Before going on to the other strategies for dealing with large numbers of variables, we want to make one more pitch for using the Think FIML strategy. First, why would one want to impute more variables? One reason might be to take advantage of the benefits of using an inclusive model (i.e., less bias, more power). However, the incremental benefit of adding causes of missingness and auxiliary variables falls off very quickly (e.g., as shown in Chap. 11).

A second reason for imputing a large number of variables is that one finds the imputation-analysis process so daunting that one wants to do the imputation part as few times as possible, for example, by imputing a large number of variables, and performing many different analyses on subsets of those variables. Because of the highly automated analysis programs, especially with SAS (also see the latest versions of Stata), and to a large extent with SPSS analysis with Norm and the MIAutomate utilities, it gets easier and easier to take the Think FIML, and "impute once, analyze once" approach.

## Imputing Whole Scales

We take it as an axiom that imputing at the item level is always at least as good as imputing at the scale level. However, in field research, especially in longitudinal panel studies, sometimes there are simply too many variables to impute everything at the item level. For example, with even 10 scales, each with five items, there are 50 items total. If one has five waves of data, there are $10 \times 5 \times 5 = 250$ individual variables. This number of variables would overwhelm any standard missing data routine, even with a large number of cases. Because scenarios such as this are all too common in longitudinal field research, one must be prepared to make some compromises. This chapter describes one such compromise.

The strategy involves imputing at least some scales at the scale level rather than at the individual item level. Although it is generally better to impute at the individual variable level, there are cases where the two approaches are essentially the same. Specifically, if all cases have either all data or no data for all of the individual variables making up a scale, then it makes virtually no difference whether imputation is done at the individual variable or the scale level (assuming, of course, that the ultimate goal is to perform analyses on scales, rather than on individual items).

However, this ideal pattern is seldom found in empirical data. So a big part of our strategy involves generating scores for some scales for individuals who have data for some, but not all of the variables comprising the scale. Creating combined scale scores when subjects are missing different items requires some relatively strong implicit assumptions. The first assumption is that the expected response for all items is identical; this assumption implies equal means and variances for all items. To see why this is true, imagine two subjects with identical scores on a scale but where the first is missing item 1 and the second is missing item 2. If the mean for item 1 is higher than the mean for item 2, the first subject would have a lower score on the combined scale than the second subject simply because he or she happened to be missing a different item. This problem is readily fixed by standardizing all items to a common mean and variance before creating summed scales. This fix is very common part of scale construction, and works well with most, though not all, types of scales.

Schafer and Graham (2002) also discussed this strategy in a general way under the heading, "Averaging the Available Items," saying that the practice "… is difficult to justify …", but that it can sometimes be useful provided the items "… form a single, well-defined domain." When the items do not form a single, well-defined domain, it is possible that items relate differentially to other variables outside the scale. Under these conditions, generating scale scores based on the average of non-missing items may cause estimation bias and is not recommended.

Identifying whether the items form a single, well-defined domain is something that must be done if one is to employ the strategy of generating scale scores based on partial data. However, there are no absolute criteria to help one determine whether the items form a single, well-defined domain. One of the main purposes of this chapter is to develop reasonable decision rules about when a scale may reasonably be thought of as forming a single, well-defined domain (we will hereafter refer to this as a "homogeneous" scale), and for dealing with the situation whether or not the scale has been judged to be homogeneous.

## *Determining Whether a Scale Is Homogeneous or Heterogeneous*

Our operational definition of whether a scale is homogeneous or not will be based on a one-factor factor analysis and on coefficient alpha. It is best in this context to make use of common factors analysis (principal axis factoring with iterations), or structural equation modeling (SEM). Other, comparable models might also make sense. Ideally this factor analysis would be based directly on an EM covariance matrix, on a single data set imputed from EM parameters (e.g., with Norm or Proc MI; see Chaps. 3 and 7), or on some other form of ML estimation with missing data.

For now, we will define the scale to be homogeneous as long as the difference between the largest and smallest factor loadings is no more than .20. However, this factor loading criterion is a necessary, but not sufficient condition for describing the scale as homogeneous. In order for a scale to be homogeneous, the .20 difference rule for factor loadings must apply, and coefficient alpha must also be at least .70.[1]

Table 9.1 presents the correlation matrix, factor loading matrix, and coefficient alpha for several different scenarios involving four scale items. These scenarios show different patterns ranging from clearly homogeneous to clearly heterogeneous. Below, we make judgments about appropriate handling with each scenario. Our judgments could certainly be used as is. However, minor deviations from our recommendations may also be justified.

---

[1] One could consider other approaches to making these judgments about unidimensionality and homogeneity. For example, one could consider using tools of exploratory factor analysis (e.g., the scree test) to verify that the items making up a scale do indeed form a single factor. One could also use the SEM framework to help make judgments about whether the scale items tap a single factor, and whether it is reasonable in a statistical sense to treat the factor loadings to be equal, that is, to be homogeneous.

**Table 9.1** Sample scenarios

*Scenario A1: homogeneous with high factor loadings (very high alpha)*

Correlation matrix

| | | | |
|---|---|---|---|
| 1.00 | | | |
| .70 | 1.00 | | |
| .70 | .70 | 1.00 | |
| .70 | .70 | .70 | 1.00 |

Factor loadings (SEM)

| | |
|---|---|
| A | .84 |
| B | .84 |
| C | .84 |
| D | .84 |

coefficient **alpha = .90**

*Scenario A2: homogeneous with good factor loadings (good alpha)*

Correlation matrix

| | | | |
|---|---|---|---|
| 1.00 | | | |
| .50 | 1.00 | | |
| .50 | .50 | 1.00 | |
| .50 | .50 | .50 | 1.00 |

Factor loadings (SEM)

| | |
|---|---|
| A | .71 |
| B | .71 |
| C | .71 |
| D | .71 |

coefficient **alpha = .80**

*Scenario A3: homogeneous, but with moderate factor loadings (moderate alpha)*

Correlation matrix

| | | | |
|---|---|---|---|
| 1.00 | | | |
| .40 | 1.00 | | |
| .40 | .40 | 1.00 | |
| .40 | .40 | .40 | 1.00 |

Factor loadings (SEM)

| | |
|---|---|
| A | .63 |
| B | .63 |
| C | .63 |
| D | .63 |

coefficient **alpha = .73**

*Scenario A4: homogeneous, but with lowish factor loadings (lowish alpha)*

Correlation matrix

| | | | |
|---|---|---|---|
| 1.00 | | | |
| .30 | 1.00 | | |
| .30 | .30 | 1.00 | |
| .30 | .30 | .30 | 1.00 |

Factor loadings (SEM)

| | |
|---|---|
| A | .55 |
| B | .55 |
| C | .55 |
| D | .55 |

coefficient **alpha = .63**

(continued)

**Table 9.1** (continued)

*Scenario A5: homogeneous, but with low factor loadings (low alpha)*
Correlation matrix
| | | | |
|---|---|---|---|
| 1.00 | | | |
| .20 | 1.00 | | |
| .20 | .20 | 1.00 | |
| .20 | .20 | .20 | 1.00 |

Factor loadings (SEM)
| | |
|---|---|
| A | .45 |
| B | .45 |
| C | .45 |
| D | .45 |

coefficient **alpha = .50**

*Scenario A6: homogeneous, but with very low factor loadings (very low alpha)*
Correlation matrix
| | | | |
|---|---|---|---|
| 1.00 | | | |
| .15 | 1.00 | | |
| .15 | .15 | 1.00 | |
| .15 | .15 | .15 | 1.00 |

Factor loadings (SEM)
| | |
|---|---|
| A | .39 |
| B | .39 |
| C | .39 |
| D | .39 |

coefficient **alpha = .41**

*Scenario B1: Heterogeneous, with three good and one very low factor loading*
Correlation Matrix
| | | | |
|---|---|---|---|
| 1.00 | | | |
| .70 | 1.00 | | |
| .70 | .70 | 1.00 | |
| .20 | .20 | .20 | 1.00 |

Factor Loadings (SEM)
| | |
|---|---|
| A | .84 |
| B | .84 |
| C | .84 |
| **D** | **.24** |

coefficient **alpha = .77**

*Scenario B2: heterogeneous, with three good and one low factor loading*
Correlation matrix
| | | | |
|---|---|---|---|
| 1.00 | | | |
| .70 | 1.00 | | |
| .70 | .70 | 1.00 | |
| .30 | .30 | .30 | 1.00 |

Factor loadings (SEM)
| | |
|---|---|
| A | .84 |
| B | .84 |
| C | .84 |
| **D** | **.36** |

coefficient **alpha = .80**

(continued)

**Table 9.1** (continued)

***Scenario B3: heterogeneous, with three good and one lowish factor loading***

Correlation Matrix

| | | | |
|---|---|---|---|
| 1.00 | | | |
| .70 | 1.00 | | |
| .70 | .70 | 1.00 | |
| .40 | .40 | .40 | 1.00 |

Factor loadings (SEM)

| | |
|---|---|
| A | .84 |
| B | .84 |
| C | .84 |
| **D** | **.48** |

coefficient **alpha = .83**

perfect fit

***Scenario B4: heterogeneous, with two good and two lowish factor loadings***

Correlation matrix

| | | | |
|---|---|---|---|
| 1.00 | | | |
| .70 | 1.00 | | |
| .40 | .40 | 1.00 | |
| .40 | .40 | .40 | 1.00 |

Factor loadings (SEM)

| | |
|---|---|
| A | .83 |
| B | .83 |
| **C** | **.50** |
| **D** | **.50** |

coefficient **alpha = .77**

***Scenario B5: heterogeneous, two dimensional scale***

Correlation matrix

| | | | |
|---|---|---|---|
| 1.00 | | | |
| .70 | 1.00 | | |
| .40 | .40 | 1.00 | |
| .40 | .40 | .70 | 1.00 |

Factor loadings (SEM)

| | |
|---|---|
| A | .80 |
| B | .80 |
| **C** | **.59** |
| **D** | **.59** |

coefficient **alpha = .80**

## *Decision Rules for These Scenarios*

### Scenario A1 (Homogeneous Loadings = .84, Alpha = .90)

This is a good candidate for generating a scale score based on partial data. With this scenario, we would feel comfortable generating a scale score based on just half the items making up the scale. Forming a scale score with 2 of 4 items or 3 of 6 would seem to be acceptable in this instance.

### Scenario A2 (Homogeneous Loadings = .71, Alpha = .80)

This is also a good candidate for generating a scale score based on partial data. With this scenario, however, we would prefer to have a majority of the items with data before forming the scale score. Forming a scale score with 3 of 4, 3 of 5, or 4 of 6 items would seem to be acceptable. Forming a scale score with 3 of 6 seems a little risky.

### Scenario A3 (Homogeneous Loadings = .63, Alpha = .73)

With this scenario, we might be willing to form a scale score with 3 of 4, 4 of 5, or 5 of 6 items, but would feel a little uncomfortable in this instance forming a scale score with 3 of 5 or 4 of 6 items.

### Scenario A4 (Homogeneous Loadings = .55, Alpha = .63)

Starting with this scenario, we would feel uncomfortable forming a scale score with anything less than all of the items. In this instance (as with scenarios A5 and A6), the items seem to tap rather different constructs. They are balanced, to be sure, but in this instance, despite that balance, omitting one item might have a rather different substantive meaning than dropping another item. For scenarios A4, A5, and A6, we would require that all of the items have data before forming a scale score.

### Scenarios B1, B2, B3 (Heterogeneous Loadings, Three Good = .83, One Lower, Alpha Good)

These scenarios all violate the requirement for homogeneous factor loadings (maximum loading difference greater than .20). Thus in these three scenarios, we would require that all items have data for forming a scale score. Another option in this instance is to rethink the scale. It is possible to drop the item with the low loading, retaining the three or more items with solid (homogeneous) loadings. Alternatively, it might be possible to separate the items into parts for imputation and recombine them later. That is, one could treat the three (or more) items with homogeneous loadings and the item(s) with lower loadings as separate subscales for imputation. Then, after imputation, the two subscales could be recombined (weighting the subscales appropriately). One would have to be very careful with the logistics of this approach, but it does seem to be a reasonable strategy that would serve to reduce the estimation load during imputation.

**Scenario B4 (Heterogeneous Loadings, Two Good = .83, Two Lowish = .50, Alpha Good)**

We would treat this scenario the same as the previous ones; begin by considering dropping the two low-loading items. Alternatively, we might treat the parts of this scale separately for imputation and recombine the subscales after imputation. In this instance, however, one would need to form three subscales (items A and B, item C, item D). If dropping the two low-loading items is not an option, we would prefer to impute at the scale level (requiring that all items have data, discarding any partial data) or impute at the individual item level.

**Scenario B5 (Heterogeneous Loadings, Two-Dimensional Scale)**

This would be a case where separating the items into two scales might be the best strategy. However, with this scenario, the researcher could consider separating the two dimensions for imputation (following the rules described above for the A scenarios) and recombine the parts into a full scale after imputation.

## *Decisions About Throwing Away Partial Data Versus Imputing at the Item Level*

In the previous sections, we outlined some strategies for determining how many of the scale items must have data before we feel comfortable forming a scale score. At one extreme, we argued that some scales must be formed only when all items have data. At the other extreme, we argued that some scales may be formed when at least half of the items have data. But even with these decision rules, one must still decide whether it is better (a) to impute scale scores, and discard any partial data for which the rules for forming a scale score have not been met, or (b) to go ahead and impute at the individual item level. We address this latter issue in this section.

### Missing Data Patterns for Scale Items

A major bit of relevant information comes from examination of the patterns of missing and nonmissing values among the items making up the scale. For example,

# Imputing Whole Scales

Table 9.2 Sample missing data patterns

| Pattern | Item A | B | C | D | Frequency (%) |
|---|---|---|---|---|---|
| 1 | 1 | 1 | 1 | 1 | 96 |
| 2 | 1 | 0 | 1 | 1 | 1 |
| 3 | 0 | 0 | 1 | 1 | 0.5 |
| 4 | 1 | 0 | 0 | 1 | 0.5 |
| 5 | 0 | 0 | 0 | 0 | 2 |

Table 9.3 Sample SAS syntax for producing table of missing data patterns

```
data a;set in.mydata;
      if A=. then ra=0;else ra=1;
      if B=. then rb=0;else rb=1;
      if C=. then rc=0;else rc=1;
      if D=. then rd=0;else rd=1;
run;
proc freq;tables ra*rb*rc*rd/list;
run;
```

the pattern of missing and nonmissing values might look like that shown in Table 9.2 for a 4-item scale, where 1 = data point observed and 0 = data point missing.

The kind of information shown in Table 9.2 can be prepared in a number of ways. Preprocessing the items from the scale with the Norm program (Schafer 1997) will produce this type of table (see Chap. 3). Just select the variables of interest and then run the Summary feature in Norm. The following SAS code (see Table 9.3) may also be used to obtain this information.

The rules here apply pretty much the same to all of the scenarios outlined above. We start with the basic pattern of missing and nonmissing values as shown in Table 9.2. Let us define the three important parts of these patterns as (a) complete data (including patterns that are complete enough to form a scale score by the rules described above), (b) entirely missing data (pattern 5 in Table 9.2), and (c) partial data that do not conform to rules described above (e.g., patterns 3 and 4 in Table 9.2).

Also important are the percentages of people falling into these three categories. Especially important is the percentage of people falling into category (c); these are the cases whose data must be deemed missing for imputing the whole scale. Let us assume that the pattern shown in Table 9.2 was based on a scenario in which we could form a scale score based on having data for 3 of the 4 items. Thus, under these circumstances, we can form a scale score for 97 % of the cases, and 2 % of the cases have no data and must be imputed. That means that in this instance, 1 % of the cases have partial data not conforming to our rules, and the partial data must be discarded.

An important part of this process is for the researcher to ask at this point, "How do I feel about discarding the partial data for 1 % of the cases?" Only the researcher can make this decision. 1 % may seem ok, but 2 % may seem to be too much.

## Issues Regarding Decision Rules

In employing this strategy, one must make some tough choices. The options (listed in approximately the order of the data quality they yield) are these:

(a) Impute at the item level.
(b) Impute whole scales using decision rules described above that involve discarding partial data not conforming to the rules.
(c) Use more lenient decision rules for forming scale scores with partial data, thereby retaining more of the partial data.

Option (a) is clearly the best option for data quality. However, if the model to be tested is even moderately large, the researcher simply may not be able to impute all scales at the item level.

Option (b) has the undesirable characteristic of discarding some data. Unless one's back is against the wall, it is often difficult to do this. However, with this option, there are minimal biases associated with discarding these data. Estimation may be very slightly less precise, but in most instances of this sort, there will be no appreciable estimation bias with discarding the data from these cases.

Option (c) has the desirable characteristic of making use of more data. However, it has the undesirable characteristic of increasing estimation bias. The situations that make this strategy improper are much more likely to exist when the rules described above are violated in order to include more data. It is important that with the previous option (b), the disadvantage of the option is that there is more **random** error. The disadvantage with this option (c) is that there is likely to be more **systematic** error, that is, bias. Because it is generally be more desirable in science to err on the side of increasing random error rather than systematic error, option (b) will generally be preferred to option (c).

On the other hand, it should still be possible to get everything possible out of the data. One important fact here is that you will almost certainly have some flexibility in most situations. For example, suppose you had 10 scales at each of five waves, with four items per scale. That is, $10 \times 4 \times 5 = 200$ items. Or, think of it as 50 scales $\times$ 4 items = 200 items. If you were able to impute at the scale level for 6 of 10 scales at each wave, that would be 30 scales + $16 \times 4 = 64$ individual items = 94 variables in the imputation model.

Also, even when the data do not conform perfectly to the decision rules described above, you may be able to achieve partial benefit of combining items before imputation. For example, in scenarios B1, B2, B3, and B5 described above, it is possible to use a hybrid decision rule by breaking the scale's items into subscales before imputation and then reassembling the scale after imputation. This option makes sense when the scales are on the large side. For example, it might make some sense to break a 4-item scale into two subscales. This would still reduce the number of items for imputation from 4 to 2. But it makes less sense to employ this approach (e.g., with scenario B4) when three subscales are needed to deal with a four-item scale.

Table 9.4 Sample missing data pattern matrix

| Pattern | Item | | | | Frequency (%) |
|---|---|---|---|---|---|
| | A | B | C | D | |
| 1 | 1 | 1 | 1 | 1 | 80 |
| 2 | 1 | 1 | 1 | 0 | 17 |
| 3 | 0 | 0 | 1 | 1 | 0.5 |
| 4 | 1 | 0 | 0 | 1 | 0.5 |
| 5 | 0 | 0 | 0 | 0 | 2 |

This general approach may also be used with scenarios A4, A5, and A6. For example, suppose one had a missingness scenario depicted in Table 9.4. With scenario A5, for example, we have recommended that the scale score be formed only when all the items have data. In the situation depicted in Table 9.4, it would be good to think of the 4-item scale as two subscales: items A, B, and C as one subscale and item D as a separate subscale. The data for people with patterns 1 and 2 (97 % of the sample) have complete data for the subscale made up of items A, B, and C. For those with pattern 2, data for item D only would be imputed.

## Splitting Variable Set for Multiple-Pass Multiple Imputation

Situations do arise in which the strategy of imputing scales is not a good solution. One such situation arises when the researcher wants to make use of the individual variables, for example, with latent variable analysis. In this situation, medium to large models might well involve more than the recommended 100 variables. If the study involves just 10 constructs, each measured at four times with four items, the researcher has 160 variables. With just a few demographic and other background variables, this number would be even higher. If the data have been collected with a nested structure (e.g., students within schools), this could add even more variables easily bringing the total to more than 200 variables. This number of variables could be a problem for a multiple imputation analysis, even if the research has thousands of cases.

A second situation may arise in which the number of variables is no more than 100, but the number of cases is small enough to make even that number inadvisable. The basic problem is that one often needs to impute more individual variables than can reasonably be handled by the software.

One solution to the problem is to break the variables into parts. For example, if the researcher has 200 variables, he or she could do two sets of multiple imputation analyses, each involving, say, 100 variables. The problem with this solution is that the two separate sets of variables are each imputed under the model that all variables in one set are correlated $r=0$ with all the variables in the other set. This is hardly a desirable solution.

## *A Solution That Makes Sense*

Following up with our example, suppose we have 200 variables. Set 1 contains 100 variables, and Set 2 contains the remaining 100 variables. If the variables in Set 1 really are uncorrelated with those in Set 2, then we can go ahead and impute the two sets separately.

Of course, it will virtually never be the case in empirical data that the between-set correlations are exactly $r=0$. However, it might well be the case that the correlations between variables from one set to the other are so small as to make any biases tolerably small. Any biases involved in imputing separately in two sets of variables can be reduced further if at least some of the information from set 1 can be used for imputing set 2 and vice versa. The strategy outlined below accomplishes this goal.

**Overview**

The five steps of the process, shown below, are these:

Step 1: Principal components analysis to identify the two sets of variables.
Step 2: Impute single data set from EM parameters in each variable set.
Step 3: Generate 10 principal components factor scores for each variable set.
Step 4: Do MI with set 1 variables and set 2 factor scores; and with set 2 variables and set 1 factor scores.
Step 5: Combine the two sets of imputations, dropping the factor scores.

**Solution Step 1**

The first step is to create two sets of variables that are roughly equal in size, and that are as uncorrelated as possible. One can do this with principal components analysis. Because there are too many variables to do multiple imputation, there are likely too many variables to perform the EM algorithm as well. Thus, at this step, we suggest using pairwise deletion. Although this is not generally an acceptable solution (e.g., see Graham and Hofer 2000; Graham 2009), it is acceptable in this one context.

The following SAS code achieves this:

```
proc corr out=ds1 noprint;var x1-x200;
run;
proc factor data=ds1(type=corr) method=prin rotate=promax
     nfact=2 reorder;
   var x1-x200;
run;
```

For SPSS, click on Analyze, Dimension Reduction, and Factor. Select the desired variables (e.g., ×1, ×2, ×3 … ×200). Under Extraction, select Principal Components (the default), and click on Fix number of factors (enter 2). Under Rotation, click on Promax. Under Options, choose Exclude cases pairwise, and click on Sorted by size.

The following SPSS syntax also performs this analysis:

```
DATASET ACTIVATE DataSet1.
FACTOR
   /VARIABLES x1 x2 x3 ... x200 [apparently you must list all
   variables]
   /MISSING PAIRWISE
   /ANALYSIS x1 x2 x3 ... x200 [again, list them all]
   /PRINT INITIAL EXTRACTION ROTATION
   /FORMAT SORT
   /CRITERIA FACTORS(2) ITERATE(25)
   /EXTRACTION PC
   /CRITERIA ITERATE(25)
   /ROTATION PROMAX(4)
   /METHOD=CORRELATION.
```

The results of this analysis will divide the data into two sets that are maximally uncorrelated. However, there are two possible drawbacks to the results based on this first principal components analysis. First, it is likely than some, even many variables will load highly on neither factor. Second, it may well happen that many more items load more highly on factor 1 than on factor 2.

The first problem is not really a problem. This is not a factor (or principal components) analysis in the usual sense. We are just trying to get two sets of variables that are maximally uncorrelated. If a particular variable loads about the same on the two factors, that is ok. Just put it with the factor for which it loads slightly higher. This also applies if a particular item load is near zero on both factors. Just put it with the factor for which it loads slightly higher.

The second problem could be more serious. If the number of variables loading on the two factors is very different, we may not have achieved our goal. For example, if 150 variables load on factor 1, and only 50 load on factor 2, this may not be a good solution, because handling 150 variables all at once may be little better than handling 200 variables all at once.

If the differences are this large, one option may be to split the variables into three groups, that is, by asking for a 3-factor solution. This will almost always help the situation. On the other hand, if the differences are more modest (e.g., 115 and 85), one can probably live with the difference.

**Solution Step 2**

Once the variables have been divided into the two (or more) groups, conduct a regular missing data analysis separately for each group. Read the data in, run the EM algorithm, and then ask the program to impute a single data set from EM parameters.

For SAS users, sample code is as follows:

```
proc mi data=a nimpute=1 out=b;
   var x1-x100;
   mcmc nbiter=0 niter=0;
run;
```

For SPSS users, within the Norm program, read the data in for each set, run the EM algorithm, and then ask the program to impute a single data set from EM parameters (see Chap. 3). This data set may then be read back into SPSS using the MIAutomate utility (see Chap. 5).

This data set will have the property of having parameter estimates that are near the middle of parameter space. It is not good for hypothesis testing, because there is no way to estimate standard errors, however it is a very good way to perform analyses, for which hypothesis testing is typically not done, for example, for exploratory factor analysis (see Graham et al. 2003). In addition, this singly imputed data set is good in that factor scores may be written out (factor scores can be written only if there are complete data).

## Solution Step 3

Perform principal components analysis on each of the sets of variables identified in Step 1, using the data sets created in Step 2.

Sample SAS code for performing these analyses is as follows (note that the factor scores will have no missing data in these analyses):

```
proc mi data=a nimpute=1 out=b1;
    var x1-x100;
    mcmc nbiter=0 niter=0;
run;
proc factor method=prin rotate=promax score out=c1 nfact=10;
    var x1-x100;
run;
data d1;set c1;
        setA1=factor1;
        setA2=factor2;
        setA3=factor3;
            *** and so on ***;
    keep ID x101-x200 setA1-setA10;
run;
proc mi data=a nimpute=1 out=b2;
    var x101-x200;
    mcmc nbiter=0 niter=0;
run;
proc factor method=prin rotate=promax score out=c2 nfact=10;
    var x101-x200;
run;
data d2;set c2;
        setB1=factor1;
        setB2=factor2;
        setB3=factor3;
            *** and so on ***;
    keep ID x1-x100 setB1-setB10;
run;
```

# Splitting Variable Set for Multiple-Pass Multiple Imputation 227

In SPSS, the logic is the same, but the imputation steps should be carried out in NORM, and imported into SPSS using the MIAutomate utility for the principal components and analysis and writing of factor scores.

## Solution Step 4

Impute the two data sets separately, asking for, say, 40 imputed data sets for each.
Sample SAS code is given below:

```
proc mi data=d1 nimpute=40 out=e1;
   var x101-x200 setA1-setA10;
   mcmc nbiter=* niter=*;
run;
*** The nbiter and niter values will be set according to the
performance of EM -- see Chapter 7 ***;
proc mi data=d2 nimpute=40 out=e2;
      var x1-x100 setB1-setB10;
      mcmc nbiter=* niter=*;
run;
```

In SPSS the logic is the same, except that the imputation steps are carried out in NORM (see Chap. 3) and the results are imported into SPSS by the MIAutomate utility (see Chap. 5).

## Solution Step 5

Combine the two sets of imputed data sets (merge them), discarding the two sets of factor scores.
Sample SAS code is given below:

```
data x1;set e1;
   keep ID _imputation_ x101-x200;
run;
proc sort;by _imputation_ ID;
run;
data x2;set e2;
   keep ID _imputation_ x1-x100;
run;
proc sort;by _imputation_ ID;
run;
data x;merge x1 x2;by _imputation_ ID;
run;
```

## Comments

As we stated at the outset of this section, the problem with imputing two sets of variables separately is that the imputation is done under the model that all correlations are $r=0$ between the variables in one set and the variables in the other set. The data sets created using this procedure will have been imputed under a different model. First, the actual correlation between the two sets will be minimized by selecting the variable sets with principal components analysis. Second, the variables in Set A are not unrepresented in the imputation of variables in Set B and vice versa. They are represented by the factor scores.

It could be argued that this is not an optimal solution to the problem of having too many variables for the multiple imputation programs to handle all at once. Although this may be true, it is, at present, the only solution we have. Further, although simulations remain to be conducted to test the performance of this procedure, our intuition is that it will work very well in real empirical data.

One alternative to procedures such as this is simply to impute all the variables at once. Imputing large numbers of variables (e.g., $k=200$ or greater) will work, in theory. Well-behaved (e.g., normally distributed) simulation data based on large numbers of variables should, for example, produce results that are as unbiased and efficient as are results based on smaller numbers of variables. But problems arise with this approach. Most importantly, the imputation process can take a long time. Stories exist, for example, of imputation models taking weeks to be complete. Two issues arise here. First, when the imputation model is churning and churning, there is no guarantee that it will ultimately be successful. It takes enormous faith, for example, to wait 1 or 2 months for the imputation results. Add to that the enormous task of double-checking the data augmentation (or MCMC) diagnostic plots, and we have a very difficult situation. Second, and perhaps more importantly, it would be virtually impossible to perform a simulation to verify that these very large MI problems do, in fact, produce proper, usable solutions. If one replication of the simulation takes 2 months, then even with very fast computers, the simulation with 1,000 replications would take 2,000 months (167 years). Even with massively distributed processing, this task would be daunting.

## References

Graham, J. W. (2009). Missing data analysis: making it work in the real world. *Annual Review of Psychology, 60,* 549–576.

Graham, J. W., & Hofer, S. M. (2000). Multiple imputation in multivariate research. In T. D. Little, K. U. Schnabel, & J. Baumert, (Eds.), *Modeling longitudinal and multiple-group data: Practical issues, applied approaches, and specific examples.* (pp. 201–218). Hillsdale, NJ: Erlbaum.

Graham, J. W., Cumsille, P. E., & Elek-Fisk, E. (2003). Methods for handling missing data. In J. A. Schinka & W. F. Velicer (Eds.). *Research Methods in Psychology* (pp. 87–114). Volume 2 of *Handbook of Psychology* (I. B. Weiner, Editor-in-Chief). New York: John Wiley & Sons.

Schafer, J. L. (1997). *Analysis of Incomplete Multivariate Data.* New York: Chapman and Hall.

Schafer, J. L., & Graham, J. W. (2002). Missing data: our view of the state of the art. *Psychological Methods, 7,* 147–177.

# Chapter 10
# Simulations with Missing Data

## Who Should Read This Chapter?

If you have some experience with simulation work, then much of what I say here in the early part of this chapter should be a review. However, even if you do have prior experience with this topic, I believe it will be good to see my take on the more traditional Monte Carlo approach to missing data. Also important is that having a good sense of the traditional Monte Carlo approach to simulations will be a good setup for the non-Monte Carlo simulations I describe toward the end of this chapter.

If you have no prior experience with simulation work, I believe you will also find this chapter useful. You should be able to pick up enough basic knowledge in this chapter to allow you to begin to do at least some simulation work. However, if you are in this category, it may be good to find a general introduction to doing simulation studies (e.g., see Fan et al. 2002).

At the very least, having a sense of how the non-Monte Carlo simulations work will be valuable in other chapters in this book (Chaps. 11 and 13).

## Background

As computers have become more and more powerful, researchers have begun to rely more and more heavily on simulations to address their questions. In this chapter, I talk about simulations, particularly those relating to the study and analysis of missing data. The most commonly used simulations are usually called Monte Carlo simulations. I will start here by describing the rudiments of this kind of simulation. I will include what I feel are important admonitions regarding the conduct of simulations.

A less used approach to simulation work will also be covered in this chapter. This approach starts with one of the first accessible methods for analysis of missing data (Allison 1987; Muthen et al. 1987), an approach that made use of the multiple group

(MG) capabilities of structural equation modeling (SEM) programs (e.g., LISREL; Jöreskog and Sörbom 1996).

The key feature of this approach, which I refer to as MGSEM, is that one can work with the population covariance matrix, thereby obviating the need to generate thousands of data sets as with the Monte Carlo approach. As I will point out in a later section of this chapter, this difference in approaches amounts to a 200-fold difference in the time it takes to complete a simulation.

Studies that have made use of this MGSEM approach to simulations (e.g., Graham et al. 2001; Graham et al. 2006) have always made the assumption that the missingness was MCAR, which, with planned missing data designs is a good assumption. In this chapter, however, I also describe the nontrivial extension of working with population covariance matrices to MAR (and NMAR) missingness. In so doing, I demonstrate how one might employ this much more compact MGSEM approach to address simulation questions that heretofore have been handled using the Monte Carlo simulation approach.

## General Issues to Consider with Simulations

### What Are the Goals of Your Simulation?

Be absolutely clear and explicit about the goals of your simulation.

### What Other Approaches Are Available to Achieve Your Goals?

The best reason for using a Monte Carlo simulation is that a closed-form solution is not possible for your question. This may often be the case, but I think researchers are a bit too quick these days to ignore the possibility that there may be an algebraic solution to the problem. Remember that a Monte Carlo solution is, by its very nature, only an approximate solution. That is, the results from Monte Carlo simulations are fully stable only when the procedure is repeated an infinite number of times. Thus, even when the procedure is replicated, say, 1,000 times, there are still some differences between average parameter estimates over the first 1,000 replications, and the parameter estimates over a second 1,000 replication. I refer to such differences as simulation "wobble." It is true that results from a good simulation can be immensely valuable; but would not it be even more valuable, not to mention elegant, if a closed-form solution were possible?

In a later section of this chapter, I describe a non-Monte Carlo simulation approach that may, in some circumstances, provides results that are as good in many respects as a closed-form solution. I will describe this approach for MCAR

## What Should the Simulation Parameters Be?

Some simulations attempt to cover a broad range of parameters. For example, Collins et al. (2001) examined $\mu_Y$ (the mean of Y, the variable with missing values), $\sigma_Y^2$ (the variance of Y), $\beta_{YX}$ (the regression coefficient for X, an important substantive variable, predicting Y), $\beta_{XY}$ (the regression coefficient for Y predicting X, and $\rho_{XY}$ (the correlation between X and Y). Alternatively, the simulation may be more focused. For example, if the simulation is meant to apply to evaluations of interventions, then it could be that fewer parameters are needed. Under these more focused circumstances, it could be that one would examine just $\beta_{YX}$, or under some circumstances, perhaps $\beta_{YX}$ and $\mu_Y$. Either the broad or more focused approach can prove to be valuable.

Several parameters relate to missingness, per se. One variable often studied is whether the missingness is MCAR, MAR, or NMAR (see Chap. 1). Within MCAR missingness, the major variable is the percent missing. Another possible variable in this context is the pattern of missingness (e.g., missing on one variable; missing on several variables within the same individuals; more complex missingness patterns). Within MAR missingness, Collins et al. (2001) studied three different kinds of MAR missingness: "MAR Linear," "MAR Convex," and "MAR Sinister" (see Collins et al. 2001; also see Chap. 1, and later in this chapter for more details). Also important within MAR missingness are (a) percent missing; (b) $\rho_{XY}$; (c) $\rho_{YZ}$ (where Z is the "cause" of missingness); and (d) $\rho_{YR}$, where R is a dichotomous variable representing missingness, per se ($R=0$ if Y is missing; $R=1$ if Y is not missing; see Chap. 1). MAR missingness typically involves including Z in the missing data model. NMAR missingness is generally the same as MAR, except that Z is excluded from the missing data model.

## What Should the Range of Parameter Values Be?

I believe that these choices are hugely important. I think one of the biggest mistakes simulation researchers make is to select parameter values, or ranges of parameters, that are not representative of the substantive research domain to which the simulation should apply.

The big issue here is to tie the range of parameter values (a) to the research question, and (b) to reality. Be able to argue why it is that this particular range of parameter values (and these parameters) helps one address the goals of the simulation. Also, be able to provide solid evidence from the relevant empirical literature to support the use of one parameter range or other.

## Monte Carlo Simulations

As I stated at the outset of this chapter, my discussion of Monte Carlo simulations is intended to be review for readers who already have some experience with these methods. Readers who do not have experience with Monte Carlo methods will find enough material here to get started using these methods. All readers will find this material a good lead-in for the non-Monte Carlo methods described in a later section.

### *Start with a Population and Generate Samples*

A simple Monte Carlo simulation starts with population values for several parameters, for example, means, variances, and correlations. From those parameters, one generates raw data (with normal or nonnormal distributions), such that a large sample (e.g., $N = 1,000,000$) will produce values very close to the population values. When one wishes to study some aspect of missing data or analysis with missing data, the procedure often begins this way.

There are several ways to conceive of the population. One way is to think of the population parameters described above as the population. With this strategy, one can generate numerous samples from that population. With this approach, one might generate numerous samples of, say, $N = 500$, using a data generation program. I often use an old program associated with LISREL 8 (Jöreskog and Sörbom 1996) called GENRAW.

A second approach is to start with the population parameters as described above, but rather than generating the numerous samples directly, one might first generate a single large sample (e.g., $N = 1,000,000$), and then call that the population, and draw random samples from that. The good thing about the first strategy is that the expected value for all parameters over a large number of samples will be the population parameter values. One bad thing about that strategy, however, relates to the fact that the next step, degrading the data set, creates some issues with population parameter values. This happens because some strategies for degrading the data set often require that at least one variable have a distribution other than normal (e.g., a 4-level variable with uniform distribution; see below). Thus the second approach may be preferred, because it may be possible to come very close to the desired population parameter values (especially correlations) in a population of a specific size, even when one or more of the variables are not normally distributed. Another advantage of this strategy is that one may use more standard software (e.g., SAS) to generate the "population" using standard SAS functions.

▶ **Sample Data**. The following SAS code provides a very simple model for generating a smallish population ($N = 100,000$) of the sort just described. The code shown below generates two variables (X and Y) that are correlated approximately $r = .50$. One can fiddle with the code, for example, by using differential weighting, to produce different correlations. The code also shows a way to draw a random sample of $N = 500$ from the population.

```
data a;*** step 1: generate the population ***;
    do i=1 to 100000;
        a = normal(0);
        X = a + normal(0);
        Y = a + normal(0);
        output;
    end;
run;
data b;set a;
    rx = uniform(0); *** step 2: sort the population by a new
    random variable ***;
run;
proc sort;by rx;
run;
data c;set b; *** step 3: generate the random sample of N = 500
***;
    if _n_ < = 500;
run;
```

With this approach, one should generate the population once and save it to a permanent file. Then each subsequent step is drawn from the same population with known parameter values.

A variant of this second approach starts with a "population" based on real empirical data. In one Monte Carlo simulation study, for example, our "population" was defined as a sample of $N=12,000$, from which we drew repeated samples of $N=100$ or $N=50$ (Graham and Schafer 1999). The nice thing about this variant is that the population parameter estimates are very realistic (because they come from real empirical data). Another nice thing about this approach is that the distributions of the variables are realistic. One drawback with this approach, however, is that the researcher has little control over the population parameter values or the distributions used.

Using any of these approaches, the key is that the population parameter values (and distributions) are known. This means that the results of any analysis can be compared against a meaningful gold standard.

## *Degrading the Sample*

The next step with a Monte Carlo simulation with missing data is to degrade the sample data set, that is, create the missing data. For starters, one must decide whether the missingness mechanism will be MCAR, MAR, or NMAR, or some combination of these mechanisms. Let me begin with the simplest case in which missingness is MCAR, and a single variable has missing values.

## MCAR Missingness

MCAR is actually very easy to accomplish. If you start with a sample of $N=500$, and want 50 % missing on a variable, say "Y", you can simply set Y to missing for the first 250 cases of the sample data set. Because the generated data were a random sample from the population, the first 250 cases of that sample represent a random sample of the sample.

▶ **Sample Data.** The following SAS code shows one way to degrade the data set just described. This code sets the variable Y to be missing for a random 50 % of the sample.

```
data d;set c;
    if _n_ < = 250 then Y=.;
run;
```

## MAR Missingness

MAR is also not difficult. Recall that MAR missingness on Y may be due to some variable you have measured, but it is not due to a variable you have not measured. In this case, I have a simple model in which the missingness on Y is due to X. But what is the form of the MAR missingness? I generally use ***MAR-linear*** to generate my missing data. But as I indicated above (also see Chap. 1), other forms of MAR are possible.

▶ **Sample Data.** The SAS code for a simple degrading of the sample data set using MAR-linear is given below. Note that for degrading the sample with MAR-linear missingness, I first change the variable X to be a four-category variable with a uniform distribution.

```
proc rank data=c out=d groups=4;var X;
    *** note that this code produces a new version of X that has
    values 0, 1, 2, and 3. Missingness on Y will be MAR if this
    new version of X is used in the missing data analysis model
    (e.g., the MI model). Note also that the correlation with Y
    will be somewhat lower ***;
run;
data e;set d;
    rx = uniform(0);
    if X = 0 and rx < .20 then Y=.;
    if X = 1 and rx < .40 then Y=.;
    if X = 2 and rx < .60 then Y=.;
    if X = 3 and rx < .80 then Y=.;
run;
```

# Monte Carlo Simulations

The IF statements shown above have a rather strong "lever" on missingness (Graham 2009). That is, with these statements, the correlation between X and *missingness* itself (a dichotomous variable, often called "R", with 0 if Y is missing and 1 if Y is present; see Chap. 1) is $r_{XR}=.447$. But an even stronger effect on missingness is possible:

```
if X = 0 and rx < .05 then Y=.;
if X = 1 and rx < .35 then Y=.;
if X = 2 and rx < .65 then Y=.;
if X = 3 and rx < .95 then Y=.;
```

These statements produce $r_{XR}=.671$, which is nearly the strongest MAR-linear effect possible. It is also easy to have IF statements that would produce a much weaker effect on missingness:

```
if X = 0 and rx < .35 then Y=.;
if X = 1 and rx < .45 then Y=.;
if X = 2 and rx < .55 then Y=.;
if X = 3 and rx < .65 then Y=.;
```

These statements produce $r_{XR}=.224$. And an even weaker effect ($r_{XR}=.045$) would be produced with these IF statements.

```
if X = 0 and rx < .47 then Y=.;
if X = 1 and rx < .49 then Y=.;
if X = 2 and rx < .51 then Y=.;
if X = 3 and rx < .53 then Y=.;
```

The important thing to consider about the strength of the "lever" on missingness relates to what is reasonable with respect to what is known from the relevant literature. I will discuss this more a bit later in this chapter, but the bottom line is that the strength of the lever used in a simulation should not be selected arbitrarily.

Another point to make about the IF statements shown above is that they all produce 50 % missingness on Y (look at the average of the four probabilities given in each case). For 25 % missingness, the IF statements might look like this:

```
if X = 0 and rx < .10 then Y=.;
if X = 1 and rx < .20 then Y=.;
if X = 2 and rx < .30 then Y=.;
if X = 3 and rx < .40 then Y=.;
```

This produces one of the stronger "levers" on missingness possible with 25 % missingness (although somewhat stronger levers are possible), but $r_{XR}=.224$. With the weaker lever shown below, $r_{XR}=.075$.

```
if X = 0 and rx < .200 then Y=.;
if X = 1 and rx < .233 then Y=.;
if X = 2 and rx < .267 then Y=.;
if X = 3 and rx < .300 then Y=.;
```

This illustrates that two things happen with less missingness. First, the smaller amount of missing data has a milder impact on statistical conclusions even under the worst conditions. Second, the correlation $r_{XR}$ is also smaller, rendering the effect on statistical conclusions even less problematic.

## MAR-Convex Missingness

MAR-Convex missingness, as described by Collins et al. (2001) was produced with IF statements like the following:

```
if X = 0 and rx < .80 then Y=.;
if X = 1 and rx < .20 then Y=.;
if X = 2 and rx < .20 then Y=.;
if X = 3 and rx < .80 then Y=.;
```

## NMAR-Linear Missingness

NMAR-linear missingness can also be relatively straightforward. Recall that missingness on Y is NMAR if the missingness is due to some variable that has not been measured (or is simply not used in the missing data analysis model). The two ways this can occur are (a) if the cause of missingness on Y (Z) is a variable that is correlated with Y, but that has not been measured (or simply not used in the missing data analysis model), and (b) if the Y itself (or a version of it) is the cause of its own missingness.

An example of the first case is that the variable Rebelliousness is a cause of missingness on Drug Use in a prevention study. And Rebelliousness (Z) and Drug Use (Y) are correlated $r_{YZ}=\sim.40$. An example of the second case is the Drug Use (Y) is the cause of its own missingness. That is, Z=Y. Note that in this latter case, it is not necessarily the case that Z and Y are perfectly correlated, $r_{YZ}=1.0$. In fact, one of the most straightforward ways of generating missing data of this form is to create a normally distributed Y variable as shown above, and then create a uniformly distributed, 4-category version of Y with the Proc Rank, for example:

```
proc rank data=c out=d groups=4;var y;ranks z;
    *** note that this code produces a new version of y (Z) that
    has values 0, 1, 2, and 3. Note also that the correlation
    with Y will be somewhat lower: r  =~.925 rather than r  =1.;
                                    yz                    yz
run;
```

```
data e;set d;
   rx=uniform(0);
   if Z=0 and rx<.20 then Y=.;
   if Z=1 and rx<.40 then Y=.;
   if Z=2 and rx<.60 then Y=.;
   if Z=3 and rx<.80 then Y=.;
run;
```

As with MAR-linear missingness, with NMAR-linear missingness, even when $r_{YZ} > .9$, the correlation $r_{ZR}$ need not be large. The IF statements shown above reflect a rather strong lever on missingness ($r_{ZR} = .447$). Most importantly, the strength of this lever (i.e., the magnitude of $r_{ZR}$) is independent of the $r_{YZ}$, the correlation between the cause of missingness (Z) and the main outcome variable (Y), which is sometimes missing. That is, a strong lever on missingness (i.e., a large value of $r_{ZR}$) is no more likely with NMAR missingness than it is with MAR missingness and is no more likely with large values of $r_{YZ}$ than with small values of $r_{YZ}$.

## Automation Strategies

Automation is essential in Monte Carlo simulations. The process is: generate the sample, perform analysis, and combine the results. The problem is that this process must be repeated *many* times. I have seen many situations in which 100 replications are too few even to have a glimpse of reality. I have seen situations where results do not begin to stabilize adequately until I got to 20,000 replications. In any event, simulations are time intensive even with automation and are simply impossible without automation.

### SAS and Other Full-Featured Software

Some simulations are pretty easy within the SAS framework (see Fan et al. 2002). I can generate the data in a DATA step (producing population parameters close to desired levels), degrade the data, perform the analysis, and combine the results, all in a single SAS syntax file. The last part, combining the results, is very nice in the SAS environment, because it is always the case with SAS PROCs that the parameters and standard errors may be output to a SAS data set. In addition, PROC MI allows one to perform multiple imputation analysis as part of the process if that is what one wants. Finally, the SAS Macro language allows for relatively simple automation of the process.

Statisticians and others commonly use the R or S-plus packages for Monte Carlo simulation work. These packages are not in common use in the social and behavioral sciences, but they provide an excellent framework for generating, degrading, and analyzing data, and for combining the results from thousands of replications of the simulation.

**Stand-Alone Simulation Software**

Another approach I take to doing Monte Carlo simulations is to write my own automation software. This is especially valuable when the analysis I want to do is not available in SAS (e.g., LISREL or HLM, etc.). With this approach, it is important to be able to write code in one of the programming languages. It is best if you can write in C++ or even FORTRAN. I happen to write my code in the ancient BASIC language (using an equally ancient BASIC compiler to produce stand-alone \*\*\*.exe files). With this approach, just as with any approach to Monte Carlo simulations, the key steps are:

Data generation
Degrading the data
Analysis
Combining results

**Simulations Involving Multiple Imputation**

For simulations involving MI, per se, for example, when MI inference with some number of imputations is part of the question to be addressed by the simulation (e.g., see Graham et al. 2007), I find that using SAS (or equivalent full-featured statistical package, such as R or S-plus) is recommended.

**Simulations Involving EM Algorithm**

On the other hand, some simulations focus on parameter estimation and do not necessarily need the overhead connected with obtaining standard errors via MI inference. For simulations like this, it is often useful simply to employ a stand-alone EM algorithm program (e.g., EMCOV; Graham and Hofer 1992; Graham and Donaldson 1993; Graham et al. 1996). Simulations such as these would simply insert additional lines of code to run the EM program.

## *Technical Issues to Consider in Monte Carlo Simulations*

**Random Number Generators**

One issue that comes up in Monte Carlo simulations relates to what constitutes randomness. Random selection has as its primary rule that all elements in the population have an equal probability of being selected. The problem with this is that many random number generators violate this basic rule. Random number generators that are based on the computer's clock to generating a starting seed, for example, are not truly random, because the clock values represent only a subset of all possible starting seeds. The bottom line is that you should find a random number generator that conforms to standards of randomness. One good one is the program from Numerical Recipes (see Press et al. 2007; also see http://www.nr.com).

**Simulation "Convergence"**

By simulation "convergence," I mean that the key parameter estimates of the simulation have stabilized sufficiently to allow you to draw good conclusions. *All* Monte Carlo simulations have what I call "simulation wobble." That is, even after tens of thousands of replications, the plots of key simulation parameters over variations in parameter values will not be perfectly smooth. The point is that a large enough number of replications must be run so that such plots (or equivalent tabled values) are smooth enough that good conclusions can be made.

One area of particular concern is the monotonicity of certain findings over variations of one parameter. For example, given a particular sample size, as the percent of missing data increases on a key variable, the amount of bias in NMAR models must increase. Similarly, the amount of estimation bias over variations of $r_{YZ}$ (the correlation between the cause of missingness, Z, and the variable that is sometimes missing, Y) must be monotonic. If a simulation seems to be showing that the amount of estimation bias is not monotonic in these (and other) cases, then there were too few replications in the simulation.

Granted, missing data theory is not always correct. But if the goal of your simulation is to demonstrate that missing data theory is wrong in one way or other, you had better demonstrate first that you have done your simulation completely correctly. I would suggest that you also have a theoretical argument as to why missing data theory was incorrect in that instance.

# Non-Monte Carlo Simulation with the MGSEM Procedure

This section describes procedures that make use of multiple group SEM analysis. In order to follow everything I present in this section, you must have at least some experience with multiple group SEM analysis. I happen to use the LISREL program, but I present the material in this section in a more generic way, so experience with any SEM package will be fine.

On the other hand, if you do not have experience with multiple group SEM analysis, or with any kind of SEM analysis, you can still follow the main points presented in this section. An important benefit of using this approach is that one is able to work with the population covariance matrix directly. Because of this, where this procedure is applicable, one is able to obtain parameter estimates and standard errors for the population, without having to conduct tens of thousands of replications that are needed with Monte Carlo methods.

**Table 10.1** Patterns of missingness

| Group | X | Y | Z | N |
|---|---|---|---|---|
| 1 | 1 | 1 | 1 | 500 |
| 2 | 1 | 0 | 1 | 500 |

**Table 10.2** Covariance matrix for Group 1

|   | X | Y | Z |
|---|---|---|---|
| X | 1.00 | | |
| Y | .10 | 1.00 | |
| Z | .10 | .60 | 1.00 |
| Means | 0.00 | 0.00 | 0.00 |

## *The Multiple Group SEM Procedure for MCAR Missingness: Overview*

What I am calling the MGSEM procedure was described by Allison (1987) and by Muthen et al. (1987). One begins by dividing up the sample into groups representing different patterns of missing and nonmissing values. Let me begin with a simple model in which there are three variables, X (the independent variable in a simple regression model), Y (the dependent variable in the regression model), and Z (an auxiliary variable, i.e., a variable that is correlated with Y, but not part of the analysis model).

To start, I assume that X and Z are never missing, but that Y is missing for 50 % of the cases. I assume further that any missingness on Y is purely of the MCAR variety. That is, I assume that the group with complete data on the three variables is a random sample of the total sample. Under these assumptions, I have the patterns of missing and observed values shown in Table 10.1.

If missingness on Y is purely MCAR, then I can assume that the covariance matrices and means in the two groups are the same. For example, suppose that the covariance matrix and means in Group 1 are as shown in Table 10.2.

In its simplest form, the MGSEM procedure is a two-group SEM model. Group 1 is set up in the usual way. Group 2 begins with a special covariance matrix (and means) as input. Where covariances are estimable, they appear as they did in Group 1. Where data are missing for a particular covariance, that element is given as "0" in the input matrix. Variances for nonmissing data are given the same as in Group 1. Variances for missing values are given as "1" in Group 2. Means for missing variables are given as "0" in Group 2. The Group 2 covariance matrix and vector of means would look as shown in Table 10.3 for the current example.

The SEM setup in Group 2 is the same as in a normal two-group model with some exceptions. The factor-level parameters (factor variances and covariances, factor regressions, factor means) are all set to be invariant in the two groups. Where

**Table 10.3** Covariance matrix for Group 2

|       | X    | Y    | Z    |
|-------|------|------|------|
| X     | 1.00 |      |      |
| Y     | .00  | 1.00 |      |
| Z     | .10  | .00  | 1.00 |
| Means | 0.00 | 0.00 | 0.00 |

item-level parameters (e.g., factor loadings and item residual variances) have data in Group 2, the parameters are estimated, and constrained to be equal to the same parameter in Group 1. If a factor loading is associated with a missing value, it is given as "0" in Group 2 (even if the value was fixed at "1" in Group 1). If an item residual variance is associated with a missing value, it is given as "1" in Group 2 (even if it is fixed at "0" in Group 1).

## *Examples of Good Uses of the MGSEM Procedure for MCAR Missingness*

Chapter 11 describes the statistical power benefits of including one or more auxiliary variables in the missing data model. That work was all done under the assumption that the missingness on Y was MCAR (please see Chap. 11 for details). Chapter 13 describes a planned missing data design that my colleagues and I have called "two-method measurement" (Graham et al. 2006). This design involves collecting data using two different approaches to measure a key construct. One measure is relatively cheap and is administered to all participants. The other measure is much more expensive and is administered only to a random sample of the participants. Thus, missingness on the more expensive measure is MCAR (please see Chap. 13 for details).

## *Overview of MGSEM Procedure for MAR/NMAR Missingness*

With MCAR missingness on Y, those with complete cases on X, Y, and Z can be thought of as a random sample of the total sample. Thus, under MCAR, it makes sense that the means, variances, and correlations in Groups 1 and 2 (see above) are all the same (where there are data in Group 2). However, with MAR missingness on Y, this is not true. But at least at a theoretical level, one can conceive of the two sets of parameters (means, variances, and correlations) in these two groups, even under MAR missingness. For example, it would certainly be possible to use the Monte Carlo simulation approach described above to generate a large number of cases, and then degrade that data set such that Y was missing, due to Z, in, say, 50 % of the cases.

It would then be possible to calculate the means, variances, and correlations in the two groups to see how they differ.

Of course, doing this in the general case would amount to nothing less than a full Monte Carlo simulation. The parameter estimates one would get from any one replication of such a simulation, even with very large sample sizes (e.g., $N = 10,000,000$), would still just approximate the true population parameter values. However, once these approximate population values are known, it may be possible to see, in a closed-form sense, what those population parameter values should be under certain assumptions.

In this chapter, I describe MAR missingness of the sort described by Collins et al. (2001) as **MAR-linear** missingness. The IF statements such as those shown below would produce MAR-linear missingness. In this case, Z has uniform distribution with the four values, 0, 1, 2, and 3.

```
data e;set d;
    rx = uniform(0);
    if Z = 0 and rx < .20 then Y=.;
    if Z = 1 and rx < .40 then Y=.;
    if Z = 2 and rx < .60 then Y=.;
    if Z = 3 and rx < .80 then Y=.;
run;
```

In this chapter, I describe MAR missingness of this sort (MAR-linear) when there is 50 % missingness on Y, and where the variances of the three variables (X, Y, and Z) are equal.

Under these conditions, some very interesting things emerge. Before getting to these things, however, I first need to define the **Range** as the difference between the smallest and largest probabilities in the MAR-linear IF statements of the sort shown above. For example, in the IF statements shown above, the highest probability is .8 and the lowest is .2, so the Range in this instance would be .6. Second the subscript "1", below, refers to the parameter value in Group 1, the group with complete data on the three variables. The subscript "2" refers to the parameter value in Group 2, the group with missing data on the variable Y. Finally, all parameter values are shown below, even though all Group 2 parameter values relating to Y would not normally be known.

## Means in Groups 1 and 2

The change in the mean of Z is a function of the Range for the IF statements, the variance of Z, and a constant (2/3). Note that the mean in Group 1 is lower by this function, and the mean in Group 2 is higher by the same function. The change in the mean of X is a function of the Range, the variance of X, the constant (2/3), and the correlation between X and Z. The change in the mean of Y is a function of the Range, the variance of Y, the constant (2/3), and the correlation between Y and Z.

$$\mu_{Z1} = \mu_Z - \text{Range} * \sigma^2_Z * (2/3)$$
$$\mu_{Z2} = \mu_Z + \text{Range} * \sigma^2_Z * (2/3)$$

$$\mu_{X1} = \mu_X - \text{Range} * \sigma^2_X * (2/3) * \rho_{XZ}$$
$$\mu_{X2} = \mu_X + \text{Range} * \sigma^2_X * (2/3) * \rho_{XZ}$$

$$\mu_{Y1} = \mu_Y - \text{Range} * \sigma^2_Y * (2/3) * \rho_{YZ}$$
$$\mu_{Y2} = \mu_Y + \text{Range} * \sigma^2_Y * (2/3) * \rho_{YZ}$$

**Variances in Groups 1 and 2**

The change in each variance is the square of the change in the corresponding mean. Note that variances are the same in both groups.

$$\sigma^2_{Z1} = \sigma^2_{Z2} = \sigma^2_Z - \left[\text{Range} * \sigma^2_Z * (2/3)\right]^2$$
$$\sigma^2_{Y1} = \sigma^2_{Y2} = \sigma^2_Y - \left[\text{Range} * \sigma^2_Y * (2/3) * \rho_{YZ}\right]^2$$
$$\sigma^2_{X1} = \sigma^2_{X2} = \sigma^2_X - \left[\text{Range} * \sigma^2_X * (2/3) * \rho_{XZ}\right]^2$$

**Correlations in Groups 1 and 2**

Note that the correlations are the same in the two groups. The correlations involving Z can be calculated using one of the formulas for the regression coefficient.

$$\rho_{XZ1} = \rho_{XZ2} = \rho_{XZ} * (\sigma_{Z1}/\sigma_{X1})$$
$$\rho_{YZ1} = \rho_{YZ2} = \rho_{YZ} * (\sigma_{Z1}/\sigma_{Y1})$$

The formula for the correlation not involving Z can be calculated using the formula for the partial correlation.

$$\rho_{XY1} = \rho_{XY2} = \rho_{XY.Z} * \left((1-\rho_{XZ1}^2)^{.5}\right) * \left((1-\rho_{YZ1}^2)^{.5}\right) + (\rho_{XZ1} * \rho_{YZ1})$$

where $\rho_{XY.Z}$ is the partial correlation of $\rho_{XY}$ partialling Z.

**Running the MGSEM Model with MAR Missingness**

Running the MGSEM model with MAR missingness is the same as described above. The only exception is that the two correlation matrices (means and standard deviations) are as calculated in this section. MGSEM analysis with MAR missingness involves all three variables (i.e., including the cause of missingness, Z). This analysis yields parameter estimates that are the same as the original population parameter values. Note that parameter estimates from the MGSEM analysis may, due to rounding error, be very slightly different from the original population values. However, one can obtain parameter estimates as precise as desired simply by estimating the parameter values in the two groups with greater precision. For example, in my experience, rounding the parameter values in the two groups to five decimal places yields MGSEM parameter estimates that are precise to at least four decimal places.

This MAR analysis yields, in a single analysis, parameter estimates and standard errors that are the same as what one would obtain from an infinite number of replications of the comparable Monte Carlo simulation.

**Running the MGSEM Model with NMAR Missingness**

Running the MGSEM model with NMAR missingness is that same as described above, except that the model omits the cause of missingness, Z. That is, the analysis involves just X and Y. Because the cause of missingness, Z, is omitted, the key parameter estimates (e.g., the regression coefficient for X predicting Y) is biased as a function of several factors, including $\rho_{YZ}$ and the percent missing on Y (Collins et al. 2001), and $\rho_{ZR}$, which is a function of the Range of the IF statements used to generate the missing data (Graham et al. 2008). This NMAR analysis yields, in a single analysis, parameter estimates and standard errors that are the same as what one would obtain from an infinite number of replications of the comparable Monte Carlo simulation.

## *Examples of Good Uses of the MGSEM Procedure for MAR/ NMAR Missingness*

The MGSEM procedure for MAR/NMAR missingness may be used in place of Monte Carlo simulations to address many missing data questions. One use would be to establish the degree to which $\rho_{YZ}$ (Collins et al. 2001) and $\rho_{ZR}$ (Graham et al. 2008) actually affect estimation bias, for example, in terms of the standardized bias (SB; e.g., see Collins et al. 2001):

$$SB = \frac{\text{Parameter Estimate - Population Value}}{\text{Standard Error}} \times 100$$

At this point, I would ideally compare the SB estimate obtained from the MGSEM procedure described here with simulation results that have already been published. Unfortunately, the current implementation of the MGSEM automation utility requires equal variances across the three variables in the simulation. Although this is not a serious limiting factor for performing a new simulation, it does make it

**Table 10.4** Standardized bias for Monte Carlo and MGSEM simulations for $r_{XY} = .60$

| Probability of missing on Y for quartiles of Z | Range | Standardized bias | | Diff |
|---|---|---|---|---|
| | | MonteCarlo | MGSEM | |
| .10, .367, .633, .90 | .80 | $-271.9^{10K}$ | −292.7 | −20.8 |
| .15, .383, .617, .85 | .70 | $-203.9^{10K}$ | −210.4 | −6.5 |
| .20, .400, .600, .80 | .60 | $-145.0^{10K}$ | −147.0 | −2.0 |
| .25, .417, .583, .75 | .50 | $-100.9^{10K}$ | −98.0 | 2.9 |
| .30, .433, .567, .70 | .40 | $-64.5^{10K}$ | −60.8 | 3.7 |
| .35, .450, .550, .65 | .30 | $-39.0^{10K}$ | −33.4 | 5.6 |
| .40, .467, .533, .60 | .20 | $-18.7^{10K}$ | −14.6 | 4.1 |
| .45, .483, .517, .55 | .10 | $-6.6^{10K}$ | −3.6 | 3.0 |

*Note*: For all of these patterns, there was 50% missingness on Y and $\rho_{ZY} = .925$. These tabled values are based on variances = 1.25 for all three variables, and the .555, .60, .925 correlations. For the Monte Carlo simulation, there were 10,000 replications for each cell shown. Diff = MGSEM estimate − Monte Carlo estimate

**Table 10.5** Standardized bias for Monte Carlo and MGSEM simulations for $r_{XY} = .124$

| Probability of missing on Y for quartiles of Z | Range | Standardized bias | | Diff |
|---|---|---|---|---|
| | | MonteCarlo | MGSEM | |
| .10, .367, .633, .90 | .80 | $-69.4^{10K}$ | −71.0 | −1.6 |
| .15, .383, .617, .85 | .70 | $-50.7^{10K}$ | −51.7 | −1.0 |
| .20, .400, .600, .80 | .60 | $-36.1^{10K}$ | −36.5 | −0.4 |
| .25, .417, .583, .75 | .50 | $-25.8^{10K}$ | −24.6 | −1.2 |
| .30, .433, .567, .70 | .40 | $-15.6^{10K}$ | −15.4 | 0.2 |
| .35, .450, .550, .65 | .30 | $-8.4^{10K}$ | −8.5 | −0.1 |
| .40, .467, .533, .60 | .20 | $-1.8^{10K}$ | −3.7 | −1.9 |
| .45, .483, .517, .55 | .10 | $-1.8^{10K}$ | −0.9 | 0.9 |

*Note*: For all of these patterns, there was 50% missingness on Y and $\rho_{ZY} = .925$. These tabled values are based on variances = 1.25 for all three variables, and the .1147, .124, .925 correlations. For the Monte Carlo simulation, there were 10,000 replications for each cell shown. Diff = MGSEM estimate − Monte Carlo estimate

difficult to compare results with any already-published simulation in which variances happened not to be equal (e.g., that described by Collins et al. 2001).

Graham et al. (2008), in extending the Collins et al. (2001) simulation, examined the degree to which Range of IF statements (see above) affected the SB. Although the original Graham et al. simulation did not have equal variances, I was able to rerun parts of that simulation using equal variances (1.25) for all three variables. The results of this simulation for $\rho_{XY} = .60$ (same as in Collins et al. 2001) appear in Table 10.4. A replication of this simulation, but with smaller $\rho_{XY}$ ($\rho_{XY} = .124$), appears in Table 10.5.

The results for the MGSEM procedure are comparable to those obtained with the Monte Carlo procedure. For each level of $\rho_{XY}$ (.60 and .124), the correlation between the two sets of SB estimates was $r=.999$. Further, although the Monte Carlo simulation results for $\rho_{XY}=.60$ appeared to be rather stable with 10,000 replications per cell, the Monte Carlo simulation results for $\rho_{XY}=.124$ were less stable, even with 10,000 replications per cell. Most notable was the fact that SB was estimated to be $-1.79$ for Range $=.10$ and $-1.78$ for Range $=.20$. The difference in SB between these two cells is small, to be sure, and the conclusion for both ranges would be that estimation bias is not large. However, this is an example of a nonmonotonic change in the SB estimates over monotonic changes in the Range variable. That is, it is an example of a simulation that has failed to converge, even with 10,000 replications.

The most important difference between the two approaches was the amount of time to complete the simulation. For example, it took virtually an entire workday to complete the Monte Carlo simulation described in Table 10.5, whereas the MGSEM figures shown in Table 10.5 were calculated in just under 2 minutes. That is more than a 200-fold difference in simulation time.

The MARSimulate automation utility, which is available from our website (http://methodology.psu.edu) asks for several bits of information, including $r_{XY}$, $r_{XZ}$, and $r_{YZ}$, the means and variances of X, Y, and Z, and the value for the Range variable. The utility then automatically generates LISREL code for performing the two-group analyses and automatically calls LISREL (the location of your version of the LISREL executable must also be provided). The user does not need to know, understand, or write the LISREL code in order to run this utility. In fact, the free student version of LISREL also works with this automation utility.

Given how little time it takes to perform the MGSEM calculations (with the automation utility), it is an easy matter to explore other factors that affect bias. For example, what is the effect of different means? What is the effect of different variances? What is effect of different values of $\rho_{XY}$ given that $\rho_{YZ}=.925$, and given that $\rho_{XZ}=\rho_{XY}\times\rho_{XZ}$? These questions may all be addressed in minutes with great precision.

**Effect of Different Means**

The long and short of it is that means do not matter. The results presented in Table 10.6 shown that the SB was constant when means changed, but correlations, variances, and Range all remained constant.

**Effect of Different Variances**

Table 10.7 displays the results for the situation in which correlations, means, and Range were constant, but variances for the three variables changed. The bottom line here is that variances do matter. SB increased with larger variances. And the increase was not linear. When variances were 2.0, SB was 2.24 greater than in the situation in which variances were all 1.0. When the three variances were 3.0, SB was 3.83 greater than in the situation in which variances were all 1.0. Also, when the three

**Table 10.6** Standardized bias from MGSEM simulations with different means

| $\rho_{XZ}$ | $\rho_{XY}$ | $\rho_{YZ}$ | $\mu_X$ | $\mu_Y$ | $\mu_Z$ | $\sigma_X^2$ | $\sigma_Y^2$ | $\sigma_Z^2$ | Range | SB |
|---|---|---|---|---|---|---|---|---|---|---|
| .555 | .600 | .925 | 1 | 1 | 1 | 1.25 | 1.25 | 1.25 | .60 | −147.0 |
| .555 | .600 | .925 | 2 | 2 | 2 | 1.25 | 1.25 | 1.25 | .60 | −147.0 |
| .555 | .600 | .925 | 1 | 2 | 2 | 1.25 | 1.25 | 1.25 | .60 | −147.0 |
| .555 | .600 | .925 | 2 | 1 | 2 | 1.25 | 1.25 | 1.25 | .60 | −147.0 |
| .555 | .600 | .925 | 2 | 2 | 1 | 1.25 | 1.25 | 1.25 | .60 | −147.0 |

**Table 10.7** Standardized bias from MGSEM simulations for different variances

| $\rho_{XZ}$ | $\rho_{XY}$ | $\rho_{YZ}$ | $\mu_X$ | $\mu_Y$ | $\mu_Z$ | $\sigma_X^2$ | $\sigma_Y^2$ | $\sigma_Z^2$ | Range | SB |
|---|---|---|---|---|---|---|---|---|---|---|
| .555 | .600 | .925 | 1 | 1 | 1 | 1.00 | 1.00 | 1.00 | .60 | −114.5 |
| .555 | .600 | .925 | 1 | 1 | 1 | 1.25 | 1.25 | 1.25 | .60 | −147.0 |
| .555 | .600 | .925 | 1 | 1 | 1 | 1.50 | 1.50 | 1.50 | .60 | −181.3 |
| .555 | .600 | .925 | 1 | 1 | 1 | 1.75 | 1.75 | 1.75 | .60 | −217.7 |
| .555 | .600 | .925 | 1 | 1 | 1 | 2.00 | 2.00 | 2.00 | .60 | −256.3 |
| .555 | .600 | .925 | 1 | 1 | 1 | 3.00 | 3.00 | 3.00 | .60 | −439.0 |
| .555 | .600 | .925 | 1 | 1 | 1 | 4.00 | 4.00 | 4.00 | .60 | −688.2 |

variances were 4.0, SB was 2.69 greater than the situation in which the three variances were 2.0.

It was already known that SB increases as a function of sample size. This new finding relating to variances further challenges the potential usefulness of SB as an indicator of the problems associated with nonignorable missingness. Because variances appear to matter so much in the level of SB, I recommend, as a starting place, that variances always be set to 1.0 as kind of standard for evaluating the impact of NMAR missingness.

## Effect of Different Values of Range and $\rho_{XY}$

Table 10.8 presents the results for varying $\rho_{XY}$, while keeping $\rho_{YZ}$, means, variances, and Range constant at the values shown. Table 10.8 also presents the results for holding $\rho_{XY}$ constant and varying Range. For these calculations, $\rho_{XZ} = \rho_{XY} \times \rho_{YZ}$. Reading down any column of Table 10.8 shows that SB is much smaller for smaller effect sizes. For example, for the column with Range = .60, for moderate to large effect sizes ($\rho_{XY}$ = .30–.50; Cohen 1977), bias from NMAR missingness had an appreciable effect on statistical conclusions. However, for small effect sizes ($\rho_{XY}$ = .10), bias due to NMAR missingness was tolerably low. Now read down a column of Table 10.8 with a more modest Range (e.g., Range = .30), that is, if the probabilities of missingness on Y for the four quartiles of Z were .35, .45, .55, and .65. In this case, SB was tolerably low for all effect sizes examined.

One can also examine the rows of Table 10.8. Holding $r_{XY}$ constant, it is easy to see the effect of changing the range variable. The top row in Table 10.8 ($r_{XY}$ = .60) gives information similar to what is shown in Table 10.4, except that figures shown in Table 10.8 are based on variances set to 1.0, rather than the 1.25 used in Table 10.4.

**Table 10.8** Standardized bias for MGSEM simulations for levels of $\rho_{XY}$ and range

| $\rho_{XY}$ | Range | | | | | | | | |
|---|---|---|---|---|---|---|---|---|---|
| | .90 | .80 | .70 | .60 | .50 | .40 | .30 | .20 | .10 |
| .60 | 297.4 | 221.9 | 162.0 | 114.5 | 77.0 | 48.1 | **26.5** | **11.6** | **2.9** |
| .50 | 263.4 | 197.3 | 144.6 | 102.5 | 69.1 | 43.2 | **23.9** | **10.5** | **2.6** |
| .40 | 219.7 | 165.1 | 121.3 | 86.2 | 58.3 | *36.5* | **20.2** | **8.9** | **2.2** |
| .30 | 169.6 | 127.8 | 94.1 | 67.0 | 45.3 | *28.4* | **15.8** | **6.9** | **1.7** |
| .20 | 115.2 | 86.9 | 64.1 | 45.7 | *31.0* | *19.4* | **10.8** | **4.7** | **1.2** |
| .10 | 58.2 | 44.0 | *32.5* | *23.2* | *15.7* | **9.9** | **5.5** | **2.4** | **0.6** |

*Note*: All SB values are negative. All variances are fixed at 1; $r_{XZ} = r_{XY} \times r_{YZ}$; and $r_{YZ} = .925$. SB values in italics (SB > 40) suggest concern for statistical inference by the standard used by Collins et al. 2001. SB values in Bold (SB < 40) suggest bias that is tolerably low by the standard used by Collins et al. 2001

When $r_{XY} = .60$ (very large effect in Cohen's terms), Range values of 40 or greater produced levels of bias that could affect statistical conclusions by the standard suggested by Collins et al. 2001. However, for Range values of .30 or less (actually .36 or less) produces, bias is tolerably low by the standard used by Collins et al. (SB < 40). However, for small effects in Cohen's (1977) terms ($r_{XY} = .10$), all but the largest (and least probable) values of the Range variable produced bias that was tolerably small by the standard used by Collins et al. (2001).

### Effect of Different Values of $\rho_{XY}$, $\rho_{YZ}$, and Range ($\rho_{ZR}$)

Finally, Table 10.9 presents results when all the relevant quantities are varied ($\rho_{XZ} = \rho_{XY} \times \rho_{YZ}$). All panels of Table 10.9 look at several levels of $\rho_{YZ}$ (.925, .7, .5, .3, .1), and several levels of Range (.90–.10 in increments of .10; corresponding $\rho_{ZR} = .67–.08$). Panel (A) examines $\rho_{XY} = .10$; Panel (B) examines $\rho_{XY} = .20$; Panel (C) examines $\rho_{XY} = .30$; and Panel (D) examines $\rho_{XY} = .40$.

With small effects (i.e., when $\rho_{XY} = .10$), estimation bias was tolerably low (by the standard of Collins et al. 2001) for all but the most extreme values of $\rho_{YZ}$ and Range. Even with medium to large effects ($\rho_{XY} = .40$), estimation bias was tolerably low under a wide range of values of $\rho_{YZ}$ and Range. In fact, for $\rho_{XY} = .40$, Range < .42 OR $\rho_{YZ} < .43$ produces tolerably low bias; for $\rho_{XY} = .30$, Range < .48 OR $\rho_{YZ} < .48$ produces tolerably low bias; for $\rho_{XY} = .20$, Range < .57 OR $\rho_{YZ} < .58$ produces tolerably low bias; for $\rho_{XY} = .10$, Range < .77 OR $\rho_{YZ} < .79$ produces tolerably low bias.

## *What Simulations Cannot Be Addressed with the MGSEM Procedures?*

Graham et al. (2007) recently conducted a Monte Carlo simulation examining the performance of multiple imputation with different numbers of imputations and compared the results against the comparable FIML model. In this instance, the goal

**Table 10.9** Standardized bias for MGSEM simulations for levels of $\rho_{XY}$, $\rho_{YZ}$, and range ($\rho_{ZR}$)

| (A) | $\rho_{XY}$ | 0.1 | 0.1 | 0.1 | 0.1 | 0.1 |
|---|---|---|---|---|---|---|
|  | $\rho_{XZ}$ | 0.0925 | 0.07 | 0.05 | 0.03 | 0.01 |
|  | $\rho_{YZ}$ | **0.925** | **0.7** | **0.5** | **0.3** | **0.1** |
| **range** | $\rho_{ZR}$ | | | Standardized bias | | |
| 0.9 | 0.671 | *58.2* | **30.5** | **14.8** | **5.2** | * |
| 0.8 | 0.596 | *44.0* | **23.6** | **11.6** | * | * |
| 0.7 | 0.522 | **32.5** | **17.7** | **8.8** | * | * |
| 0.6 | 0.447 | **23.2** | **12.8** | **6.4** | * | * |
| 0.5 | 0.373 | **15.7** | **8.8** | * | * | * |
| 0.4 | 0.298 | **9.9** | **5.6** | * | * | * |
| 0.3 | 0.224 | **5.5** | * | * | * | * |
| 0.2 | 0.149 | * | * | * | * | * |
| 0.1 | 0.075 | * | * | * | * | * |

| (B) | $\rho_{XY}$ | 0.2 | 0.2 | 0.2 | 0.2 | 0.2 |
|---|---|---|---|---|---|---|
|  | $\rho_{XZ}$ | 0.185 | 0.14 | 0.1 | 0.06 | 0.02 |
|  | $\rho_{YZ}$ | **0.925** | **0.7** | **0.5** | **0.3** | **0.1** |
| **range** | $\rho_{ZR}$ | | | Standardized bias | | |
| 0.9 | 0.671 | *115.2* | *60.3* | **29.2** | **10.2** | * |
| 0.8 | 0.596 | *86.9* | *46.6* | **22.8** | **8.0** | * |
| 0.7 | 0.522 | *64.1* | **35.0** | **17.3** | **6.1** | * |
| 0.6 | 0.447 | *45.7* | **25.3** | **12.6** | * | * |
| 0.5 | 0.373 | **31.0** | **17.3** | **8.7** | * | * |
| 0.4 | 0.298 | **19.4** | **11.0** | **5.5** | * | * |
| 0.3 | 0.224 | **10.8** | **6.1** | * | * | * |
| 0.2 | 0.149 | * | * | * | * | * |
| 0.1 | 0.075 | * | * | * | * | * |

| (C) | $\rho_{XY}$ | 0.3 | 0.3 | 0.3 | 0.3 | 0.3 |
|---|---|---|---|---|---|---|
|  | $\rho_{XZ}$ | 0.2775 | 0.21 | 0.15 | 0.09 | 0.03 |
|  | $\rho_{YZ}$ | **0.925** | **0.7** | **0.5** | **0.3** | **0.1** |
| **range** | $\rho_{ZR}$ | | | Standardized bias | | |
| 0.9 | 0.671 | *169.6* | *88.5* | *42.8* | **14.9** | * |
| 0.8 | 0.596 | *127.8* | *68.3* | *33.4* | **11.7** | * |
| 0.7 | 0.522 | *94.1* | *51.2* | **25.3** | **8.9** | * |
| 0.6 | 0.447 | *67.0* | *37.0* | **18.5** | **6.6** | * |
| 0.5 | 0.373 | *45.3* | **25.3** | **−12.7** | * | * |
| 0.4 | 0.298 | **28.4** | **16.0** | **8.1** | * | * |
| 0.3 | 0.224 | **15.8** | **8.9** | * | * | * |
| 0.2 | 0.149 | **6.9** | * | * | * | * |
| 0.1 | 0.075 | * | * | * | * | * |

(continued)

Table 10.9 (continued)

| (D) | $\rho_{XY}$ | 0.4 | 0.4 | 0.4 | 0.4 | 0.4 |
|---|---|---|---|---|---|---|
|  | $\rho_{XZ}$ | 0.37 | 0.28 | 0.20 | 0.12 | 0.04 |
|  | $\rho_{YZ}$ | 0.925 | 0.7 | 0.5 | 0.3 | 0.1 |
| range | $\rho_{ZR}$ | \multicolumn{5}{c}{Standardized bias} | | | | |
| 0.9 | 0.671 | 219.7 | 114.1 | 55.0 | 19.1 | * |
| 0.8 | 0.596 | 165.1 | 87.9 | 42.9 | 15.0 | * |
| 0.7 | 0.522 | 121.3 | 65.9 | 32.5 | 11.5 | * |
| 0.6 | 0.447 | 86.2 | 47.5 | 23.7 | 8.4 | * |
| 0.5 | 0.373 | 58.3 | 32.5 | 16.3 | 5.8 | * |
| 0.4 | 0.298 | 36.5 | 20.6 | 10.4 | * | * |
| 0.3 | 0.224 | 20.2 | 11.5 | 5.8 | * | * |
| 0.2 | 0.149 | 8.9 | 5.1 | * | * | * |
| 0.1 | 0.075 | * | * | * | * | * |

*Note*: All variances are fixed at 1. $\rho_{XZ} = \rho_{XY} \times \rho_{YZ}$. All SB values are negative. An * signifies SB < 5. SB values in italics (SB > 40) suggest concern for statistical inference by the standard used by Collins et al. (2001). SB values in Bold (SB < 40) suggest bias that is tolerably low by the standard used by Collins et al. (2001)

of the analysis was to examine the standard errors and statistical conclusions from various MI models. Thus in this case, there is no way to simulate those results with the MGSEM procedure; one must use a Monte Carlo simulation in this instance.

## *Other Considerations with the MGSEM Procedures for MAR/NMAR Missingness*

Examining the results, especially those shown in Table 10.4, an interesting pattern seemed to emerge. For higher values of the Range variable, the SB with the MC approach was slightly smaller than the SB with MGSEM. But with lower values of the Range variable, the effect was reversed: The SB with the MC approach was slightly larger than the SB with the MGSEM approach.

That pattern of results may or may not be real. For example, it could be that the pattern is simply the result of simulation wobble; it is much less clear that results shown in Table 10.5 show a similar pattern. But if the pattern is real, one might be tempted to speculate about which approach yielded the "correct" results. An important point here is that it is quite possible that both approaches are correct, but that they are simply different in some small way. One way they could be different, for example, relates to the way the Z variable works in the Monte Carlo simulations. Even if Z starts out as a variable with a normal distribution, the fact that it is "quartilized" (divided into quartiles) to generate MAR missingness changes it. With the MGSEM procedure, however, the Z variable has some elements of the quartilized variable, but some elements of a continuous variable (in that the population correlations are being dealt with directly).

My tentative conclusion is that the Monte Carlo simulations and the MGSEM procedures described in this chapter are subtly different. In most instances, these differences will not change the main findings of either type of simulation. Future research will explore these minor differences in more detail.

# References

Allison, P. D. (1987). Estimation of linear models with incomplete data. In C. Clogg (Ed.), *Sociological Methodology 1987* (pp. 71–103). San Francisco: Jossey Bass.

Cohen, J. (1977). *Statistical power analysis for the behavioral sciences.* New York: Academic Press.

Collins, L. M., Schafer, J. L., & Kam, C. M. (2001). A comparison of inclusive and restrictive strategies in modern missing data procedures. Psychological Methods, 6, 330–351.

Fan, X., Felsovalyi, A., Sivo, S. A., & Keenan, S. C. (2002). *SAS for Monte Carlo studies: A guide for quantitative researchers.* Cary, NC: SAS Press.

Graham, J. W. (2009). Missing data analysis: making it work in the real world. *Annual Review of Psychology, 60*, 549–576.

Graham, J. W., & Hofer, S. M. (1992). *EMCOV User's Guide.* Unpublished manuscript, University of Southern California.

Graham, J. W., & Donaldson, S. I. (1993). Evaluating interventions with differential attrition: The importance of nonresponse mechanisms and use of followup data. *Journal of Applied Psychology, 78*, 119–128.

Graham, J. W., Hofer, S. M., & MacKinnon, D. P. (1996). Maximizing the usefulness of data obtained with planned missing value patterns: An application of maximum likelihood procedures. *Multivariate Behavioral Research, 31*, 197–218.

Graham, J. W., Olchowski, A. E., & Gilreath, T. D. (2007). How Many Imputations are Really Needed? Some Practical Clarifications of Multiple Imputation Theory. *Prevention Science, 8*, 206–213.

Graham, J. W., & Schafer, J. L. (1999). On the performance of multiple imputation for multivariate data with small sample size. In R. Hoyle (Ed.) *Statistical Strategies for Small Sample Research*, (pp. 1–29). Thousand Oaks, CA: Sage.

Graham, J. W., Palen, L. A., Smith, E. A., and Caldwell, L. L. (2008). Attrition: MAR and MNAR Missingness, and Estimation Bias. Poster presented at the 16th Annual Meetings of the Society for Prevention Research, San Francisco, CA, May 2008.

Graham, J. W., Taylor, B. J., & Cumsille, P. E. (2001). Planned missing data designs in analysis of change. In L. Collins & A. Sayer (Eds.), New methods for the analysis of change, (pp. 335–353). Washington, DC: American Psychological Association.

Graham, J. W., Taylor, B. J., Olchowski, A. E., & Cumsille, P. E. (2006). Planned missing data designs in psychological research. *Psychological Methods, 11*, 323–343.

Jöreskog, K. G., & Sörbom, D. (1996). LISREL 8 User's Reference Guide. Chicago, IL: Scientific Software, Inc.

Muthen, B., Kaplan, D., & Hollis, M. (1987). On structural equation modeling with data that are not missing completely at random. *Psychometrika, 52*, 431–462.

Press, W. H., Teukolsky, S. A., Vetterling, W. T., and Flannery, B. P. (2007). Numerical Recipes 3rd Edition: The Art of Scientific Computing. New York: Cambridge University Press.

# Chapter 11
# Using Modern Missing Data Methods with Auxiliary Variables to Mitigate the Effects of Attrition on Statistical Power

John W. Graham and Linda M. Collins

Missing data in a field experiment may arise from a number of sources. Participants may skip over questions inadvertently or refuse to answer them; they may offer an illegible response; they may fail to complete a questionnaire; or they may be absent from an entire measurement session in a longitudinal study. The last is often called wave nonresponse. Many participants who are unavailable for one or more occasions of measurement are available at later occasions. We define attrition is a special case of wave nonresponse in which a participant drops out of a study after a certain time and is no longer available at any subsequent wave of data collection.

We focus on attrition in this chapter because it continues to be a major issue in longitudinal field experiments. Despite the best efforts of researchers, most longitudinal studies have attrition. Attrition tends to occur more frequently in transient populations, so research is particularly susceptible when based on the high-risk populations in which intervention scientists are often most interested. Furthermore, it is common in intervention research for key outcomes to be measured several years after the beginning of the study, say in a third or fourth follow-up wave of measurement (e.g., a school-based drug abuse prevention program in which a pretest takes place in seventh grade but the key outcome is drug use in tenth grade). As more time goes by, there is more opportunity for attrition. If even a modest number of participants drop out at each wave of measurement, by the time the key outcome is measured the cumulative amount of attrition can be substantial.

Although attrition must be taken seriously and should be minimized, the damage it does in intervention research today is much less than it once was, provided that modern missing data procedures such as multiple imputation (MI) or maximum likelihood (ML) methods are used. Attrition raises two concerns in evaluation of an intervention. The first is that attrition may produce estimation bias, which will affect the internal and external validity of the study. To the extent that the Missing at Random (MAR) assumption is met, modern missing data approaches deal effectively with estimation biases introduced by attrition and other forms of missing data. Even when the MAR assumption is not fully met, modern missing data procedures are a distinct improvement over the ad hoc and unprincipled approaches formerly used, such as casewise deletion and mean substitution. Thus even if estimation bias cannot be eliminated completely, it can be greatly reduced, often to acceptable levels (Collins et al. 2001; also see extensive discussions of this topic in Chaps. 1 and 10).

The second concern that attrition raises is that the loss of data will result in loss of statistical power, possibly reducing power to unacceptable levels. Modern missing data procedures help with this concern as well. In addition to mitigating estimation bias, modern missing data procedures recover some of the statistical power that would otherwise be lost due to attrition. In fact, we suggest that loss of power due to attrition has frequently been overestimated because the impact of modern missing data procedures on power has not been considered.

Intervention scientists often base power analyses on the sample size expected after attrition has taken its toll. Such a power analysis assumes that any data provided by dropouts before they leave the study are unavailable to later statistical analysis. However, modern missing data procedures can readily make use of the partial data provided by these individuals. In fact, if one pays careful attention to the missing data model, using modern missing data procedures can lead to smaller standard errors and, therefore, to increased statistical power. That is, with these methods, statistical power lost to attrition can be restored to an extent.

## Effective Sample Size

We find it helpful to quantify the level of statistical power achieved by use of modern missing data procedures in terms of the effective sample size ($N_{EFF}$). Suppose a statistical analysis is to be performed on a set of variables that have been subject to attrition, and modern missing data procedures are to be used. This analysis is associated with a particular level of statistical power. The $N_{EFF}$ is the size of the sample of complete cases that would provide the same statistical power. The $N_{EFF}$ always falls somewhere between the sample size after attrition (which is the sample size that would result if all incomplete cases were discarded, i.e., the sample size with complete cases: $N_{CC}$) and the original total sample size ($N_{TOT}$). How close the $N_{EFF}$ is to $N_{TOT}$ is a reflection of how successful the missing data procedure has been at restoring power lost due to attrition.

Of course, intervention scientists would prefer to achieve an $N_{EFF}$ as close as possible to $N_{TOT}$. This can be accomplished by making use of ideas from Collins et al. (2001), who showed that both reduction of estimation bias and recovery of lost power are desirable consequences of using an inclusive missing data strategy. An inclusive missing data strategy is one that makes use of auxiliary variables, that is, variables that are not a part of the substantive analysis model being fit but are included in order to increase the effectiveness of the missing data procedure. All else being equal, auxiliary variables increase the effectiveness of the missing data procedure more when they are highly correlated with the variables that are subject to missingness. Fortunately, good, effective auxiliary variables are almost always available in multi-wave prevention studies.

The purpose of this chapter is to show how modern missing data procedures can be used to mitigate the impact of attrition on statistical power. There are two issues here. The first issue relates to how one includes auxiliary variables in the missing data analysis (MI or ML) models. The second issue relates to detailing exactly what the benefits are for including auxiliary variables, and how to predict what effect a candidate auxiliary variable will have.

The first issue, how one includes an auxiliary variable in one's missing data analysis model, is largely a trivial one. When that missing data analysis model is normal model MI, for example, one simply adds any auxiliary variables to the list of variables included in the MI model. Although adding auxiliary variables in ML/FIML models is a little more complicated, Graham (2003) has also shown how auxiliary variables may efficiently be added to FIML models in a way that has the equivalent benefit enjoyed by MI models. At least one FIML program (Mplus; Muthén and Muthén 2010) has recently added a feature in which the addition of auxiliary variables has been automated. Because of the relative ease of including auxiliary variables in these missing data analysis models, we do not spend time with this issue in this chapter.

The second issue, on the other hand, needs much more elaboration. Researchers have in the past included auxiliary variables to "help" with the imputation. But it was never made explicit what this "help" was. Collins et al. (2001) provided some initial insights as to how these auxiliary variables were a benefit. The purpose of this chapter is to expand on those ideas as they relate to statistical power benefits that accrue from including auxiliary variables in the model. The chapter has four main goals. First, we begin by demonstrating how using a modern missing data procedure with a single auxiliary variable can improve power; for this we use a simple artificial data example as an illustration. The remaining goals focus on the benefit intervention scientists can expect when missing data procedures are used with more complex, and more realistic, attrition patterns.

Second, we demonstrate the benefit of a single auxiliary variable with the more complicated (and more realistic) scenario in which fewer than 100 % of the eligible subjects (those missing on Y) have data for the auxiliary variable. Third, we demonstrate the auxiliary variable benefit in the still more complicated (and realistic) scenario in which one has two auxiliary variables, possibly with different $r_{YZ}$'s (correlations between the auxiliary variable, Z, and the main dependent variable, Y), and different percentages of eligible subjects having data for the two auxiliary variables. Finally, we provide intervention scientists simple guidance for estimating the auxiliary variable benefit they might enjoy in their own empirical data. We do this by providing an automation utility designed to work with any version of LISREL 8 (including the free, downloadable, student version). The user does NOT need to be a LISREL user. The utility asks a few basic questions about the data, and then automatically writes the LISREL code, runs the analyses required, and prints the primary results to the screen.

## An Artificial Data Demonstration of Improving Power Using a Missing Data Model with Auxiliary Variables

The $N_{EFF}$ can be determined by means of a straightforward simulation based on the multiple group structural equation modeling (MGSEM) missing data procedure suggested by Allison (1987) and Muthén et al. (1987). Note that although we refer to this as a simulation, it was not a Monte Carlo simulation (please see Chap. 10 for a detailed discussion of this approach to simulation work). Rather, the MGSEM procedure allows one to make use of the population covariance matrices for those with complete and partial data. Because of this, each cell of the simulation may be carried out with just a single analysis (rather than the thousands of analyses required with Monte Carlo simulations).

### *Details of MGSEM Procedure*

In order to estimate the relevant $N_{EFF}$, we test a simple correlation model involving three variables: X, always observed (think of X as the independent variable of substantive interest), Y, sometimes missing (think of Y as the main dependent variable of substantive interest), and Z, always observed (Z is an auxiliary variable, correlated with Y, but not necessarily of direct substantive interest). We examined the standard error (SE) for the key parameter estimate ($r_{XY}$) from several models.

We started by estimating the SE in a baseline model; attrition but with no auxiliary variables. Given the simple models we tested, this SE was similar to a complete cases analysis. But note that this model is technically not a complete cases model. Even in this simple, two-variable, case (X always observed, Y sometimes missing), and even when the missingness on Y is MCAR, there is a small difference in $r_{XY}$ between the complete cases analysis and an analysis based on appropriate missing data methods (e.g., an ML method such as EM algorithm). This difference applies to the estimate of $r_{XY}$, but as pointed out in Graham and Donaldson (1993), the regression coefficients for X predicting Y are always identical in this simplistic case between complete cases and ML analyses.

Second, we introduced the auxiliary variable with specified properties and noted the SE for that model. These SEs were smaller than the SE in the baseline model. Third, we repeated the first model, but with the larger sample size that produced the same SE as the second model.[1] This new, larger sample size was the $N_{EFF}$.

To estimate the relevant SEs, we made use of the multiple group capabilities of LISREL 8.5 (Jöreskog and Sörbom 1996). Using the missing data procedure described by Allison (1987) and Muthén et al. (1987), one is able to partition

---

[1] This last step involved a simple trial and error process: Try a particular sample size; if the SE was too large, increase the sample size and try again.

**Table 11.1** LISREL code: Model 1 (baseline model)

```
mapping auxiliary variables group 1 (complete data)
da no=500 ni=2 ma=cm ng=2
labels
x y
cm sy
1.00
 .10 1.00
mo ny=2 ne=2 ly=fu,fi ps=sy,fr te=di,fi
le
X Y
ma ly
1 0
0 1
ou nd=5
mapping auxiliary variables group 2 (Y missing)
da no=500 ni=2 ma=cm ng=2
labels
x y
cm sy
1.00
 .00 1.00
mo ny=2 ne=2 ly=fu,fi ps=in te=di,fi
le
X Y
ma ly
1 0
0 0
ma te
0 1
ou nd=5
```

the data into groups that correspond to the different patterns of missing and non-missing values in one's data set. Normally, one would simply make use of one of the full information maximum likelihood (FIML) procedures (e.g., in alphabetical order, Amos, EQS 6.1, LISREL 8.5+, Mplus, Mx) to perform SEM analyses with missing data. However, in the present context, the multiple group SEM procedure has proven to be a useful replacement for Monte Carlo simulation studies (e.g., Graham et al. 2001; Graham et al. 2006; also see Chap. 10).[2]

---

[2] The MGSEM procedure makes use of the covariance matrix as input. When the covariance matrix is analyzed in this manner, one may simply change the sample size indicated in model being tested without changing the input covariance matrix. The more commonly used FIML approach cannot do this. With that approach, raw data must be input. And with raw-data input, the sample size is tied directly to the data being input (e.g., with $N=500$, 500 cases are read from the raw data file). Thus with the FIML methods, changing the sample size changes the data being read, thereby producing changes in the results.

The LISREL code for the baseline, two-group, model is presented in Table 11.1. In this simple application of the MGSEM procedure, we specified the input (population) correlation matrix in Group 1 to be:

|   | X    | Y    |
|---|------|------|
| X | 1.00 |      |
| Y | .10  | 1.00 |

In most respects, Group 1 of the LISREL model (see Table 11.1) was set up like a regular one-group model with manifest variables.

Group 2 (see Table 11.1) was set up the same as Group 1, with the following exceptions: First, the input correlation matrix was:

|   | X    | Y    |
|---|------|------|
| X | 1.00 |      |
| Y | .00  | 1.00 |

Following Allison (1987), the variance is set to 1.0 for any variable with missing values in this group, and all covariances relating to this variable are set to 0.0. In addition, all of the factor variance and covariance parameters for Group 2 were set to be equal to those in Group 1. Further, all factor loadings involving the missing variable are fixed at 0.0 in Group 2, and all residual item variances in Group 2 are fixed at 1.0 (see Table 11.1).

▶ **Sample Data.** Running the LISREL code shown in Table 11.1 produces the following output under LISREL Estimates of Group 2. The output shown is for the PSI matrix, the matrix of factor variances and covariances. In our simplistic examples, the key parameter estimate is the correlation between X and Y.

```
PSI
            X             Y
          -----         -----
X      1.00000
      (0.04477)
      22.33831


Y      0.10000       1.00000
      (0.04477)     (0.06331)
       2.23383       15.79596
```

The top quantity in each element is the parameter estimate. The middle quantity (in parentheses) is the standard error. The bottom quantity is often referred to as the critical ratio (parameter estimate divided by its standard error). This bottom quantity is largely unused in these analyses. Note two things about the output. First, the parameter estimate for $r_{XY}=.10000$. That is, not surprisingly, the parameter estimate in the model is exactly the same as in the population

**Table 11.2** LISREL code: Model 2 (MGSEM model with auxiliary variable)

```
mapping auxiliary variables group 1 (complete data)
da no=500 ni=3 ma=cm ng=2
labels
x y z
cm sy
1.00
 .10 1.00
 .10  .60 1.00
mo ny=3 ne=3 ly=fu,fi ps=sy,fr te=di,fi
le
X Y Z
ma ly
1 0 0
0 1 0
0 0 1
ou nd=5
mapping auxiliary variables group 2 (Y missing)
da no=500 ni=3 ma=cm ng=2
labels
x y z
cm sy
1.00
 .00 1.00
 .10  .00 1.00
mo ny=3 ne=3 ly=fu,fi ps=in te=di,fi
le
X Y Z
ma ly
1 0 0
0 0 0
0 0 1
ma te
0 1 0
ou nd=5
```

covariance matrix.[3] The key quantity in this example is the standard error for $r_{XY}$ (.04477).

The second MGSEM model was much the same as the baseline model. The LISREL code for this second model appears in Table 11.2. The correlation $r_{YZ}$, shown as ".60" in the Table 11.2 for illustration purposes, was varied from $r_{YZ}=.10$ to $r_{YZ}=.95$ in increments of .05. Group 1 of the LISREL model (see Table 11.2) was again set up much like a regular one-group model with manifest variables. The input

---

[3] One can safely ignore the "W_A_R_N_I_N_G" in the LISREL output that "LAMBDA-Y does not have full column rank". It is a necessary byproduct of this analysis.

covariance matrix for Model 2 has three variables and includes correlations for the auxiliary variable, Z.

|   | X    | Y    | Z    |
|---|------|------|------|
| X | 1.00 |      |      |
| Y | .10  | 1.00 |      |
| Z | .10  | .60  | 1.00 |

As with the baseline model, the variance in the input covariance matrix is set to 1.0 for any variable with missing values in this group, and all covariances relating to this variable are set to 0.0.

|   | X    | Y    | Z    |
|---|------|------|------|
| X | 1.00 |      |      |
| Y | .00  | 1.00 |      |
| Z | .10  | .00  | 1.00 |

In addition, all of the factor variance and covariance parameters for Group 2 were set to be equal to those in Group 1, and all factor loadings involving the missing variable were fixed at 0.0 in Group 2. All residual item variances in Group 2 were fixed at 1.0 (see Table 11.2).

▶ **Sample Data.** Running the LISREL code shown in Table 11.2 produced the following output under LISREL Estimates for Group 2. The output shown is for the PSI matrix, the matrix of factor variances and covariances. In our simplistic example, the key parameter estimate was again the correlation between X and Y.

```
PSI
              X           Y           Z
           --------    --------    --------
X         1.00000
         (0.04477)
          22.33831

Y         0.10000     1.00000
         (0.04064)   (0.06120)
          2.46057     16.33874

Z         0.10000     0.60000     1.00000
         (0.03181)   (0.04475)   (0.04477)
          3.14344     13.40840    22.33831
```

▶ **Sample Data.** Note again that all parameter estimates were exactly the same as those in the input population variance-covariance matrix. Note that standard error for $r_{XY}=.04064$ for this model. This SE is rather smaller than the SE for the baseline model (.04477).

The third MGSEM model was the same as the baseline model, except that we modified the sample size ("no=") in Groups 1 and 2. We increased the sample size in Group 1 by some amount and decreased the sample size in Group 2 by the same amount so that the total sample size remained $N_{TOT}=1{,}000$.

▶ **Sample Data.** Running the LISREL code shown in Table 11.1, but increasing the $N$ for Group 1 to 550, and decreasing the $N$ for Group 2 to 450, yielded a somewhat smaller SE for $r_{XY}$ (.04270). Although smaller than the SE for the baseline model, this value was still larger than the SE we observed for Model 2, which included the auxiliary variable. Changing the N to 600 for Group 1 and 400 for Group 2 yielded an even smaller SE for $r_{XY}$ (.04090). Although still smaller, this SE was still somewhat larger than that observed for Model 2. When we changed the $N$ to 608 for Group 1 and 392 for Group 2, the resulting SE for $r_{XY}$ (.04063) was as close as we could get to the SE observed for Model 2.

The conclusion is that a standard missing data model with $N_{CC}=608$ is equivalent, in terms of statistical power, to an auxiliary variable model with $N_{CC}=500$. That is, $N_{EFF}=608$ in this case.

## Artificial Data Example for One Auxiliary Variable, 100 % of Eligible Subjects with Data

The procedure described above was repeated several times. We varied the value of $r_{YZ}$ from .10 to .90 in increments of .10. We also included $r_{YZ}=.95$. For all of these artificial data examples, we fixed $r_{XY}=.10$, and $r_{XZ}=.10$.[4] First, we examined the scenario in which the total N, $N_{TOT}=1{,}000$, and the complete cases N, $N_{TOT}=500$ (that is, 50 % attrition). The results of those analyses appear as the bottom curve in Fig. 11.1. In the figure, the values for $r_{YZ}$ are on the X-axis, and the corresponding $N_{EFF}$ is on the Y-axis.

Using this procedure (with $N_{TOT}=1{,}000$, $N_{CC}=500$), we were able to estimate the standard error for $r_{XY}$ for the various values of the $r_{YZ}$. For example, when $r_{YZ}=.10$, $SE(r_{XY})=.04467$, which corresponds to $N_{EFF}=502$; when $r_{YZ}=.60$, $SE(r_{XY})=.04064$, which corresponds to $N_{EFF}=608$. We also examined the scenario with $N_{TOT}=1{,}000$ and $N_{CC}=667$ (33 % attrition; the middle curve in Fig. 11.1), and the scenario with $N_{TOT}=1{,}000$ and $N_{CC}=750$ (25 % attrition; the top curve in Fig. 11.1).

It is evident from Fig. 11.1 that for any amount of missing data, as $r_{YZ}$ increases, $N_{EFF}$ also increases. In addition, as $r_{YZ}$ increases the increase in $N_{EFF}$ accelerates. For example, with 50 % missing on Y, increasing $r_{YZ}$ from .3 to .4 increased $N_{EFF}$ by 20,

---

[4] We chose $r_{XY}=.10$ because the issue of $N_{EFF}$ becomes most important with small effect sizes. This is closely related to the issue of determining statistical power with varying effect sizes. With large effect sizes, especially in field experiments, it is often possible to find significant effects, even with relatively small sample sizes. It is often the case that sample size is an issue only with smaller effect sizes. We address the issue of other values of $r_{XY}$ later in this chapter.

We arbitrarily chose $r_{XZ}=.10$. In our experience, this value always tends to be rather similar to $r_{XY}$. We address the issue of different values of $r_{XZ}$ later in this chapter.

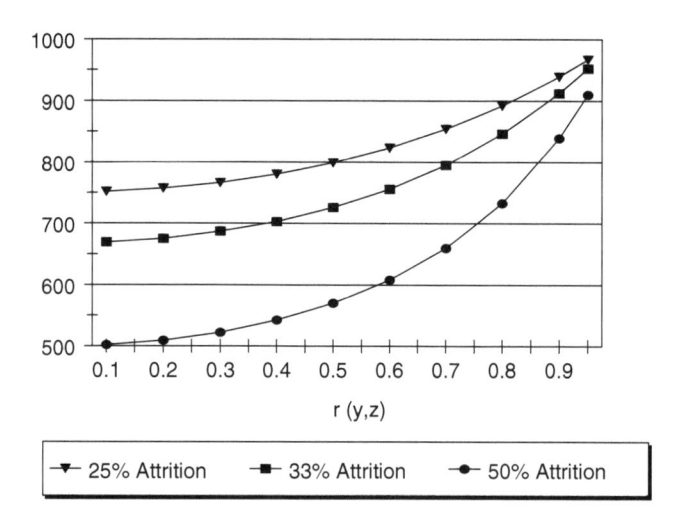

**Fig. 11.1** Effective sample size ($N_{EFF}$) for varying levels of $r_{YZ}$

whereas increasing $r_{YZ}$ from .6 to .7 increased $N_{EFF}$ by 52. This acceleration is less pronounced with less missingness.

Figure 11.1 also shows the magnitude of the recovery in absolute terms. For example, with 50 % missing data on Y and $r_{YZ}=.7$, $N_{EFF}=660$. Compared to an analysis that deletes all subjects with incomplete data, this represents an increase of power equivalent to adding 160 subjects with complete data.

## Artificial Data Demonstrations with More Realistic Attrition Patterns

### *Less than 100 % of Eligible Subjects with Data for the One Auxiliary Variable*

The patterns shown in Fig. 11.1 offer great promise for using an auxiliary variable in intervention evaluation research. However, the numbers in Fig. 11.1 are based on the idea that 100 % of those missing on the main dependent variable (DV) have data for the auxiliary variable. But consider the scenario in which there is an intervention in seventh grade ($X_7$), and the main DV is measured at two follow-up waves, eighth grade ($Y_8$) and ninth grade ($Y_9$). Given that all participants have data for the program variable ($X_7$), the three key patterns of missing and nonmissing values are shown below in Table 11.3.

Table 11.3 Missing data patterns

| Pattern | $X_7$ | $Y_8$ | $Y_9$ | N with pattern |
|---|---|---|---|---|
| 1 | 1 | 1 | 1 | 500 |
| 2 | 1 | 1 | 0 | 375 |
| 3 | 1 | 0 | 0 | 125 |

1 = data present; 0 = data missing

**Table 11.4** Effective sample size ($N_{EFF}$) for auxiliary variable model for various levels of $r_{YZ}$ and percent with data for auxiliary variables: one auxiliary variable

| | Percent of eligible cases having data for auxiliary variable | | | | | | | |
|---|---|---|---|---|---|---|---|---|
| | 100 % | | 75 % | | 50 % | | 25 % | |
| $r_{YZ}$ | $N_{EFF}$ | Statistical power for $r_{XY}=.10$ | $N_{EFF}$ | Statistical power for $r_{XY}=.10$ | $N_{EFF}$ | Statistical power for $r_{XY}=.10$ | $N_{EFF}$ | Statistical power for $r_{XY}=.10$ |
| 0.1 | 502 | .61 | 502 | .61 | 501 | .61 | 501 | .61 |
| 0.2 | 509 | .62 | 508 | .62 | 506 | .62 | 504 | .61 |
| 0.3 | 522 | .63 | 519 | .63 | 515 | .62 | 509 | .62 |
| 0.4 | 542 | .64 | 536 | .64 | 527 | .63 | 516 | .62 |
| 0.5 | 570 | .66 | 559 | .66 | 544 | .65 | 526 | .63 |
| 0.6 | 608 | .69 | 590 | .68 | 567 | .66 | 538 | .64 |
| 0.7 | 660 | .73 | 631 | .71 | 596 | .69 | 554 | .65 |
| 0.8 | 733 | .77 | 687 | .75 | 634 | .71 | 573 | .67 |
| 0.9 | 839 | .83 | 764 | .79 | 684 | .75 | 596 | .69 |
| 0.95 | 910 | .86 | 814 | .82 | 714 | .76 | 609 | .70 |

$r_{XY}=r_{XZ}=.10$ for all cells. Cases are "eligible" if they have missing data for the main DV (Y).
$N=1,000$ for X and Z; $N=500$ for Y

In the scenario depicted in Table 11.3, 500 cases have complete data; 375 cases have missing data for the main DV ($Y_9$), but do have data for the auxiliary variable ($Y_8$). Another 125 cases have missing data for both $Y_9$ and $Y_8$. In this instance, 75 % of those eligible (i.e., 75 % of those with missing data on the main DV) have data for the auxiliary variable. We refer to this percentage as %Z=75 %.

Our artificial data illustration again looked at values of $r_{YZ}$ from .10 to .90 in increments of .10, plus $r_{YZ}=.95$. In this illustration, $r_{XY}=.10$, $r_{XZ}=.10$, $N_{TOT}=1,000$, and $N_{CC}=500$. Also in this illustration, we examined the situations in which 75 %, 50 %, and 25 % of the eligible cases (those missing on the main DV) had data for the auxiliary variable, that is, %Z=75 %, 50 %, and 25 %.

The results of this artificial data illustration appear in Table 11.4. For comparison, also shown in Table 11.4 are figures for the situation in which 100 % of the eligible participants have data for the auxiliary variable (these figures correspond to the bottom curve in Fig. 11.1). Scanning the tabled results for $r_{YZ}=.95$, we see that the increment of $N_{EFF}$ over $N_{CC}$ was 409, 313, 214, and 109, respectively, for %Z=100 %, 75 %, 50 %, and 25 %. For the 75 %, 50 %, and 25 % cases, respectively, the benefit was 76.5 %, 52.3 %, and 26.7 % of the benefit for %Z=100 %.

These percentages are at least similar to what might be expected. However, the tabled values for $r_{YZ}=.50$ are a bit different. The benefits compared to $\%Z=100\%$ are 82.9 %, 62.9 %, and 37.1 %, respectively, for $\%Z=75\%$, 50 %, and 25 %.

## Two Auxiliary Variables

Another way in which the situation is more complex arises if one has more than one auxiliary variable. Even with two auxiliary variables, there are numerous new factors to consider. With just one auxiliary variable, one must consider six factors:

$N_{TOT}$, $N_{CC}$, $r_{XY}$, $r_{XZ}$, $r_{YZ}$, and % of eligible with data for Z

With just two auxiliary variables, one must consider these 11 factors:

$N_{TOT}$, $N_{CC}$, $r_{XY}$, $r_{X,Z1}$, $r_{Y,Z1}$, $r_{X,Z2}$, $r_{Y,Z2}$, $r_{Z1,Z2}$
Percent of eligible with data for $Z_1$ only ($\%Z_1$)
Percent of eligible with data for $Z_2$ only ($\%Z_2$)
Percent of eligible with data for both $Z_1$ and $Z_2$ ($\%Z_1Z_2$)

For now, we reduced the number of factors to consider by making certain assumptions. First, we assumed that $r_{XY}=r_{X,Z1}=r_{X,Z2}=.10$. The rationale for $r_{XY}=.10$ is that sample size, and any possible benefits in $N_{EFF}$ due to auxiliary variables, will be most critical for small effect sizes. Second, to the extent that a variable, Z, is a good auxiliary variable for Y, it is expected to be correlated similarly with X. This second point applies to both $r_{XZ1}$ and to $r_{X,Z2}$, which, in this case, were also set to .10. Third, we made the assumption that once one has one auxiliary variable with a particular $r_{YZ}$, adding a second auxiliary variable with a lower $r_{YZ}$ will generally add only trivially to the $N_{EFF}$ benefit. Thus, our strategy for now is to identify one auxiliary variable ($Z_1$), which has the larger of the two $r_{YZ}$ values. Thus, $\%Z_1$ will also include $\%Z_1Z_2$. Fourth, we made the assumption that $r_{Z1,Z2}$ was the mean of $r_{YZ1}$ and $r_{YZ2}$. Finally, for now, we cover only the situation with $N_{TOT}=1000$ and $N_{CC}=500$ (i.e., 50 % attrition). The more general case, in which all of these assumptions are relaxed, is covered later in this chapter.

## Two Auxiliary Variables with Different Values for $r_{YZ1}$, $r_{YZ2}$, $\%Z_1$, and $\%Z_2$

In longitudinal intervention data, it is common that two auxiliary variables will vary with respect to their correlation with the main DV ($r_{YZ1}$, $r_{YZ2}$), and with respect to the percent of eligible people with data ($\%Z_1$ and $\%Z_2$). One example of the variability of $\%Z_1$ and $\%Z_2$ is presented in Table 11.5, which presents the attrition patterns from one cohort of the Adolescent Alcohol Prevention Trial (AAPT; Hansen and Graham 1991).

Artificial Data Demonstrations with More Realistic Attrition Patterns

**Table 11.5** Attrition patterns over four waves of AAPT

| Pattern | Grade Prog (Seventh) | Smoking Eighth | Ninth | Tenth | N | Percent | % of those missing Smk10 |
|---|---|---|---|---|---|---|---|
| 1 | 1 | 1 | 1 | 1 | 543 | 36.7 | |
| 2 | 1 | 0 | 1 | 1 | 70 | 4.7 | |
| 3 | 1 | 1 | 0 | 1 | 125 | 8.5 | |
| 4 | 1 | 0 | 0 | 1 | 27 | 1.8 | |
| 5 | 1 | 1 | 1 | 0 | 155 | 10.5 | 21.7% |
| 6 | 1 | 0 | 1 | 0 | 45 | 3.0 | 6.3% |
| 7 | 1 | 1 | 0 | 0 | 308 | 20.8 | 43.2% |
| 8 | 1 | 0 | 0 | 0 | 205 | 13.9 | 28.8% |
| Total | | | | | 1478 | | |

Attrition patterns are based on a 3-item cigarette smoking scale. 1 = data present; 0 = data missing. All 1478 had data for the program membership dummy variable

Table 11.5 shows that 713 of 1478 participants were missing data for the main DV, smoking at tenth grade (Smk10). And in that study, there were rather complicated patterns of who had and did not have the two auxiliary variables. Just 6.3 % of those eligible had data for Smk9 only; 43.2 % of those eligible had data for Smk8 only; and 21.7 % of those eligible had data for both Smk8 and Smk9. We used our assumption that having data for both auxiliary variables is not appreciably better than having data for just the one auxiliary variable with the higher $r_{YZ}$. Thus, this problem reduces to one in which the auxiliary variable with the higher $r_{YZ}$ (Smk9) had $r_{Y,Z1} = .82$ and $\%Z_1 = .280$ $(.217 + .063)$. The other auxiliary variable (Smk8) had $r_{Y,Z2} = .66$ and $\%Z_2 = .432$.

In order to illustrate $N_{EFF}$ benefits over a range of circumstances with two auxiliary variables, we conducted another artificial data example. In order to reduce the magnitude of the problem, with this artificial data example, we examined all combinations of $r_{YZ}$ for each of two auxiliary variables, where $r_{YZ}$ ranged from .40 to .90 in increments of .10. Further, this illustration looked at scenarios in which 100 %, 75 %, or 50 % of the eligible subjects had data for some combination of the two auxiliary variables. The 100 % eligible scenario was broken down into three patterns of $\%Z_1$ and $\%Z_2$: 75 %/25 %, 50 %/50 %, and 25 %/50 %. The 75 % eligible scenario was broken down into two patterns of $\%Z_1$ and $\%Z_2$: 50 %/25 %, and 25 %/50 %. The 50 % eligible scenario had just one pattern for $\%Z_1$ and $\%Z_2$: 25 %/25 %.

Table 11.6 presents the results for this artificial data example. Several interesting patterns emerge in the table. First, it is not surprising that when $r_{Y,Z1} = r_{Y,Z2}$, $N_{EFF}$ values in the .75/.25 column are the same as those in the .25/.75 column. When $r_{Y,Z1} = r_{Y,Z2}$, these two columns mean the same thing. Also note that when $r_{Y,Z1} = r_{Y,Z2}$, $N_{EFF}$ values in the .50/.50 column are slightly higher than in the .75/.25 and .25/.75 columns. Also of note is the fact that the $N_{EFF}$ values in the .75/.25 column get larger faster as $r_{Y,Z1}$ increases, compared to the values in the .50/.50 and .25/.75 columns. Again, this is to be expected.

**Table 11.6** Effective sample size ($N_{EFF}$) for auxiliary variable model for various levels of $r_{YZ}$ and percent with data for auxiliary variables: two auxiliary variables

| Higher $r_{YZ}$ | Lower $r_{YZ}$ | Percent with higher/lower $r_{YZ}$: .75/.25 | Percent with higher/lower $r_{YZ}$: .50/.50 | Percent with higher/lower $r_{YZ}$: .25/.75 | Percent with higher/lower $r_{YZ}$: .50/.25 | Percent with higher/lower $r_{YZ}$: .25/.50 | Percent with higher/lower $r_{YZ}$: .25/.25 |
|---|---|---|---|---|---|---|---|
| .4 | .4 | 548 | 550 | 548 | 541 | 541 | 530 |
| .5 | .4 | 570 | 566 | 557 | 557 | 549 | 539 |
| .6 | .4 | 600 | 587 | 568 | 578 | 561 | 551 |
| .7 | .4 | 640 | 614 | 582 | 607 | 575 | 566 |
| .8 | .4 | 694 | 650 | 599 | 643 | 593 | 585 |
| .9 | .4 | 770 | 697 | 621 | 691 | 615 | 607 |
| .5 | .5 | 578 | 581 | 578 | 566 | 566 | 549 |
| .6 | .5 | 608 | 602 | 589 | 587 | 577 | 560 |
| .7 | .5 | 648 | 629 | 604 | 615 | 591 | 575 |
| .8 | .5 | 702 | 665 | 621 | 652 | 609 | 593 |
| .9 | .5 | 777 | 712 | 642 | 700 | 631 | 616 |
| .6 | .6 | 619 | 623 | 619 | 598 | 598 | 572 |
| .7 | .6 | 659 | 650 | 633 | 627 | 613 | 587 |
| .8 | .6 | 713 | 686 | 651 | 663 | 631 | 605 |
| .9 | .6 | 788 | 733 | 672 | 711 | 653 | 628 |
| .7 | .7 | 673 | 678 | 673 | 641 | 641 | 602 |
| .8 | .7 | 728 | 714 | 691 | 678 | 660 | 621 |
| .9 | .7 | 803 | 762 | 714 | 727 | 682 | 644 |
| .8 | .8 | 747 | 751 | 747 | 697 | 697 | 640 |
| .9 | .8 | 823 | 800 | 770 | 747 | 721 | 663 |
| .9 | .9 | 849 | 852 | 849 | 772 | 772 | 687 |

Percent with higher/lower $r_{YZ}$ means the percent of eligible people (those missing the main DV) with data for the auxiliary variables with higher and lower values for $r_{YZ}$. For all cells, $r_{Z1,Z2} = (r_{YZ1} + r_{YZ2})/2$

Perhaps one of the most interesting findings in Table 11.6 relates to the comparison with $N_{EFF}$ values in Table 11.4. Look at the %Z = 100 % column in Table 11.4 and compare those values with the .50/.50 column in Table 11.6 where $r_{Y,Z1} = r_{Y,Z2}$. Note that the values in Table 11.6 are always somewhat larger, ranging from a $N_{EFF}$ difference of 8 for $r_{YZ} = .40$ to a $N_{EFF}$ difference of 14 when $r_{YZ} = .90$. These differences occur because $r_{Z1,Z2}$ in the two auxiliary variable case is not $r = 1.0$, as it is in the one auxiliary variable case. Recall that $r_{Z1,Z2}$ in Table 11.6 were set to be the average of $r_{YZ1}$ and $r_{YZ2}$. When this value is set to $r = .99$, the $N_{EFF}$ values in Table 11.6 are the same as the corresponding values in Table 11.4.

## Estimating $N_{EFF}$ with One or Two Auxiliary Variables: The General Case

It is possible to estimate the $N_{EFF}$ in complex, two auxiliary variable scenarios, based on combinations of tabled values, and interpolation of tabled values for one auxiliary variable (Table 11.4). However, this approach is complicated, somewhat tedious and error prone, and at best provides only a rough approximation of the $N_{EFF}$ in complex, two auxiliary variable scenarios. A closed-form solution may also be possible for calculating the $N_{EFF}$ in all one- and two auxiliary variable scenarios. However, the closed-form solution is not currently available.

We have taken a third approach here. Using an automation utility, similar in many ways to the other automation utilities described in this book (see especially Chap. 10), it is possible to generate the LISREL code required to obtain exact estimates of the $N_{EFF}$ in all one- and two auxiliary variable scenarios. We now describe this utility.

### Automation Utility for Estimating $N_{EFF}$ in All One Auxiliary Variable Scenarios

The tables provided in this chapter go a long way toward helping investigators determine the benefit they might realize by including auxiliary variables in their missing data and analysis models. However, the tables cannot hope to provide the kind of detail researchers are likely to find in many studies.

As we noted above, with just one auxiliary variable, one must take six factors into account ($N_{TOT}$, $N_{CC}$, $r_{XY}$, $r_{XZ}$, $r_{YZ}$, and %Z). Although Table 11.4 provides good insights about the benefit one can realize with one auxiliary variable, many possible scenarios fall between the values provided in the tables.

Our automation utility, AuxMARSimulate, allows researchers to calculate the precise benefit from including one auxiliary variable. The utility is a Windows Java application. The user supplies some basic information and the utility automatically writes the multiple group LISREL syntax that will perform the analyses needed to calculate the exact $N_{EFF}$ benefit. Of course, in order for the utility to work, one must already have LISREL installed on the computer to be used. Fortunately, pretty much

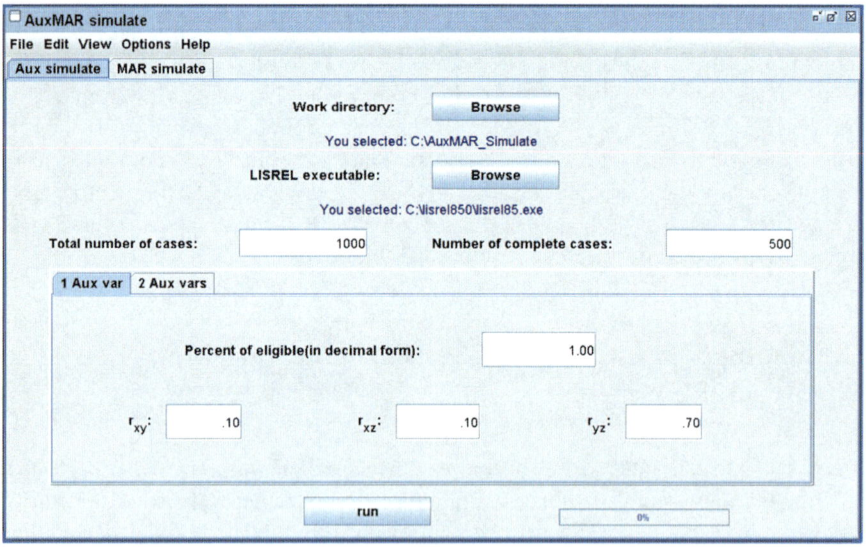

**Fig. 11.2** AuxMARSimulate (automation utility) window. This utility calculates the benefits of adding one auxiliary variable with the parameters shown in the figure

any version of LISREL will work, as far back as LISREL 7. In fact, even the free, downloadable, student version of LISREL 8.8 will work with this utility. Further, those using the utility need have virtually no knowledge of LISREL. The utility handles the writing of LISREL syntax, and running the program, all automatically.

**Running AuxMARSimulate Utility**

Download the AuxMARSimulate.exe utility from our website (http://methodology.psu.edu). This utility can be placed into any Windows folder that is convenient (e.g., on the desktop).

Locate the AuxMARSimulate.exe utility and run it. A picture of the utility window for auxiliary variables is shown in Fig. 11.2.

Click on the Browse button and specify the Work directory. All work files and the output file will go to the specified folder. The folder selected will appear in blue below the Browse button.

Click on the Browse button for the LISREL executable. This file may be located in the folder Program Files, but it may also be located in a LISREL file off the root directory. The location of your LISREL executable will appear in blue under the Browse button, as illustrated in Fig. 11.2.

Specify the total number of cases and the number of complete cases.

Specify the percent of eligible cases with data (in decimal form). 100 % is entered as 1.00 as shown in Fig. 11.2. 85 % would be shown as .85.

Table 11.7 Output for AuxMARSimulate utility

```
Output for Aux simulate Utility
target SE = 0.039014
Current SE = 0.039017
SE diff = 0.000003
Ntot = 1000
OrigNcc = 500
Neff = 660
Neff percent benefit = 32.0%
```

The "Neff percent benefit" is the percent of the way from Ncc to Ntot. This output corresponds to input values shown in Fig. 11.2

Specify the values for the three correlations, $r_{XY}$, $r_{XZ}$, and $r_{YZ}$.
Click on the run button.

At the conclusion of the iterations, the output from the utility is written to a file called "AuxOut.txt", and will automatically appear in a Notepad window. For example, the parameters appearing in Fig. 11.2 produced the output shown in Table 11.7. Note that changes may be made to any parameter shown in the AuxMARSimulate window, and the utility may be rerun without changing the other parameters.

## Automation Utility for Estimating $N_{EFF}$ in All Two Auxiliary Variable Scenarios

The AuxMARSimulate.exe utility can also handle all scenarios involving two auxiliary variables. For this version of the utility, one may specify any desired values for these 11 factors: $N_{TOT}$, $N_{CC}$, $r_{XY}$, $r_{XZ1}$, $r_{YZ1}$, $r_{XZ2}$, $r_{YZ2}$, $r_{Z1Z2}$, $\%Z_1$, $\%Z_2$, and $\%Z_1Z_2$ (some of these factors have default values in the utility).

To run the two-auxiliary-variable version of the utility, just click on the "2 Aux vars" tab. A picture of the window for this version of the utility appears in Fig. 11.3. The steps for running this version of the utility are virtually the same as described above. The only differences are (a) that there are more quantities to be entered, and (b) the sum of the three percents cannot exceed 100 % (i.e., 1.0; however, the sum of the three percents may be less than 100 %). The output from this version of the utility, using the parameter values shown in Fig. 11.3, appears in Table 11.8.

## Implications of $N_{EFF}$ for Statistical Power Calculations

When planning research, intervention scientists frequently conduct power analyses in order to decide on a target sample size. These power analyses have traditionally been based on the sample size after attrition, without considering the impact of the

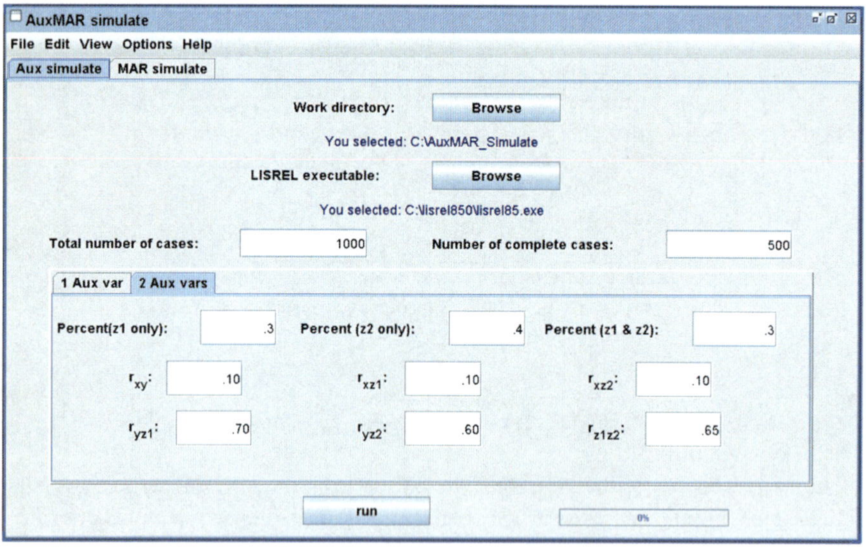

**Fig. 11.3** AuxMARSimulate (automation utility) window. This utility calculates the benefits of adding two auxiliary variables with the parameters shown in the figure

**Table 11.8** Output for AuxMARSimulate utility

```
Output for Aux simulate Utility
target SE = 0.039133
Current SE = 0.039134
SE diff = 0.000002
Ntot = 1000
OrigNcc = 500
Neff = 656
Neff percent benefit = 31.2%
```

The "Neff percent benefit" is the percent of the way from Ncc to Ntot. This output corresponds to input values shown in Fig. 11.3

missing data approach. As a way of maintaining power, researchers have often ensured a sufficiently large sample size at the end of a study by increasing the starting sample size to compensate for an expected attrition rate. For example, the researcher who expects a 10 % attrition rate per year might increase the starting sample size to $N = 1372$ in order to ensure power corresponding to a target $N = 1,000$ at the third follow-up measure. In this chapter, we propose that when modern missing data methods are used, the target for statistical power assessment can be $N_{EFF}$ rather than $N_{CC}$. This means that in evaluating the resource demands of a planned study, not only the expected attrition rate per se but also the missing data model, including possible auxiliary variables, should be considered. Collecting data on a useful set of auxiliary variables ultimately may maintain statistical power as well as or better than increasing the starting sample size to compensate for anticipated attrition. This strategy may also be less costly and more efficient.

It should be stressed that this possibility can be realized only if modern missing data methods, such as MI or ML methods, are used. There is no way to achieve the $N_{EFF}$ benefits with older methods such as analysis of complete cases.[5] A key to achieving a strong missing data model is a set of auxiliary variables that together are highly predictive of the outcome variable. Researchers planning studies may wish to consider what auxiliary variables to collect. Prior measures of the outcome variable, such as those available in most multi-wave longitudinal prevention studies, will often be useful auxiliary variables. Depending on the circumstances, other variables may also be useful.

## Loose Ends

### *What Happens When Pretest Covariates Are Included in the Model?*

To keep the examples simple, the models tested in this chapter involved a program variable predicting an outcome without a covariate (an after-only design). To be sure, including a covariate in the analysis model would change the degree to which adding an auxiliary variable would produce an $N_{EFF}$ benefit. However, that change is relatively easily calculated. A good approximation of the benefit of adding a particular auxiliary variable when a covariate is part of the model is to use, in place of $r_{YZ}$, the partial correlation, $r_{YZ}$, partialling the covariate. For example, in the AAPT study used as the main empirical example in this chapter, the correlation between the auxiliary variable Smk9 and the main DV, Smk10, was $r_{YZ}=.82$. The partial correlation between these two variables, partialling the pretest score (Smk7) was $r=.74$. Thus the $N_{EFF}$ benefit expected if Smk7 were included in the analysis model would be looked up for $r_{YZ}=.74$.

### *Multilevel Models*

Many intervention studies are conducted with individuals who come from intact units, for example, students within schools. That is, many intervention studies can

---

[5] This is true unless the variables acting as auxiliary variables happen to be part of the analysis model. The only analysis that fits this requirement well is growth modeling. That is, even when there are missing values in the growth part of the model, the growth model can be estimated making use of partial data. Although the results of this analysis are not maximum likelihood, they do tend to be unbiased and efficient.

be thought of as group randomized trials (GRT; e.g., see Murray 1998). The $N_{EFF}$ benefit from inclusion of auxiliary variables is, to be sure, more complicated in such studies. However, the $N_{EFF}$ benefits in such studies can be approximated in a straightforward way. One method for estimating power in GRT research is by estimating the program effect and standard error without taking the cluster structure into account and then adjusting that standard error by the design effect (DEFF; Murray 1998). It is also an easy matter to recalculate the effective sample size in these studies after taking the DEFF into account. In this kind of study, the sample size used prior to estimating the DEFF would be the $N_{EFF}$ (after taking auxiliary variables into account), rather than the nominal sample size normally used.

## *"Highly Inclusive" Versus "Selectively Inclusive" Models*

As part of their research, Collins et al. (2001) conducted simulations demonstrating that there could be a benefit of including many auxiliary variables in a model, and that there was no known harm in doing so. Since their article was published, however, many researchers have begun to notice that highly inclusive imputation models that consist of 100 or more variables can present serious logistical problems in the imputation and analysis phases of their research (see Chap. 9). For example, with the currently available (2012) software, including more than 100 variables in an imputation model often leads to problems such as EM convergence taking 1,000 or more iterations; imputation models that take up to 2 months to run; and analysis models that take days or even weeks to run, especially if a large number of imputations are used (e.g., see Graham et al. 2007). The results produced can have questionable validity. This problem should fade in the future as software and hardware increase in capability. However, the fact remains that although there may be no theoretical limits on the number of auxiliary variables included in the model, today there are practical limits.

Also important is the fact that one reaches the point of diminishing returns rather quickly when adding auxiliary variables to one's model. The relevant correlations for demonstrating this concept are $r_{Y,Z1}$, $r_{Y,Z2}$, and $r_{Z1,Z2}$.[6] One way to demonstrate the point would be to examine all possible combinations of the three correlations. A serious drawback to this approach, however, is that some unusual combinations of the correlations produce unbelievable results. For example, with a single auxiliary variable with $r_{Y,Z1} = .82$, $N_{EFF} = 750$. However, adding a second auxiliary variable with $r_{Y,Z2} = .001$ and $r_{Z1,Z2} = .517$ yields $N_{EFF} = 922$. Although there could be a plausible explanation for this finding (e.g., relating to suppressor effects), we feel it would be better to stay with more typical configurations of these three correlations. For this reason, we believe that the best approach here is to show a range of correlations from real empirical data.

---

[6] For this demonstration, we will stay with the scenario in which $N_{TOT} = 1,000$, $N_{CC} = 500$, and %Z = 100 % for both auxiliary variables.

**Table 11.9** Incremental $N_{EFF}$ benefit of adding a second auxiliary variable

| Variable | Measured at Grades | $r_{Y,Z1}$ | $r_{Y,Z2}$ | $r_{Z1,Z2}$ | $N_{EFF}$ 1 Aux. Var. | 2 Aux. Vars. | Increase |
|---|---|---|---|---|---|---|---|
| Alcohol | 7, 8, 9 | .56 | .44 | .57 | 591 | 598 | 7 |
| Alcohol | 8. 9, 10 | .57 | .48 | .56 | 595 | 608 | 13 |
| Alcohol | 9, 10, 11 | .63 | .44 | .57 | 621 | 625 | 4 |
| Drunk | 7, 8, 9 | .60 | .45 | .57 | 608 | 614 | 6 |
| Drunk | 8. 9, 10 | .67 | .50 | .60 | 642 | 648 | 6 |
| Drunk | 9, 10, 11 | .77 | .57 | .67 | 708 | 711 | 3 |
| Smoking | 7, 8, 9 | .62 | .48 | .58 | 617 | 625 | 8 |
| Smoking | 8. 9, 10 | .72 | .57 | .62 | 672 | 684 | 12 |
| Smoking | 9, 10, 11 | .76 | .63 | .72 | 700 | 707 | 7 |
| Marijuana | 7, 8, 9 | .50 | .30 | .38 | 570 | 574 | 4 |
| Marijuana | 8. 9, 10 | .54 | .36 | .50 | 583 | 587 | 4 |
| Marijuana | 9, 10, 11 | .62 | .42 | .54 | 617 | 620 | 3 |
| Peer Use | 7, 8, 9 | .52 | .41 | .46 | 576 | 588 | 12 |
| Peer Use | 8. 9, 10 | .56 | .41 | .52 | 591 | 598 | 7 |
| Peer Use | 9, 10, 11 | .63 | .48 | .56 | 621 | 630 | 9 |

| Variables and grades | $r_{Y,Z1}$ | $r_{Y,Z2}$ | $r_{Z1,Z2}$ | $N_{EFF}$ 1 Aux. Var. | 2 Aux. Vars. | Increase |
|---|---|---|---|---|---|---|
| Smk9, Smk8, Reb8 | .62 | .33 | .37 | 617 | 621 | 4 |
| Smk9, Smk8, Peer8 | .62 | .24 | .34 | 617 | 617 | 0 |
| Smk10, Smk9, Posatt9 | .72 | .41 | .43 | 672 | 678 | 6 |
| Smk8, Smk7, Likepar7 | .58 | .17 | .23 | 599 | 599 | 0 |
| Smk9, Smk8, Likepar8 | .62 | .22 | .20 | 617 | 620 | 3 |

*Top panel*: the third variable in each set is the main DV (Y); the second variable is the auxiliary variable $Z_1$; the first variable is the auxiliary variable $Z_2$
*Bottom Panel*: Grade is shown at the end of each variable. The first variable in each set is the main DV (Y); the second variable is the auxiliary variable $Z_1$; the third variable is the auxiliary variable $Z_2$. "Smk" = Smoking; "Reb" = Rebelliousness; "Peer" = Perceptions of Peer Use; "Posatt" = Beliefs about the positive consequences of alcohol use; "Likepar" = Relationship with Parents

Let us consider two scenarios. First, let us consider the scenario in which one has a dependent variable measured at three consecutive posttest waves. The measure at the third posttest wave represents the main DV. The measure at the second posttest wave (one wave removed from the main DV) represents the auxiliary variable with the best $r_{YZ}$ ($r_{Y,Z1}$). The measure at the first posttest wave (two waves removed from the main DV) represents an auxiliary variable with a somewhat lower $r_{YZ}$ ($r_{Y,Z2}$). Data from the AAPT study can be used to illustrate the effects of the three relevant correlations: $r_{Y,Z1}$, $r_{Y,Z2}$, and $r_{Z1,Z2}$.

AAPT data for this scenario appear in the top panel of Table 11.9. Note that for each of these variables there was a small increment in $N_{EFF}$ when the second auxiliary variable was added. The average increment in $N_{EFF}$ was 7.0 for this scenario.

The average $N_{EFF} = 620.8$ ($N_{EFF}$ benefit of 120.8) with the first auxiliary variable, so this increment represents just a 5.8 % incremental benefit ($127.8/120.8 = 1.058$).

**Bottom Panel**

Grade is shown at the end of each variable. The first variable in each set is the main DV (Y); the second variable is the auxiliary variable $Z_1$; the third variable is the auxiliary variable $Z_2$. "Smk" = Smoking; "Reb" = Rebelliousness; "Peer" = Perceptions of Peer Use; "Posatt" = Beliefs about the positive consequences of alcohol use; "Likepar" = Relationship with Parents.

The second scenario involves the main dependent variable (Smoking in this case) at one grade. The first auxiliary variable ($Z_1$) is the same variable measured at the previous wave. The second auxiliary variable ($Z_2$) is another variable measured at the same wave as $Z_1$. The AAPT results for this scenario are presented in the lower panel of Table 11.9. The second auxiliary variable in this illustration was one of these: Rebelliousness (Rebel), Perceived Peer Use (Peer), Beliefs about the Positive Consequences of Alcohol Use (Posatt), or Relationship with Parents (Likepar). These variables were meant to be like the kinds of variables that researchers often consider as auxiliary variables: They are different from the main DV, but are variables that are reasonably highly correlated (in real-world terms) with the main dependent variable.

Note that the average increment in $N_{EFF}$ for this scenario was only 2.6. The average $N_{EFF} = 624.4$ ($N_{EFF}$ benefit of 124.4) with the first auxiliary variable only. Thus, the increment of adding the second auxiliary variable represents just a 2.1 % incremental benefit ($127.0/124.4 = 1.021$).

The results shown in Table 11.9 do illustrate the point that there will often be relatively little gain in adding a second auxiliary variable with $r_{YZ}$ lower than the first auxiliary variable already in the model. This does not mean that one should never include a second (or third or fourth) auxiliary variable in the model. It just means that one should be aware of the trade-offs. If one is testing a relatively small model, that is one with relatively few variables, then one can easily afford to include a few extra auxiliary variables, even if the incremental $N_{EFF}$ benefit is relatively small. However, when the number of variables is large, one must be more judicious in selecting auxiliary variables.

It is true that the empirical data shown in Table 11.9 do not represent a wide range of values researchers will encounter. It may well be that a researcher will find that the incremental benefit of adding a second (or third or fourth) auxiliary variable to the model will be much larger than implied by the results shown here. The automation utility described above for calculating the $N_{EFF}$ benefit given any combination of factors will help researchers calculate the benefit they can expect in their particular situation.

One last point here is that the relatively small gains for adding a second auxiliary variable described in Table 11.9 were based on the idea that 100 % of subjects missing on Y have data for both auxiliary variables. With other missing data patterns, adding a second auxiliary variable will be much more beneficial. For example, although not shown here, consider the scenario in which 33 %, 33 %, and 34 % of the eligible subjects have data, respectively, for $Z_1$ only, $Z_2$ only, and $Z_1$ plus $Z_2$. Given the same correlations shown in Table 11.9, this new scenario yields $N_{EFF}$ benefits that are roughly triple those shown above.

## What Other Factors May Affect the True $N_{EFF}$ Benefit?

The models used in the artificial examples in this chapter assumed data were normally distributed. Empirical data generally deviate rather substantially from normal. This very likely will affect the actual $N_{EFF}$ to an extent. It is possible that theoretical estimates of $N_{EFF}$ will be more accurate for nonnormal data if bootstrap methods are used to obtain standard errors.

There is some evidence that MAR missingness that deviates substantially from MCAR may yield somewhat lower $N_{EFF}$ benefits. However, we have every reason to believe that the missingness in many mainstream intervention studies deviate from MCAR in a much more mild way.

## References

Allison, P. D. (1987). Estimation of linear models with incomplete data. In C. Clogg (Ed.), Sociological Methodology 1987 (pp. 71–103). San Francisco: Jossey Bass.

Collins, L. M., Schafer, J. L., & Kam, C. M. (2001). A comparison of inclusive and restrictive strategies in modern missing data procedures. Psychological Methods, 6, 330–351.

Graham, J. W. (2003). Adding missing-data relevant variables to FIML-based structural equation models. *Structural Equation Modeling*, 10, 80–100.

Graham, J. W., & Donaldson, S. I. (1993). Evaluating interventions with differential attrition: The importance of nonresponse mechanisms and use of followup data. Journal of Applied Psychology, 78, 119–128.

Graham, J. W., Olchowski, A. E., & Gilreath, T. D. (2007). How Many Imputations are Really Needed? Some Practical Clarifications of Multiple Imputation Theory. Prevention Science, 8, 206–213.

Graham, J. W., Taylor, B. J., & Cumsille, P. E. (2001). Planned missing data designs in analysis of change. In L. Collins & A. Sayer (Eds.), *New methods for the analysis of change*, (pp. 335–353). Washington, DC: American Psychological Association.

Graham, J. W., Taylor, B. J., Olchowski, A. E., & Cumsille, P. E. (2006). Planned missing data designs in psychological research. Psychological Methods, 11, 323–343.

Hansen, W. B., & Graham, J. W. (1991). Preventing alcohol, marijuana, and cigarette use among adolescents: Peer pressure resistance training versus establishing conservative norms. Preventive Medicine, 20, 414–430.

Jöreskog, K. G., & Sörbom, D. (1996). LISREL 8 User's Reference Guide. Chicago, IL: Scientific Software, Inc.

Murray, D. M. (1998). Design and analysis of group-randomized trials. New York: Oxford University Press.

Muthén, B., Kaplan, D., & Hollis, M. (1987). On structural equation modeling with data that are not missing completely at random. Psychometrika, 52, 431–462.

Muthén, L. K., & Muthén, B. O. (2010). *Mplus User's Guide. (6th ed.)*. Los Angeles: Author.

# Section 4
# Planned Missing Data Design

# Chapter 12
# Planned Missing Data Designs I: The 3-Form Design

## Who Should Read This Chapter?

This chapter draws heavily on the material covered in the article, "Planned missing data designs in psychological research" published in the journal, *Psychological Methods,* by Graham et al. (2006). Early in that article, we made this statement:

> The value of the planned missing data designs presented in this article hinges on one's ability to make use of analysis procedures that handle missing data.

I believe this statement. It does seem to imply that one should not tackle this chapter until one has mastered the analysis of missing data, which is covered in detail in earlier chapters of this book. But let us take a closer look. What are the reasons why one should and should not use a planned missing data design such as the 3-form design?

## *Reasons for Not Using the 3-Form Design*

### Lack Missing Data Analysis Skills

Certainly one reason for not using a measurement design that increases missing data is that one lacks the skills for performing the required missing data analysis. Having data from the 3-form design (and other related designs) does increase the need to have missing data analysis abilities.

However, I do not see this as a legitimate reason for not using this design. Missing data analysis skills are also needed for handling other kinds of missing data. In longitudinal studies, for example, it is relatively rare for there not to be a substantial amount of missing data due to attrition. Further, using the recommended procedures, such as those described in this book, is becoming the norm. And it is getting more and more difficult to publish empirical articles in top journals without using these procedures.

**Happy with Data Collected**

A second reason for not using the 3-form design is that there is simply no need. If the researcher is completely happy with the number of questions that can be addressed at each wave of measurement with a particular population, then there is no need to make use of a design whose main feature is increasing the number of questions that can be asked. I agree that this is a legitimate reason for not making use of the 3-form design.

## *Reasons for Using the 3-Form Design*

There is just one reason for using the 3-form design. That reason, the need to ask more questions than seems possible, is embodied in these two scenarios:

> Scenario 1: The researchers would very much like to ask 133 questions of their research participants. But, as is often the case, the participants are willing or able to answer only 100 questions given the time (and/or payment) available to them.
> In this scenario, only option seems to be to ask fewer questions.

> Scenario 2: In a longitudinal study, the researchers have been asking their participants questions requiring 60 minutes of work at every wave of measurement. Now, however, the data collection manager tells them that the gate keepers (e.g., school administrators) can provide only 45 minutes for questionnaire completion.
> In this scenario, the only option seems to be to ask fewer questions than asked in previous waves, so that the participants can complete the survey in 25 % less time.

In both of these scenarios, conditions seem to require that the researchers ask fewer questions than they would like to ask. The 3-form design was designed to address this very problem; it was designed to give researchers another option in these two scenarios.

## The 3-Form Design: History, Layout, Design Advantages

The 3-form design is a measurement design that falls under the general heading of ***matrix sampling*** designs. Matrix sampling designs can be thought of as one of several kinds of ***efficiency design***. The main goal of all efficiency designs is to conduct the research in a way that provides a rigorous test of the research questions, while reducing research costs compared to alternative designs.

Perhaps the most common kind of efficiency design is random sampling of subjects (e.g., Thompson 2002). Other, commonly used efficiency designs include what has been referred to as ***optimal designs*** (e.g., Allison et al. 1997; McClelland 1997), and ***factorial designs*** (including full factorial and fractional factorial designs; e.g., Box et al. 1978; Collins et al. 2009, 2005; West and Aiken 1997). The efficiency of optimal designs and factorial designs relates to the independent

Table 12.1 Simple matrix sampling design

| Form | Item sets answered | | | |
|---|---|---|---|---|
| | 100 A | 100 B | 100 C | 100 (items within each item set) D |
| 1 | 1 | 0 | 0 | 0 |
| 2 | 0 | 1 | 0 | 0 |
| 3 | 0 | 0 | 1 | 0 |
| 4 | 0 | 0 | 0 | 1 |

1: respondents received questions; 0: respondents did not receive questions

variable in experiments. Matrix sampling, on the other hand, relates to measurement of the dependent variables and covariates in experimental and nonexperimental designs.

## *Matrix Sampling: Early Designs*

The main goal of subject sampling designs is, of course, to sample which subjects will be included in the study. The main goal of optimal and factorial designs is to sample which experimental effects will be studied. The main goal of matrix sampling is a little different. Matrix sampling samples which items will be offered to which respondents. In the earliest days of matrix sampling (e.g., Lord 1962; Shoemaker 1973; Munger and Loyd 1988), the focus of the studies was on obtaining meaningful estimates of means and standard deviations for a large number of items, but without taxing individual respondents too much. An example of this kind of design is shown in Table 12.1.

The example design shown in Table 12.1 is best at reducing the load on the individual respondents. For example, suppose each item set (A, B, C, D) included 100 items as shown in the table. That would mean that means and standard deviations could be estimated for 400 individual items, and yet each respondent would respond to just 100 items. An important limitation of this kind of design is that correlations can be estimated only for the items within each set. That is, with this type of design, correlations cannot be estimated for two items from different item sets.

## *History of the 3-Form Design*

They say that need is the mother of invention. Nowhere is that truer than with the original development of the 3-form design. In 1982, I was working in a research group that eventually became known as the Institute for Prevention Research (IPR) at the University of Southern California. We were working on the first, large-scale multiple substance abuse prevention program ever funded (Project SMART;

**Table 12.2** 3-form design

| Form | Item sets answered | | | |
|---|---|---|---|---|
| | 34 | 33 | 33 | 33 (items within each item set) |
| | X | A | B | C |
| 1 | 1 | 1 | 1 | 0 |
| 2 | 1 | 1 | 0 | 1 |
| 3 | 1 | 0 | 1 | 1 |

1: respondents received questions; 0: respondents did not receive questions

Andy Johnson, Principal Investigator). The project, like many large-scale field research projects, had multiple investigators, each of whom wanted to see many favorite questions on the final version of our questionnaire. Scenario 1, given above under Reasons for Using the 3-form design was definitely true for us. Based on pilot work in our schools, we figured our students would answer approximately 125 questions in the 50 min class periods available to us. Unfortunately, our first cut through the survey netted more like 200 questions.

In our case, as in most situations like this (which I have found to be the rule, not the exception in collaborative field research), we could cut the number of questions down some, but the number did not approach the 125 questions we thought we needed. Thus, the first version of the 3-form design was born.

## *Basic Layout of the 3-Form Design*

Table 12.2 shows the basic layout of the original 3-form design. With this design (which remains the most commonly implemented version), there are four item sets: X, A, B, and C. The items in the X set are typically the questions most important for answering the central questions of the research. These questions are answered by everyone. The A, B, and C sets are then rotated such that each form omits one of the sets as shown.

## *Advantages of the 3-Form Design over Other Designs*

It is easy to see that the main advantage of the 3-form design over the 1-form design (which is the same as using Form 1 only) is that data can be collected from more questions using the 3-form design. If the item sets have the same number of questions, then the 3-form design increases the number of variables by 33 % compared to the 1-form design. For example, if each item set contains the number of items shown in Table 12.2, then each respondent sees only 100 questions, but data are collected on 133 questions in total.

The 3-form design is also better than the simple matrix sampling design shown in Table 12.1 in the sense that all correlations between variables may be estimated with the 3-form design. Data from more questions (400) can be collected using the simple matrix sampling design, but only means and standard deviations may be estimated on all of those variables; correlations (and related quantities) may estimated only for variables within each item set and only for the subsample of the population for which those variables were collected.

A key advantage of the 3-form design is that the missingness due to the design is MCAR. Of course, there is almost always at least a small amount of MAR missingness that is superimposed over the planned missing data, but for the most part, the MCAR assumption for these data is strong.

## *Disadvantages of the 3-Form Design Compared to the 1-Form Design*

The disadvantage of the 3-form design is that a particular correlation effect[1] might be nonsignificant when tested with the 3-form design, but would have been significant had the 1-form design been used. However, I find it difficult to call this a disadvantage, in that at the time one chooses between the two designs, the probability can be as low as one likes that this disadvantage will manifest itself with an important correlation effect.

Let me lay out this issue in some detail here, and at the end of this section I will revisit the question of whether it is really a disadvantage. I begin by examining the correlation effects testable with the 3-form design. These effects are summarized in Table 12.3. Going back to Table 12.2, you can see that any correlation involving two variables from the X set (referred to as XX) will be tested with the full $N$. Any correlation between two variables within the A set, B set, or C set (referred to as AA, BB, or CC) will be tested with $2N/3$. Any correlation between one variable in X and one variable in A, B, or C (referred to as XA, XB, or XC) will also be tested with $2N/3$. Finally, any correlation between one variable in A, B, or C, and another variable in one of the other sets (A, B, or C; referred to as AB, AC, or BC), will be tested with $N/3$. There are $k(k-1)/2$ correlation effects within each item set and $k^2$ effects across any two item sets, where $k$ is the number of items per set. With $k=10$ in each of the four item sets, that works out to be 45 effects within each item set, and 100 effects across any two item sets.[2] The totals are as shown in Table 12.3.

---

[1] Throughout this chapter, I talk about correlations and correlation effects. What I say certainly does apply to correlations, per se, but the points made throughout this chapter are meant to apply as well to other measures of association.

[2] I chose $k=10$ here to reflect the idea that there are approximately 10 scales within each item set. Assuming 3 or 4 individual items per scale that would be 30–40 items per item set, which is consistent with the other examples I use in this chapter. So the correlation effects I talk about here are correlations between scales, not between individual items.

**Table 12.3** Correlation effects tested with 3-form design

| | Correlation effects tested with N shown | |
| --- | --- | --- |
| | 3-form design | 1-form design |
| Tested with total N (1,000) | | |
| XX effects | 45 | 435 |
| Tested with 2N/3 (667) | | |
| AA, BB, CC effects | 135 | — |
| XA, XB, XC effects | 300 | — |
| Tested with N/3 (333) | | |
| AB, AC, BC effects | 300 | — |
| Total | 780 | 435 |

Figures based on total $N = 1000$, and $k = 10$ scales per item set. With the 1-form design, everyone receives Form 1 as shown in Table 12.2.

## Total Number of Effects Testable in 1- and 3-Form Designs

With $k = 10$, the 3-form design allows one to test 780 correlation effects in total, as shown in Table 12.3. The 1-form design allows one to test just 435 correlation effects. The difference is that with the 1-form design, all 435 effects are tested with the full N, whereas with the 3-form design, 45 effects are tested with the full N, 435 effects are tested with 2N/3, and 300 effects are tested with N/3.[3]

## Statistical Power for Testing Various Effects

*The Tables.* More important than the sample size is the statistical power associated with testing various effects. Following the approach taken in Graham et al. (2006), statistical power for effect sizes from $\rho = .05$ to $\rho = .30$ for two different study sample sizes are given in Tables 12.4 and 12.5. Graham et al. (2006) provided tables for study $N = 300$. In Tables 12.4 and 12.5, I present tables for Study $N = 600$ and 1,000.[4]

In Tables 12.4 and 12.5, the ✘ mark indicates an effect that is better with the 1-form design, that is, an effect that has power ≥ .80 with the 1-form design and power < .80 with the 3-form design. The ✔ indicates an effect that is better with the 3-form design, that is, an effect that has power ≥ .80 with the 3-form design, but is untestable with the 1-form design because the C questions were not asked.[5]

---

[3] These numbers assume equal numbers of items in each item set of the 3-form design.

[4] Supplementary materials from Graham et al. (2006), including the comparable tables for $N = 3,000$ can be found at: http://dx.doi.org/10.1037/1082-989X.11.4.323.supp. Supplementary tables for this book, including power tables for several different sample sizes can be found at: http://methodology.psu.edu.

[5] The column for XX effects is omitted from these tables. Note that power for XX effects is the same as 1-form design power for other effects, and that power for XX effects is the same for both designs, that is, there are no ✔ or ✘ marks in the omitted columns.

**Table 12.4** Power with various effect sizes ($N=600$)

| Effect Size ($\rho$) | XA, XB, AA, BB 1-form $N=600$ | XA, XB, XC AA, BB, CC 3-form $N=400$ | Power Ratio | AB 1-form $N=600$ | AB, AC, BC 3-form $N=200$ | Power Ratio |
|---|---|---|---|---|---|---|
| 0.05 | 0.232 | 0.170 | 1.36 | 0.232 | 0.109 | 2.13 |
| 0.06 | 0.312 | 0.224 | 1.39 | 0.312 | 0.135 | 2.31 |
| 0.07 | 0.403 | 0.288 | 1.40 | 0.403 | 0.167 | 2.41 |
| 0.08 | 0.500 | 0.360 | 1.39 | 0.500 | 0.204 | 2.45 |
| 0.09 | 0.598 | 0.437 | 1.37 | 0.598 | 0.246 | 2.43 |
| 0.10 | 0.689 | 0.517 | 1.33 | 0.689 | 0.293 | 2.35 |
| 0.11 | 0.770 | 0.596✗ | 1.29 | 0.770 | 0.344✗ | 2.24 |
| 0.12 | 0.838 | 0.672✗ | 1.25 | 0.838 | 0.397✗ | 2.11 |
| 0.13 | 0.892 | 0.741✗ | 1.20 | 0.892 | 0.453✗ | 1.97 |
| 0.14 | 0.931 | ✓0.802 | 1.16 | 0.931 | 0.510✗ | 1.83 |
| 0.15 | ** | ✓0.854 | 1.12 | ** | 0.567✗ | 1.69 |
| 0.16 | ** | ✓0.896 | 1.09 | ** | 0.622✗ | 1.57 |
| 0.17 | ** | ✓0.928 | 1.06 | ** | 0.676✗ | 1.46 |
| 0.18 | ** | ✓0.952 | 1.04 | ** | 0.726✗ | 1.37 |
| 0.19 | ** | ✓0.969 | 1.03 | ** | 0.772✗ | 1.29 |
| 0.20 | ** | ✓0.981 | 1.02 | ** | ✓0.813 | 1.23 |
| 0.21 | ** | ✓0.989 | 1.01 | ** | ✓0.850 | 1.18 |
| 0.22 | ** | ✓0.994 | 1.01 | ** | ✓0.881 | 1.13 |
| 0.23 | ** | ✓** |  | ** | ✓0.908 | 1.10 |
| 0.24 | ** | ✓** |  | ** | ✓0.930 | 1.07 |
| 0.25 | ** | ✓** |  | ** | ✓0.948 | 1.05 |
| 0.26 | ** | ✓** |  | ** | ✓0.962 | 1.04 |
| 0.27 | ** | ✓** |  | ** | ✓0.973 | 1.03 |
| 0.28 | ** | ✓** |  | ** | ✓0.981 | 1.02 |
| 0.29 | ** | ✓** |  | ** | ✓0.987 | 1.01 |
| 0.30 | ** | ✓** |  | ** | ✓0.991 | 1.01 |

** indicates power > .995. ✗ indicates an effect size for which the 1-form design has power ≥ .80, and the 3-form design has power < .80. ✓ applies to XC or CC effects on the left, and AC or BC effects on the right. ✓ indicates an effect for which the 3-form design has power ≥ .80, and the 1-form design does not allow the test. The power ratio is the power for the 1-form design divided by the power for the 3-form design. Larger ratios favor the 1-form design; smaller ratios favor the 3-form design. All power ratios for XX effects are 1.00 (equal power for the two designs)

In Table 12.4, for example, a correlation of $\rho=.12$ between a variable in the X set and a variable in the A set (an XA effect) would be tested with power = .84 with the 1-form design ($N=600$), and with power = .67 with the 3-form design ($N=400$). The power ratio (1.25) in this instance means that the power with the 1-form design is 25 % higher than the power with the 3-form design. Also, any correlation of $\rho=.14$ or greater with one variable from the X set and one from the C set (an XC effect) is tested with power ≥ .80 with the 3-form design, and because the C set does not appear, the correlation is not testable at all with the 1-form design.

**Table 12.5** Power numbers with $N=1000$

| Effect Size ® | XA, XB, AA, BB  1-form  $N=1000$ | XA, XB, XC AA, BB, CC  3-form  $N=667$ | Power Ratio | AB  1-form  $N=1000$ | AB, AC, BC  3-form  $N=333$ | Power Ratio |
|---|---|---|---|---|---|---|
| 0.05 | 0.353 | 0.252 | 1.40 | 0.353 | 0.149 | 2.33 |
| 0.06 | 0.475 | 0.341 | 1.41 | 0.475 | 0.194 | 2.53 |
| 0.07 | 0.601 | 0.440 | 1.36 | 0.601 | 0.248 | 2.40 |
| 0.08 | 0.717 | 0.543 | 1.33 | 0.717 | 0.309 | 2.32 |
| 0.09 | 0.813 | 0.643✗ | 1.27 | 0.813 | 0.376✗ | 2.13 |
| 0.10 | 0.887 | 0.735✗ | 1.20 | 0.887 | 0.447✗ | 1.98 |
| 0.11 | 0.937 | ✔0.813 | 1.16 | 0.937 | 0.520✗ | 1.81 |
| 0.12 | 0.968 | ✔0.875 | 1.10 | 0.968 | 0.593✗ | 1.64 |
| 0.13 | 0.985 | ✔0.921 | 1.08 | 0.985 | 0.662✗ | 1.50 |
| 0.14 | 0.994 | ✔0.953 | 1.04 | 0.994 | 0.727✗ | 1.36 |
| 0.15 | ** | ✔0.973 | 1.03 | ** | ✔0.785 | 1.26 |
| 0.16 | ** | ✔0.986 | 1.01 | ** | ✔0.835 | 1.19 |
| 0.17 | ** | ✔0.993 | 1.01 | ** | ✔0.877 | 1.14 |
| 0.18 | ** | ✔** | | ** | ✔0.911 | 1.10 |
| 0.19 | ** | ✔** | | ** | ✔0.938 | 1.06 |
| 0.20 | ** | ✔** | | ** | ✔0.957 | 1.04 |
| 0.21 | ** | ✔** | | ** | ✔0.972 | 1.03 |
| 0.22 | ** | ✔** | | ** | ✔0.982 | 1.02 |
| 0.23 | ** | ✔** | | ** | ✔0.989 | 1.01 |
| 0.24 | ** | ✔** | | ** | ✔0.993 | 1.01 |
| 0.25 | ** | ✔** | | ** | ✔** | |
| 0.26 | ** | ✔** | | ** | ✔** | |
| 0.27 | ** | ✔** | | ** | ✔** | |
| 0.28 | ** | ✔** | | ** | ✔** | |
| 0.29 | ** | ✔** | | ** | ✔** | |
| 0.30 | ** | ✔** | | ** | ✔** | |

** indicates power > .995. ✗ indicates an effect size for which the 1-form design has power ≥ .80, and the 3-form design has power < .80. ✔ applies to XC or CC effects on the left, and AC or BC effects on the right. ✔ indicates an effect for which the 3-form design has power ≥ .80, and the 1-form design does not allow the test. The power ratio is the power for the 1-form design divided by the power for the 3-form design. Larger ratios favor the 1-form design; smaller ratios favor the 3-form design. All power ratios for XX effects are 1.00 (equal power for the two designs)

Tables 12.4 and 12.5 can definitely be a help in deciding between the designs. However, there is a tendency for researchers to be somewhat risk averse. That is, they tend to overvalue the badness of the ✗ effects and to undervalue the goodness of the ✔ effects. Graham et al. (2006) made two counterarguments in this regard. With their first counterargument, they showed, by looking at the power ratios, that the differences in power were relatively small between effects tested with the full $N$ and effects tested with $2N/3$. This point can also be made by examining the lowest testable effect (with power = .80) with the different study sample sizes and for effects

**Table 12.6** Smallest testable effect size (with power = .80)

| Study | Sample size | | |
|---|---|---|---|
| N | N | 2N/3 | N/3 |
| 3000 | .051 | .064 | .09 |
| 1000 | .09 | .11 | .15 |
| 600 | .115 | .14 | .20 |
| 300 | .16 | .20 | .28 |

that are tested with the full $N$, $2N/3$, and $N/3$. Table 12.6 displays this information. Note that with any study $N$, the difference in the smallest testable effect is not large between effects tested with $N$ and $2N/3$.

As I have argued above, researchers have control over where items are placed into the 3-form design and thus have a great deal of control over which effects are tested with $N$ and $2N/3$. For example, if the researcher deems a particular effect to be important, but expects a small effect size, then it makes most sense to place both variables relating to the effect in the X set, making it an XX effect. If the researcher deems an effect to be important, but expects the effect size to be larger (e.g., in the $\rho = .20-.30$ range), then it makes sense to place the variables into the survey such that the effect is one of those tested with $2N/3$. The problem arises, therefore, because an effect that was expected to be somewhat larger turns out to be smaller than expected. However, when this happens, as the numbers in Table 12.6 illustrate, the researcher is still protected to a large extent. For example, with study $N=600$, an effect that was expected to be $\rho = .20$ would have to fall below $\rho = .14$ for the effect to be a problem. And even if the true effect were $\rho = .11, .12$, or $.13$ (all values for which the 1-form design would have power $\geq .80$), power, although not ideal, would still be reasonable (.60, .67, .74, respectively).

With larger study sample sizes (e.g., $N=1,000$ or $N=3,000$), the chances are slim that a problem of the type just described would actually occur. With smaller study sample sizes, there is still some protection, but as in the case of study $N=300$, it would be advisable to draw the line somewhat higher as to which effects would go into the XX part of the design, and which might go into a part of the design where effects are tested with $2N/3$. That is, with study $N=1,000$, I might feel quite comfortable placing an effect into the $2N/3$ parts of the design if the expected effect size were at least $\rho = .20$. The true effect size would have to drop below $\rho = .11$ before there would be a problem with power. However, with study $N=300$, I would almost certainly require the effect size of $\rho \geq .30$ before I would feel comfortable placing the effect in a $2N/3$ part of the design.

The bottom line with this argument is that, for the most part, effects tested with $2N/3$ (XA, XB, AA, and BB) that are marked with a ✘ are not a huge concern.

The second counterargument made by Graham et al. (2006) focuses on the effects tested with $N/3$ (i.e., AB effects). They start by noting that, in the scenario with $k=10$ scales per item set, there are just 100 AB effects. Out of the total 780 effects available with the design, this represents just 12.8 % of the total number of effects. In addition, Graham et al. noted that effects are very likely not uniformly distributed and used data from the Adolescent Alcohol Prevention Trial (AAPT; Hansen and Graham 1991) as an example. The absolute values of the 1,540 correlations described from that data set had a slightly positive skew (1.01) with a mean $r=.194$ (SD=.139; median=.17), and ranged from 0 (rounded to nearest hundredth) to $r=.77$. If we focus on the study $N=600$ (see Table 12.4), nine of the AB effects are marked with a ✗, ranging from $\rho=.11$ to $\rho=.19$. In the AAPT data, 394/1,540, correlations or 25.6 % fell in this range. Summarizing, by chance alone, the probability is 12.8 % that an effect would be in the AB part of the design, and the probability is 25.6 % that an effect would be in the range of effect sizes where there is a problem. The joint probability, then, is just 3.3 % that there would be a problem.

Next, consider the probability that the researcher even chooses to study that particular effect. Recall that these effects are, for the most part, left over after the researcher makes predictions. That is, hypotheses (correlation effects) that are considered important are typically placed in parts of the design that are tested with the full $N$ (XX effects) or $2N/3$ (XA, XB, XC, AA, BB, CC effects). This does not necessarily mean that these leftover effects are unimportant. However, it must be true that they were not important enough to place them in a part of the design tested with at least $2N/3$. I believe I am being conservative in suggesting that there is a 50 % chance that the researcher will actually choose to test the effect in question.

Finally, statistical power is itself a probability. Look again at the AB effects marked ✗ in Table 12.4. The effect sizes range from $\rho=.11$ to $\rho=.19$. Statistical power for these effects ranges from .34 to .77, with median power=.57. This means that there is a 43 % chance that an effect of this magnitude would not be found to be significant. Combine all these probabilities, and we have

$$\text{probability of "bad" effect} = 12.8\% \times 25.6\% \times 50\% \times 43\% = 0.7\%.$$

That is, taking all the factors into account, the probability is very low for finding an effect to be nonsignificant with the 3-form design that would have been significant had the researcher opted for the 1-form design.

## Effect of Study $N$ on Number of ✗ and ✔ Marks

Looking at Tables 12.4 and 12.5 (also see the comparable table for $N=300$ in Graham et al. 2006), it is easy to see that smaller sample sizes have more effects that favor the 1-form design (more ✗ and fewer ✔), and that larger sample sizes have more effects that favor the 3-form design (more ✔ and fewer ✗). The bottom line summary is presented in Table 12.7. When taking all of the factors into account as I did above, the probability of there being a problem is somewhat higher with smaller study sample sizes. However, bottom line difference between study sample sizes is not that large. Different study sample sizes yield the probabilities shown in Table 12.7.

**Table 12.7** Probability of "bad" effect with 3-form design with different study N

| Study sample size | Factor probabilities | Bottom line probability |
|---|---|---|
| 300 | 12.8 % × 31 % × 50 % × 42 % | = 0.83 % |
| 600 | 12.8 % × 25.6 % × 50 % × 43 % | = 0.70 % |
| 1,000 | 12.8 % × 18.1 % × 50 % × 44.4 % | = 0.51 % |
| 3,000 | 12.8 % × 12.2 % × 50 % × 46 % | = 0.36 % |

## *The Disadvantage of the 3-Form Design Is Not Really a Disadvantage*

The main reason why researchers may feel more comfortable having all correlation effects tested with the full N is that they cannot see into the future, and they want to guard against the possibility of wanting to test a particular correlation later on, only to discover that they have insufficient $N$ to test the effect with adequate power. This is certainly a possibility. But rather than focus on this one possibility, consider the possibilities relating to both options:

Option (a): Ask the known, important, research question XC (or CC), with good power, and forego the *possibility* of later discovering an AB effect[6] that cannot be tested with power equal to that of the 1-form design (note that with study $N=600$, any newly discovered AB effect with effect size $\rho \geq .20$ can still be tested with good power; with study $N=1,000$, any newly discovered AB effect with effect size $\rho \geq .15$ can still be tested with good power).

Option (b): Do not ask the known, important, research question XC (or CC), and retain the *possibility* of later discovering an AB effect that can be tested with the same power as the 1-form design.

The real issue behind these two options is that there is a known, important, research question (in XC or CC). This gets back to the scenarios I presented at the start of this chapter. Use the 3-form design if there are more questions you would like to ask than are possible with the 1-form design. It may seem as though the choice here is an example of the bird-in-the-hand-is-worth-two-in-the-bush concept. But look closer. Actually, it is closer to being a case of two birds in the hand being better than one in the bush. It illustrates that people would never trade away a known, important, research question in favor of the *possibility* of another research question (possibly less important) later on, especially when, as I have shown in this chapter, that the chances are so slim that there would be any disadvantage in using the 3-form design.

---

[6] Recall that the XC and CC effects (along with the AC and BC effects) are extra effects made possible by the 3-form design; these are effects that are not possible with the 1-form design. The AB effect are the main source of problems in that these effects are most likely to have power < .80 for the 3-form design, and power ≥ .80 for the 1-form design.

## 3-Form Design: Other Design Elements and Issues

### Item Order

One of the key elements of the design is that the item sets should be rotated. With the most common implementation, the three forms are laid out as shown in Table 12.8. The good thing about rotating these item sets is that a different item set is presented last with each form. Because of this, respondents who fail to complete the questionnaire do not always leave the same items blank. I often suggest this rotation of item sets even if all items are presented.

**Variant of 3-Form Design**

A sometimes useful variant of the 3-form design involves presenting all item sets to the respondents. In this variant, as shown in Table 12.8, the item sets shown in brackets are asked. Because a different item set appears last for each form, respondents who fail to complete the survey will not always leave the same questions blank. Thus, the MAR assumption is much more plausible with this design. It is probably a good idea to use this variant only when a relatively high proportion of the participants can complete the entire survey. Although the MAR assumption is very good in this context (when causes of failing to complete the survey are measured early in each form), the missingness is not MCAR with this variant of the 3-form design.

### The X Set

**Is the X Set Needed?**

One question that often arises is whether the X set is even needed? Having fewer variables in the X set does mean that more variables can be examined. At the extreme, with the example shown in Table 12.2 (133 questions total, respondents answer 100 questions), the 1-form design has just 100 questions total, the balanced 3-form design (equal numbers of variables in all item sets) has 133 questions, and the version of the 3-form design with no X set has 150 questions (0 in the X set and

**Table 12.8** 3-form design item order

| Form | Item set order |
|---|---|
| 1 | X A B [C] |
| 2 | X C A [B] |
| 3 | X B C [A] |

Item sets in brackets are typically missing

50 in each of the A, B, and C sets). So if we get more data for more questions with this version, why not drop the X set altogether?

The answer is twofold. First, having a set of items for which everyone has data is what allows researchers to protect the most important hypotheses. That is, with the balanced version of the 3-form design, a certain number of correlation hypotheses are tested with the full sample size, thereby providing best possible power for the test of these important hypotheses. Most researchers do not want to give up this feature of the design. This is especially important when these important hypotheses also have small effect sizes. Second, having a substantial set of items for which everyone has data adds stability to the missing data model.

**How Large Should the X Set Be?**

My recommendation is to have the same number of variables in each of the item sets, including the X set. I believe this strategy provides the best balance of leveraging one's resources and providing a safety net for important hypotheses with small expected effect sizes. And, as I have argued above, I believe the balanced version of the design provides advantages with minimal disadvantages. On the other hand, some researchers have too many hypotheses to protect than can be protected by the balanced version of the design. These people often prefer to have a slightly larger X set. This strategy can work very well as long as it is understood that the trade-off is that having more items in the X set means fewer items overall. From the completely balanced version of the design, for every two items added to the X set, one fewer item can be measured overall (while holding constant the number of items seen by each respondent). Of course, it is also possible to increase the total number of items asked by reducing the number of items in the X set. I do not generally recommend this strategy, but small deviations from the fully balanced version of the design should work well.

**Placement of the X Set**

The most commonly implemented version of the 3-form design has the X items first. After all, the main point of including the X set is to have some effects tested with the full $N$. Placement of X items too close to the end of the survey could undermine this goal. On the other hand, I have often found it desirable to move sections of the X items further back in the survey. Although this can create some confusion during data analysis, this can sometimes be a very useful strategy.

## *Variations of the 3-Form Design: A Family of Designs*

Graham et al. (2006) described a family of designs, each of which involved offering to respondents all possible combinations of $L$ item sets taken two at a time. The

**Table 12.9** Specifications for family of designs: 3, 6, and 10-form designs

| Design | k addressed | Sample size for | | |
|---|---|---|---|---|
| | | XX | XA, AA | AB |
| 3-form | 133 | N | 2N/3 | N/3 |
| 6-form | 166 | N | 3N/6 | N/6 |
| 10-form | 199 | N | 4N/10 | N/10 |

XX refers to a correlation based on two items from the X set; XA refers to a correlation based on one item from the X set and one item from the A set; AA refers to a correlation based on two items from the A set, and so on. XA, AA also refers to items sets XB, XC, XD, XE (where available), and BB, CC, DD, and EE (where available). AB also refers to item set combinations AC, AD, AE, BC, BD, BE, CD, CE, and DE (where available)

3-form design offers all combinations of three item sets taken two at a time (the X set does not figure into this). But there can also be a 6-form design (all combinations of four item sets taken two at a time) and a 10-form design (all combinations of five item sets taken two at a time). The 10-form design has been described as the Split Questionnaire Survey Design (SQSD; Raghunathan and Grizzle 1995).

The advantage of these larger designs is that more questions can be addressed. With 34 items in the X set, and 33 remaining sets, the 3-form design allows the one to collect data on 133 items; the 6-form design allows one to collected data on 166 items; and the SQSD (10-form design) allows one to collect data on 199 items. In each case, respondents see only 100 items.

Although the logistical issues relating to the 3-form design have proven to be quite manageable for nearly 30 years of use, the problems associated with dealing with multiple forms do compound as the number of forms increases. Also, with the larger designs, the number of cases decreases as shown in Table 12.9. The sample sizes available for the other two sets of effects (XA, AA, etc., and AB, AC, etc.) are as shown in Table 12.9. It is easy to generalize these numbers for even larger design (e.g., 15- and 21-form designs).

The key disadvantage of these larger designs is that unless the study sample size is rather large, the sample sizes available for testing effects in the middle category can be rather small. On the other hand, when sample sizes are very large, these designs could have very desirable properties.

## What About a 2-Form Design?

The "2-form design" simply drops one form and one item set from the regular 3-form design, yielding the design shown in Table 12.10. But now each remaining item set can include 50 items, because each participant sees just two item sets (X and A or X and B). Although I have seen designs like this used, I do not recommend it under any circumstances. A serious flaw with the design is that correlations cannot

# 3-Form Design: Other Design Elements and Issues

**Table 12.10** "2-form" design (do not use it)

| Form | Item sets answered | | |
|---|---|---|---|
| | 50 | 50 | 50 (items within each item set) |
| | X | A | B |
| 1 | 1 | 1 | 0 |
| 2 | 1 | 0 | 1 |

1: respondents received questions; 0: respondents did not receive questions

**Table 12.11** Strategies for working with scale items in 3-form design

| | Item set | | |
|---|---|---|---|
| Strategy | A | B | C |
| (1) Keep Items Together | $R_1 R_2 R_3$ | $S_1 S_2 S_3$ | $T_1 T_2 T_3$ |
| (2) Split Items Across Sets | $R_1 S_1 T_1$ | $R_2 S_2 T_2$ | $R_3 S_3 T_3$ |

be estimated between items in set A and those in set B. This design offers only a 12.8 % increase in items over the balanced 3-form design, and its flaws make it an undesirable alternative to the 3-form design.

## *Keeping Scale Items Within One Item Set Versus Splitting Them Across Item Sets*

This issue, which comes up a lot, is described in Table 12.11. In the first strategy, the items from the R, S, and T scales are kept together. In the second strategy, the items are split, such that each item set contains some items from each scale. Graham et al. (1996) examined the statistical properties of these two strategies. In particular, we looked at the standard errors for one scale predicting another. The clear conclusion in that article was that strategy (2) (split items across sets) produces lower (better) standard errors.

Although the results of that study clearly favored strategy (2), there are good reasons for using strategy (1) instead. Most of what I say here comes from experience with the data from a large-scale study in which we implemented the strategy (2) version of the 3-form design. Most importantly, because the items were split across forms, we found that it was nearly always necessary to perform missing data analyses at the individual item level. With that data set, we were not able to perform complete cases analysis for anything. And the number of variables in our missing data models tended to be large, even for relatively simple analyses. Also, given what we said in Chap. 9, I would be very reluctant about imputing scale scores, some of which are based on partial data, after having used strategy (2) with the 3-form design. I will also say that with strategy (1), which I have now used on several large-scale data sets, has never proven to be an analytical problem. But that one attempt at splitting items across item sets has convinced me never to do that again.

# References

Allison, D. B., Allison, R. L., Faith, M. S., Paultre, F., & Pi-Sunyer, F. X. (1997). Power and money: Designing statistically powerful studies while minimizing financial costs. *Psychological Methods, 2*, 20–33.

Box, G. E. P., Hunter, W. G., & Hunter, J. S. (1978). Statistics for experimenters: An introduction to design, data analysis, and model building. New York: Wiley.

Collins, L. M., Dziak, J. J., and Li, R. (2009). Design of Experiments With Multiple Independent Variables: A Resource Management Perspective on Complete and Reduced Factorial Designs. Psychological Methods, 14, 202–224.

Collins, L. M., Murphy, S. A., Nair, V. N., & Strecher, V. J. (2005). A strategy for optimizing and evaluating behavioral interventions. Annals of Behavioral Medicine, 30, 65–73.

Graham, J. W., Hofer, S. M., & MacKinnon, D. P. (1996). Maximizing the usefulness of data obtained with planned missing value patterns: An application of maximum likelihood procedures. *Multivariate Behavioral Research, 31*, 197–218.

Graham, J. W., Taylor, B. J., Olchowski, A. E., and Cumsille, P. E. (2006). Planned missing data designs in psychological research. *Psychological Methods, 11*, 323–343.

Hansen, W. B., & Graham, J. W. (1991). Preventing alcohol, marijuana, and cigarette use among adolescents: Peer pressure resistance training versus establishing conservative norms. *Preventive Medicine, 20*, 414–430.

Lord, F. M. (1962). Estimating norms by item sampling. *Educational and Psychological Measurement, 22*, 259–267.

McClelland, G. H. (1997). Optimal design in psychological research. *Psychological Methods, 2*, 3–19.

Munger, G. F., & Loyd, B. H. (1988). The use of multiple matrix sampling for survey research. *Journal of Experimental Education, 56*, 187–191.

Raghunathan, T., & Grizzle, J. (1995). A split questionnaire survey design. *Journal of the American Statistical Association, 90*, 54–63.

Shoemaker, D. M. (1973). *Principles and procedures of multiple matrix sampling*. Cambridge, MA: Ballinger Publishing.

Thompson, S. K. (2002). *Sampling* (2nd ed.). New York: Wiley.

West, S. G., & Aiken, L. S. (1997). Toward understanding individual effects in multicomponent prevention programs: Design and analysis strategies. In K. Bryant, M. Windle, & S. West (Eds.), *The science of prevention: Methodological advances from alcohol and substance abuse research* (pp. 167–209). Washington, DC: American Psychological Association.

# Chapter 13
# Planned Missing Data Design 2: Two-Method Measurement

**John W. Graham and Allison E. Shevock**

In the early stages of developing measures of any construct, the primary objective is to develop a reasonable measure of the construct. Thus, it is common for the early measures of a construct to be a measure that is readily available, often involving a simple self-report, or a relatively noninvasive physical, physiological, or biological approach to measurement. However, the early measures often have construct validity problems that become obvious only as the science of measurement matures for that construct. Over time, researchers develop better measures of the construct, that is, measures with considerably improved construct validity.

However, it is also common for these better measures to be much more costly than the earlier measures, in terms of time, materials or equipment required, expert technicians required, payments to participants, and invasiveness. In cigarette smoking research, simple self-reports of smoking continue to be common, but many researchers now collect saliva samples (which are analyzed for cotinine, a metabolite of nicotine, or other substances related to smoking; Etter et al. 2000; Luepker et al. 1981), or expired air samples (which is analyzed for carbon monoxide; Biglan et al. 1985). In body composition research, self-reports of height and weight are still commonly used to calculate the body mass index (BMI). More involved measures of height and weight (for BMI calculations) involve using trained technicians and well-calibrated measurement equipment. Still more involved and costly is the use of dual energy X-ray absorptometry (DEXA) to assess body composition (Avesani et al. 2004; Fisher et al. 2000; Lohman 1996; Roubenoff et al. 1993). Blood pressure (BP) measurement is most commonly conducted in health clinics; a uniformed doctor, nurse, or technician typically places the cuff on the patient during a regular visit, and within seconds has the BP reading that is copied into the patient's permanent chart. A more recent, much more valid, but much more costly approach to BP measurement is ambulatory BP measurement (Gerin et al. 2006; O'Brien et al. 1991; Verdecchia et al. 2001); a BP device is worn by the patient for 24–36 consecutive hours, and the BP readings are taken and recorded every 15 min over that period.

In short, it is common for multiple measures to exist for any one construct; and the different measures often vary (sometimes greatly) in their construct validity, and in their cost. Compared to a cheaper measure, the more expensive measure is usually thought to be a more valid measure of the construct of interest. Researchers' decisions regarding which measure(s) to use are influenced, many times, by budget constraints. In a fixed cost scenario, selecting the expensive measure over the cheaper measure limits the amount of data that can be collected. Thus, the benefit of improved construct validity is offset by the power disadvantage of a small sample size. However, the alternative is not ideal, either; collecting data using a cheaper measure may improve sample size, but the researcher will still need to address the measure's low construct validity during data analysis.

The two-method measurement (TMM) design addresses this dilemma by providing researchers with a third data collection option. With the TMM design, constructs are measured using two or more indicators of variable cost and validity. The key idea behind the TMM approach is that both cheap and expensive measures can reasonably be modeled as measures of the same construct. The TMM design takes advantage of the fact that the combination of cheap and expensive measures produces greater statistical benefits than either measure provides on its own. Because of its lower cost, the cheap measure can be collected on many respondents, thereby providing statistical power benefits. In addition, because of its greater construct validity, the expensive measure can be used to model the bias (lack of construct validity) in the cheap measure, thereby producing highly valid statistical conclusions. Most importantly, the bias-correction ability of the expensive measures remains largely unchanged, even when only a small random subset of the respondents provides data for the expensive measure.

In sum, the TMM approach offers better statistical power than is possible using the expensive measure alone, and better construct validity than is possible using the cheap measure alone.

## Definition of Response Bias

The model we describe here is a response bias-correction model. By response bias, we are not referring to estimation bias. Rather, what we mean by bias in this context relates to construct validity; we are referring to the part of the response or score that is not valid. A measure is valid (i.e., has good construct validity) if it measures what we think it measures. For example, if we were talking about a self-report measure of cigarette smoking, the valid part of the measure is the part that actually measures cigarette smoking; the biased part might be the respondent's tendency to underreport cigarette smoking (e.g., for social desirability reasons). To the extent that response bias has a similar effect on all measures of a certain kind (this has been described as "halo errors"; Hoyt 2000; or "correlational bias"; Berman and Kenny 1976; also see Graham and Collins 1991), the bias can be modeled.

## The Bias-Correction Model

The bias-correction model has roots in the tradition of SEM analysis of multitrait-multimethod data (e.g., Eid 2000; Graham and Collins 1991; Kenny and Kashy 1992). Following these models and the thinking laid out in Palmer et al. (2002), Graham et al. (2006) outlined the bias-correction model and the two-method measurement design. Before talking about the missing data part of the model, we lay out the model itself.

Two important features of the bias-correction model distinguish it from other SEM models. First, there are at least two measures of the cheap but potentially flawed measure of the construct of interest. Second, there is at least one measure of the expensive measure, which can be assumed to be a valid measure of the same construct of interest. In real-world applications, this latter assumption need not actually be correct; it need only be the case that the expensive measure is one that is universally preferred over the cheap measure.

The bias-correction model, as presented by Graham et al. (2006), is shown in Fig. 13.1. In this model, cigarette smoking predicts health. Cigarette smoking is measured using four indicators. Two self-report measures serve as the cheap smoking measures, and expired CO and saliva cotinine represent the more expensive, more valid measures. Because there were two cheap measures of cigarette smoking, it was possible to model the bias associated with the self-report measures simply by allowing those two measures to load on a separate bias factor in addition to the smoking factor (see Fig. 13.1). The presence of the expensive measures (CO and cotinine) permits estimation of the bias factor. In the absence of the expensive measures in this model, it would not have been possible to have the cheap measures load on both the smoking and bias factors. In other words, the expensive measures were

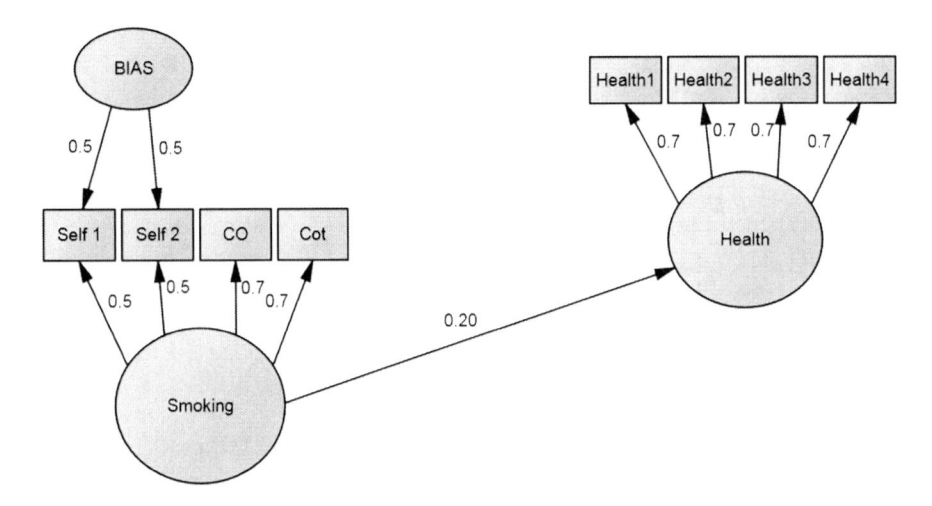

**Fig. 13.1** Bias correction model presented by Graham et al. (2006)

necessary for disentangling the valid parts of the self-report measures from the biased parts. Note that although the model presented in Fig. 13.1 involved estimating a separate bias factor, the same model may also be tested simply by estimating the residual covariance between the two cheap (self-report) items (e.g., see Kenny and Kashy 1992).

## Benefits of the Bias-Correction Model

### *The Idea of the Benefit*

Graham et al. (2006) presented results from several simulations showing the benefits of the two-method measurement design. These benefits stem from the fact that data are collected using a planned missingness approach. In other words, the researcher purposefully tailors the data collection processes so that all respondents provide data for the cheap measures, but only a random sample of those respondents also provides data for the expensive measure(s). The end result is that the majority of respondents have missing data for the expensive measures, and a smaller subsample has complete data.

Table 13.1 presents a scenario in which the cheap measures can be obtained for $4 per respondent, and the expensive measures are obtained for $20 per respondent (a 5:1 cost ratio). The first row in Table 13.1 outlines the complete case scenario; for a total of $7,200 in measurement costs, complete data can be collected from $N=300$ participants. The 5:1 cost ratio scenario outlined in this example means that for every one fewer participant presented with the expensive measure, the total sample size can be expanded by collecting cheap measure data from five additional participants. For presentation purposes, Table 13.1 summarizes sample sizes when the number of cases presented with expensive measures decreases by multiples of 20. Collecting expensive data for just 20 fewer cases means that, for the same total costs, one can collect cheap measure data for 100 additional cases, thus expanding total sample size by $N=100$.

Row 2 of Table 13.1 shows the first planned missing data collection strategy: for the same overall costs of $7,200, one can collect data for $N=400$ cheap measures and 280 expensive measures. In this second scenario, $N=120$ participants of the total sample provide partial data (cheap measures only), and the remaining $N=280$ provide complete data. In the most extreme partial data scenario, shown in the last row of Table 13.1, cheap measure data are obtained from $N=1,700$ cases, and expensive measures are obtained from just $N=20$ cases, yielding a 84:1 ratio of cases with partial to complete data.

Showing that the various designs in Table 13.1 all cost the same is only part of the picture. An interesting thing happens when we test the model of cigarette smoking predicting health using the parameters shown in Fig. 13.1 and the different sample size configurations shown in Table 13.1. As noted previously, the

**Table 13.1** Hypothetical data collection costs when expensive measures cost five times more than cheap measures

| Total $N$ | $N$ cheap | $N$ expensive | $N$ partial | $N$ complete | Total costs | Standard error | $N_{EFF}$ | $N_{EFF}$ increase factor |
|---|---|---|---|---|---|---|---|---|
| 300 | 300 | 300 | 0 | 300 | $7,200 | .0543 | 300 | |
| 400 | 400 | 280 | 120 | 280 | $7,200 | .0511 | 338 | |
| 500 | 500 | 260 | 240 | 260 | $7,200 | .0486 | 373 | |
| 600 | 600 | 240 | 360 | 240 | $7,200 | .0465 | 409 | |
| 700 | 700 | 220 | 480 | 220 | $7,200 | .0448 | 440 | |
| 800 | 800 | 200 | 600 | 200 | $7,200 | .0434 | 469 | |
| 900 | 900 | 180 | 720 | 180 | $7,200 | .0422 | 495 | |
| 1,000 | 1,000 | 160 | 840 | 160 | $7,200 | .0413 | 518 | |
| 1,100 | 1,100 | 140 | 960 | 140 | $7,200 | .0407 | 533 | |
| **1,200** | **1,200** | **120** | **1,080** | **120** | **$7,200** | **.0403** | **542** | **1.81** |
| 1,300 | 1,300 | 100 | 1,200 | 100 | $7,200 | .0404 | 540 | |
| 1,400 | 1,400 | 80 | 1,320 | 80 | $7,200 | .0410 | 525 | |
| 1,500 | 1,500 | 60 | 1,440 | 60 | $7,200 | .0425 | 489 | |
| 1,600 | 1,600 | 40 | 1,560 | 40 | $7,200 | .0463 | 412 | |
| 1,700 | 1,700 | 20 | 1,680 | 20 | $7,200 | .0573 | 269 | |

For this example, cheap and expensive measures cost $4.00 and $20.00, respectively, for each case. The standard errors shown are for the regression coefficient for smoking predicting health in the hypothetical model in Fig. 13.1. $N_{EFF}$ refers to Effective $N$. The $N_{EFF}$ Increase Factor is calculated by dividing $N_{EFF}$ by $N$ from the complete-cases model ($N = 300$ in this case)

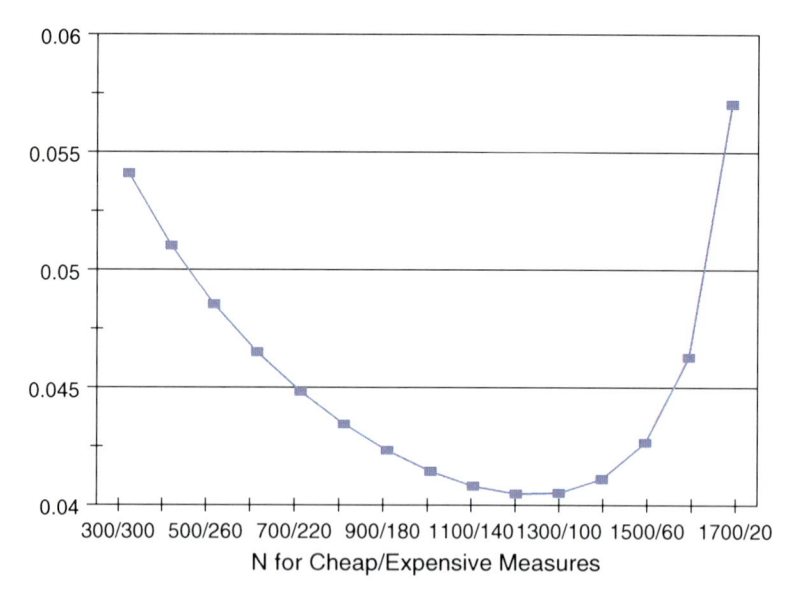

**Fig. 13.2** Standard errors for different *N* configurations

parameter estimate of most substantive importance in our model is the regression coefficient for smoking predicting health. The standard error (SE) for this regression coefficient for each sample size configuration is also shown in Table 13.1 and plotted in Fig. 13.2.

With complete cases $N$ ($N_{CC}$ = 300/300 for cheap/expensive measures), the SE for the key regression coefficient is .0543. Note that as you read down the last column in Table 13.1, the SE continues to decrease monotonically, reaching a minimum of .0403 for the sample size configuration with $N$ = 1200/120 for the cheap/expensive measures. After this configuration, the SE begins to increase.

In this scenario, the SE for the regression coefficient of main substantive interest is minimized at .0403 when $N$ = 1,200 cases provide cheap measure data and $N$ = 120 of the total sample also provide expensive measure data. If we were to test a complete-cases model with sample size increased to $N$ = 542, we would also find that SE = .0403. This means that analyzing data with the $N$ = 1,200/120 configuration yields an SE and statistical power equivalent to having $N$ = 542 complete cases. Graham et al. (2006) referred to this larger $N$ (542 in this case) as the Effective $N$ ($N_{EFF}$). In other words, in this scenario, the optimal configuration of the TMM design behaves, effectively, as if one had collected complete data from $N$ = 542 cases.

Graham et al. (2006) also provided a tool to quantify the $N_{EFF}$ benefit in comparison to the complete-cases design costing the same as the optimal TMM design configuration. As shown in Table 13.1, $N$ = 300 complete cases can be collected for \$7,200 (i.e., $N_{CC}$ = 300). The ratio of $N_{EFF}/N_{CC}$ (542/300 = 1.81 in this case) is referred to as the $N_{EFF}$ Increase Factor. In short, using the TMM design with $N$ = 1,200/120 allows one to test the key study hypothesis with power that is equivalent to a sample

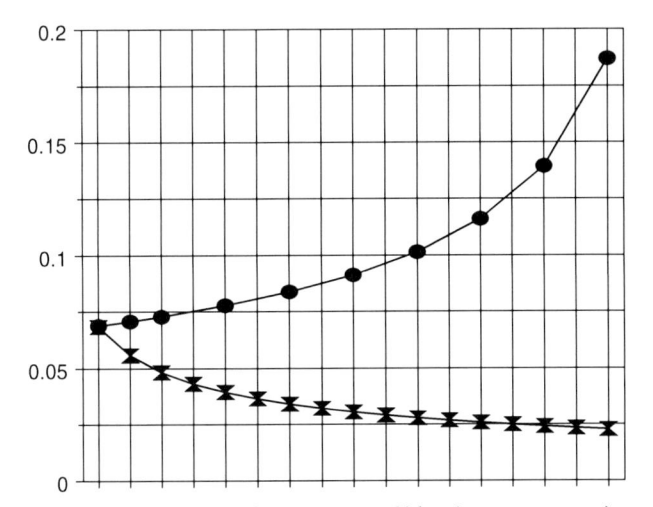

Bottom curve shows SE changes as N for cheap measures increases.
Top curve shows SE changes as N for complete cases decreases.

**Fig. 13.3** Changes in standard error as $N$ changes

size that is 1.81 times larger than the complete-cases design costing the same. Both the $N_{EFF}$ and the $N_{EFF}$ Increase Factor can be used as convenient ways to judge the level of benefit with the TMM design; higher $N_{EFF}$ and higher $N_{EFF}$ Increase Factors imply greater benefit.

## *How the Sample Size Benefit Works in Bias-Correction Model*

The sample size benefit produced by the TMM design is a function of two main factors: (a) the total sample size (i.e., the number of cases providing cheap measure data, regardless of whether they also provide expensive measure data) and (b) the ability of the bias-correction model to obtain a stable estimate of the bias-related parameters. The latter factor is determined by the number of cases with complete data. We discuss these two factors in more detail, below.

In Fig. 13.3, two SE curves illustrate the impact that the total sample size and the complete case sample size have on the power to estimate the main regression parameter in our model. The bottom curve shows how the SE for the key regression parameter estimate decreases as the sample size for the cheap measures is increased, in $N=100$ increments, when the smoking factor is defined only by the two self-report (cheap) measures. The top curve shows resulting SEs for the key regression parameter estimate as the sample size is decreased, in $N=20$ increments, for the complete case model (i.e., when the smoking factor is defined by the cheap and expensive measures). The total SE for the bias-correction model is a function of the combination of these two SEs. Although not perfect, the simple average of these two curves approximates the shape of the curve shown Fig. 13.2.

Examine the two curves in Fig. 13.3 carefully. The bottom curve changes downward rather quickly with the first increases in $N$ and then begins to flatten out as $N$ continues to grow. The top curve, however, starts out increasing at a rather slow rate as the complete case $N$ is reduced incrementally; however, as the complete-cases $N$ continues to decline, the SE curve begins to increase sharply. A key here is that the slope of the lower curve is steeper for a period than is the slope of the upper curve. Thus, for a time, the combined SE for the main parameter estimate of interest becomes smaller. At some point, the two curves in Fig. 13.3 have the same slope (one negative, one positive); at this point, the combined SE for the parameter of interest flattens out and the power increase provided by the TMM design is maximized. Then, as Ns continue to change (i.e., as the ratio of partial to complete data continues to increase), the slope of the top curve in Fig. 13.3 becomes steeper, resulting in an increase in the combined SE. Although not shown in Fig. 13.3, as the complete case sample size becomes very small, the top curve becomes very steep, asymptoting at infinity. This sharp increase in the slope of the top SE curve illustrates how the bias-related parameter estimates become very unstable with small complete case sample sizes. In the most extreme case, bias-related parameter estimates are inestimable when the expensive measures are missing altogether.

## *Factors Affecting the $N_{EFF}$ Benefit*

Graham et al. (2006) studied several factors that affected the $N_{EFF}$ benefits produced by the TMM design. The parameter estimates shown in Fig. 13.1 represent one possible scenario. In the case shown, the expensive smoking measures (CO and cotinine) were better than the cheap (self-report) measures in two important ways. First, the expensive measures had greater valid reliability (i.e., the expensive measures both had factor loadings of .70 on the smoking factor, compared to .50 loadings for the two self-report measures). Second, the expensive measures were not associated with self-report bias, whereas the cheap measures were comprised of valid variance (.50 loadings on smoking factor) as well as and self-report bias (.50 loadings on the bias factor). Other configurations are possible relating to the amounts of valid reliability and self-report bias associated with the expensive and cheap measures, respectively. However, Graham et al. (2006) found these factors to have relatively little impact on the $N_{EFF}$ benefits of the TMM design.

Other factors, however, were found to have much more impact on the benefits of the TMM design. Among these was the cost ratio between expensive and cheap measures. Graham et al. (2006) tested a model similar to that shown in Fig. 13.1, with the exception that the regression coefficient for smoking predicting health was $\beta=.40$ as opposed to $\beta=.20$; resulting $N_{EFF}$ benefits from this modified model are displayed in Table 13.2. When the cost for the expensive measures was only 1.6

**Table 13.2** $N_{EFF}$ benefits as a function of expensive-to-cheap measure cost ratio

| Cost ratio | $N_{EFF}$ increase factor |
|---|---|
| 1.6 : 1 | 1.09 |
| 2.3 : 1 | 1.18 |
| 4.1 : 1 | 1.43 |
| 10 : 1 | 1.96 |

$N_{EFF}$ increase factor is $N_{EFF}/N_{CC}$

times higher than the cost for the cheap measures, the two-method measurement design produced a $N_{EFF}$ just 9 % greater than the complete-cases model costing the same. However, when the expensive measure was ten times more expensive than the cheap measures, the $N_{EFF}$ for the TMM design was nearly double that of the complete-cases model costing the same. In other words, with a cost ratio of 1.6:1, the two-method measurement design allowed the key study hypothesis to be estimated with power equivalent to a sample size that was 9 % larger than the financially equivalent complete-cases design. However, with a more extreme cost ratio of 10:1, the key study hypothesis was tested with power that was equivalent to a sample size that was nearly double that of the financially equivalent complete-cases design.

Another factor having impact on the $N_{EFF}$ benefit was the effect size of the regression coefficient for smoking predicting health (see Table 13.3). In the model tested by Graham et al. (2006) (identical to that shown in Fig. 13.1, except that the regression coefficient of smoking predicting health was $\beta=.40$), the resulting $N_{EFF}$ benefits were the same as shown in Table 13.2 for both the 2.3:1 and 10:1 cost ratios. However, when the main regression coefficient (smoking predicting health) was reduced to $\beta=.10$, resulting $N_{EFF}$ benefits were substantially greater. Even for the modest 2.3:1 cost ratio, the $N_{EFF}$ Increase Factor for the smaller effect size ($\beta=.10$ for smoking predicting health) was 1.35, nearly double that for the 2.3:1 cost ratio with the larger effect size. For the 10:1 cost ratio, the $N_{EFF}$ with the smaller effect size was nearly three and a half times greater than the complete-cases design costing the same. These results suggest that the two-method measurement design has enormous potential in research situations where the effect sizes for the main hypotheses are expected to be small, such as in prevention intervention research.

## Real Effects on Statistical Power

As shown in Table 13.2, with a modest 2.3:1 cost ratio and an effect size of $\beta=.40$, the two-method measurement design effectively produces an 18 % increase in sample size. However, under what circumstances is this 18 % increase meaningful? To answer this and similar questions, it is important to consider the practical impact of $N_{EFF}$ benefits on statistical power.

In any study, the expected effect size of the main parameter estimates drives the desired sample sizes for the study. To see clearly what the sample size issues are in

**Table 13.3** $N_{EFF}$ benefits as a function of difference effect sizes for main regression coefficient

| Cost ratio, effect size configuration | $N_{EFF}$ Increase Factor ($N_{EFF}/N_{CC}$) | Lowest range:[a] $N_{EFF}$ and $N_{CC}$ power<.80 | Critical range:[a] $N_{EFF}$ power ≥ .80 $N_{CC}$ power<.80 | Highest range:[a] $N_{EFF}$ and $N_{CC}$ power ≥ .80 | Power ratio in critical range |
|---|---|---|---|---|---|
| 2.3:1, ρ=.40 | 1.18 | 0–38 | 39–45 | 46+ | 1.095–1.079 |
| 2.3:1, ρ=.10 | 1.35 | 0–578 | 579–772 | 773+ | 1.187–1.131 |
| 10:1, ρ=.40 | 1.96 | 0–23 | 24–45 | 46+ | 1.564–1.231 |
| 10:1, ρ=.10 | 3.47 | 0–222 | 223–772 | 773+ | 2.48–1.257 |

[a]$N$s shown are for $N_{CC}$

this context, we compare the relevant, or *operative*, sample size for the TMM design (using $N_{EFF}$) and the complete-cases design costing the same (using $N_{CC}$). In this discussion, it is useful to think of three ranges of potential sample sizes. In the first range (labeled "lowest range" in Table 13.3), the sample size is too small to yield good statistical power (power ≥ .80) with either $N_{CC}$ or with $N_{EFF}$. Within this sample size range, the choice of designs is perhaps less important; in this case, increasing the sample size takes precedence. In the second range (labeled "highest range" in Table 13.3), sample size is large enough that $N_{CC}$ and $N_{EFF}$ both yield good power (power ≥ .80). With these sample sizes, the choice of design may also be somewhat less important.

However, in the third range, which we refer to as the critical range, power ≥ .80 based on $N_{EFF}$, but power < .80 based on the same-cost $N_{CC}$. Within this critical range of sample sizes, differences in the statistical power yielded by the two designs may or may not have important implications. One way to evaluate the power implications for the two designs is to examine the critical range sample sizes in the context of both cost ratio and effect size. Each cell in the "critical range" column of Table 13.3 specifies a range of sample sizes; the lower value is the $N$ for which $N_{EFF}$ yields power = .80. The higher value (+1) is the $N$ for which $N_{CC}$ yields power = .80. When the critical range is narrow, as is the case for the first scenario in Table 13.3, the traditional complete-cases design and the TMM design do not differ much in practical terms. In that first scenario (top row of Table 13.3), the difference between $N=39$ and $N=45$ would typically have minimal impact on researchers' decisions about choices of sample size. However, when critical range is large, the difference between the competing designs is more marked.

But, the critical range of sample sizes does not tell the whole story; for example, the difference of $N=22$ in the critical range for the third scenario in Table 13.3 has more important power implications than does the difference of $N=194$ in the second scenario. Another way to look at this issue is to consider the power ratio for the competing designs. In the rightmost column of Table 13.3, we present these figures for power within the critical range. The power ratio, which is power($N_{EFF}$)/power($N_{CC}$), shows how much more power is available to the researcher who opts to use the TMM design over the financially equivalent complete-cases design.

Perhaps the best way to view the implications of these power ratios is to examine the power values for both designs (presented in Table 13.4). In the first scenario, with a cost ratio of 2.3:1 and an effect size of $\rho=.40$, the power ratio in the critical range varied from 1.095 to 1.079. With the power ratio of 1.095, the actual difference in power for the two designs was not large (.73 for $N_{CC}$ vs. .80 for $N_{EFF}$). With the power ratio of 1.079, the difference in power was even smaller (.79 for $N_{CC}$ vs. .85 for $N_{EFF}$).

Although one would always prefer better power, all things being equal, one may not be willing to give up much to obtain the higher level of power when the differences in designs are as small as those in the first scenario of Table 13.4. Thus, for this particular scenario, it is not clear that the TMM approach produces much benefit in a practical sense. In this instance, some might prefer to stay with the more traditional complete-cases design rather than assume the extra steps required for a planned missingness approach to data collection.

**Table 13.4** $N_{EFF}$ benefit details

| Cost ratio, effect size configuration | Power ratio in critical range | Critical range power ratio: upper limit | | | Critical range power ratio: lower limit | | |
|---|---|---|---|---|---|---|---|
| | | Value | Power for $N_{CC}$ | Power for $N_{EFF}$ | Value | Power for $N_{CC}$ | Power for $N_{EFF}$ |
| 2.3:1, $\rho=.40$ | 1.095–1.079 | 1.095 | .73 | .80 | 1.079 | .79 | .85 |
| 2.3:1, $\rho=.10$ | 1.187–1.131 | 1.187 | .67 | .80 | 1.131 | .79 | .90 |
| 10:1, $\rho=.40$ | 1.564–1.231 | 1.564 | .52 | .81 | 1.231 | .79 | .97 |
| 10:1, $\rho=.10$ | 2.48–1.257 | 2.48 | .32 | .80 | 1.257 | .79 | .999 |

However, for the other scenarios depicted in Table 13.4, the differences in power are such that the TMM design should be considered. For example, in the second scenario in Table 13.4, when power ratio = 1.187, the difference in power between designs (.67 for NCC vs. .80 for NEFF) is large enough that many researchers will want to consider the TMM design. For the scenarios shown in the last two rows of Table 13.4, the differences in power are large enough that most researchers would give serious consideration to the two-method measurement design. In sum, with a large cost ratio, a small effect size, or a combination of these two factors, the TMM approach should be considered.

## Potential Applications of Two-Method Measurement

A key criterion for identifying potential applications of the two-method measurement approach is that the standard measure of an important construct used in a particular research domain is flawed. Nowhere is this more clear than in the social, behavioral, and health sciences, where researchers frequently rely on self-reports as the primary mode of data collection. Self-reports, especially from self-administered questionnaires, are routinely criticized by reviewers and journal editors. Despite the fact that self-reports might often have better validity than is often feared, the criticism is common.

A second criterion is that there is another measure of the same construct that enjoys substantially more respect in these same research domains. This other measure is typically viewed as being a more objective assessment of the construct under study, whereas the self-reports are criticized as being overly subjective.

It is probably true that self-reports are often not as biased as feared, and it is certainly true that the so-called objective measures are often not as valid as believed. We will cover these issues in a later section. For now, we will accept the idea that self-reports can be exactly as biased as feared, and the objective measure can be highly valid. Here we present several research domains where these two basic criteria for the two-method measurement approach seem to be in place.

### *Cigarette Smoking Research*

Researchers studying smoking etiology, smoking prevention, and smoking cessation have commonly used self-report measures as the primary assessment of cigarette smoking. But these researchers have also been at the forefront of efforts to obtain more objective measures of the key construct (smoking). Fairly early on, researchers made use of saliva thiocyanate (SCN; e.g., Biglan et al. 1985; Luepker et al. 1981) as an objective measure of cigarette smoking. Subsequently, smoking researchers moved more toward saliva cotinine (e.g., Etter et al. 2000) and expired air carbon monoxide (CO; e.g., Biglan et al. 1985) as the primary objective indicators of cigarette smoking. Although these researchers typically used these measures as external validators of self-report indicators, this research domain seems well suited to taking the two-method measurement approach.

## Alcohol Research

Self-reports of alcohol consumption have also been criticized in the alcohol literature. Many researchers have made good use of breathalyzer devices to provide objective assessments of alcohol consumption (e.g., Glindemann et al. 2007). Unfortunately, the very short half-life of alcohol in the system means that breathalyzer data, although certainly very objective, is of limited value for validating self-reported drinking measures when drinking behavior has occurred more than 24 h in the past. However, other approaches to measuring alcohol consumption over longer periods have been successful in providing more object assessments. Sobell and Sobell (1990, 1992) have had good success with the time line follow-back (TLFB) procedure. Although itself a self-report procedure, the TLFB procedure has the advantage of helping motivated respondents overcome the memory difficulties in accurately recalling drinking behavior that has occurred as long ago as 6 months prior to data collection. Because of the intensive requirements (i.e., the expense) of collecting data via the TLFB, and because the measure has enjoyed more respect than have simpler self-report measures of past alcohol use, the TLFB can be thought of as the expensive and more valid in the TMM approach.

## Blood-Vessel Health

Cardiovascular health research has commonly involved relatively expensive measures. For example, West et al. (2004, 2005) used flow-mediated dilation to measure blood-vessel health in people with type 2 diabetes. Although reasonably noninvasive and accurate, flow-mediated dilation can be a costly measure (e.g., $150 per administration of the technique). Alternatively, it may be possible to employ simpler and cheaper (but less valid) blood-pressure techniques to approximate the results that can be obtained by flow-mediated dilation.

## Measurement of Hypertension

The standard clinical method for taking blood pressure (BP) measurements is known to be unreliable and of questionable validity (Gerin et al. 2006; O'Brien et al. 1991; Verdecchia et al. 2001). For some individuals, methods typically employed in doctors' offices often lead to a short-term, artificial elevation in BP (a situation often

Potential Applications of Two-Method Measurement 309

referred to as "white-coat hypertension"), resulting in overreporting of the person's BP. For other individuals, ironically, the same methods can produce underreporting of the person's BP (often referred to as "masked hypertension"). One solution is to collect BP continuously over a substantial period of time (e.g., 24–36 h). This is possible through the use of ambulatory BP devices which the patients wear continuously over the data collection period. Although it is substantially more expensive to use such devices, the resulting assessments of BP are much more accurate.

## *Nutrition Research*

Assessing food and nutrient intake is difficult. Brief self-report indicators of nutrient intake are highly questionable in terms of reliability and validity. Gold-standard assessments of nutrient intake do not exist, except under highly controlled circumstances. In normal living conditions, the best that can be done is to do much more expensive assessments involving extensive interview procedures or food diary assessments.

## *Measuring Body Composition/Adiposity*

Measuring body fat content can easily be accomplished using the body mass index (BMI), which is a simple function of the individual's height and weight. The least expensive method of calculating BMI is simply to include questions of height and weight on a self-administered survey. A more expensive method for measuring BMI is to use a lab technician to obtain highly accurate measures of height and weight. However, even at its best, the BMI is known to be susceptible to various biases, including the muscle-mass bias. That is, individuals with greater muscle mass have higher BMI values regardless of body fat content. For this reason, other, more accurate measures of body composition are used. One highly regarded measure, although much more expensive than BMI, is dual energy X-ray absorptometry (DEXA) technique (Avesani et al. 2004; Fisher et al. 2000; Lohman 1996; Roubenoff et al. 1993).

## *Assessment of Physical Conditioning and Physical Activity*

Measuring physical conditioning can be accomplished simply by asking respondents a few questions on a self-administered survey. A much more extensive (and expensive), but much more highly regarded measure of conditioning is the $VO_2$-max. Measuring physical activity (PA) itself has been a popular research endeavor for a number of years. But as with assessment of nutrient intake, this has proven to be a very difficult task. Numerous investigators have developed PA interviews, and others have attempted to adapt those interviews to self-administered questionnaires (e.g., for a recent review, see Sallis and Saelens 2000). Success of these self-report PA measures has been limited. Validity correlations with more objective measures (most often data from uniaxial accelerometers) have been modest at best. Self-reports with young people in ad lib conditions have often been poor. The more expensive measures of PA (the uniaxial accelerometers) are rather common in this type of research. We will explore this particular measure in more detail in a later section.

## *Survey Research*

Survey research itself has its cheaper and more expensive methods. It is very inexpensive to use mail survey procedures. But besides the typically low response rate, the unknown conditions under which respondents complete such surveys make the reliability and validity of these measures suspect. At the other end of the cost (and validity) continuum is the extensive face-to-face interview. Most researchers would prefer the face-to-face interview (with modifications of the procedure for the most sensitive questions), but the costs are often prohibitive. Other self-report approaches are available for costs ranging between these two extremes.

## *Retrospective Reports*

An interesting application of survey techniques involves the use of retrospective reports. With this approach, respondents are asked about behaviors from some period in their past. Short-term recall questions might ask about substance use over the previous 30 days. But retrospective reports might also ask about periods much further in the past. For example, respondents might be asked about their substance use over a specific 30-day period a year before. While these questions are easy to ask, data resulting from such questions have highly questionable validity. Behavior recall data from the recent past are routinely questioned (e.g., see the paragraph on the time line follow back), but data from longer-term retrospective reports have been all but dismissed as having no validity at all. Any researcher would prefer prospective reports (e.g., short-term recall of substance use behavior) over long-term retrospective reports (e.g., recall of 30-day substance use behavior from the previous year).

## Cost Ratio Issues

We have shown here and in previous work that the cost ratio between expensive and cheap measures is an important factor in determining the benefit of the two-method measurement approach. An important issue in this context is how one calculates the cost ratio. In all of our examples thus far, and in the examples described by Graham

**Table 13.5** SE benefits of the two method measurement design, hold costs constant (20:1 cost ratio)

| N total | N cheap (SR) | N expensive (TLFB) | N partial (SR only) | N complete (SR and TLFB) | Total costs | SE r=.20 | SE r=.10 |
|---|---|---|---|---|---|---|---|
| 375 | 375 | 375 | 0 | 375 | $7,875 | 0.0485 | 0.0501 |
| 875 | 875 | 350 | 525 | 350 | $7,875 | 0.0385 | 0.0383 |
| 1,875 | 1,875 | 300 | 1,575 | 300 | $7,875 | 0.0302 | 0.0287 |
| 2,875 | 2,875 | 250 | 2,625 | 250 | $7,875 | 0.0266 | 0.0249 |
| 3,875 | 3,875 | 200 | 3,675 | 200 | $7,875 | 0.0251 | 0.0223 |
| 4,875 | 4,875 | 150 | 4,725 | 150 | $7,875 | 0.0250 | 0.0209 |
| 5,875 | 5,875 | 100 | 5,775 | 100 | $7,875 | 0.0269 | 0.0205 |

et al. (2006), the cost ratios were simulated. But how does one really calculate this ratio? In the simplest case, one calculates the rather literal costs of collecting the two kinds of measures. However, it is virtually never the case that the two measures in question are being looked at in a vacuum. On the other hand, the complexity of the study involving the two variables can vary widely. At one extreme, the research is highly focused, with data collected from relatively few other variables. At the other extreme, the research is broadly focused, and the variables relating to the two-method measurement design represent only a small fraction of is the constructs being measured. Calculating the cost ratio and estimating the benefits of the two-method measurement design are rather different in these two kinds of studies.

## *Calculating Cost Ratio and Estimating Benefits in Studies with Narrow Focus*

Suppose a study was focused rather narrowly on alcohol use among college students. Asking several (e.g., six) alcohol use questions, along with a relatively few related questions would plausibly be accomplished in a large survey course, with payment for participation coming in the form of course credit. For comparison purposes, we set the cost of this study arbitrarily at $1 per subject. In this context, it would also be desirable to ask a subset of the students to attend a separate measurement session in which they would be asked to complete a more in-depth measure of their recent alcohol use (e.g., via the TLFB procedure). Although the procedure might take no more than 15–30 min, one would very likely need to pay the students $20 to get them to show up for the session. Thus, for this rather narrowly focused study, there is a 20:1 cost ratio for the two measures.

Table 13.5 presents the complete-cases design ($N_{cc}$=375) and six variants of the TMM design. In these scenarios, the cheap measures are represented by self-report alcohol use indicators, and the expensive measures are represented by the TLFB procedure. The total costs in this hypothetical example are $7,875 for each of the designs. In the last two columns of the table, we provide the SE for the key factor

**Table 13.6** Study costs when statistical power is held constant (20:1 cost ratio)

| N total | N cheap (SR) | N expensive (TLFB) | N partial (SR only) | N complete (SR and TLFB) | Total costs | SE $r=.10$ |
|---|---|---|---|---|---|---|
| 375 | 375 | 375 | 0 | 375 | $7,875 | 0.0501 |
| 406 | 406 | 300 | 106 | 300 | $6,406 | 0.0501 |
| 520 | 520 | 200 | 320 | 200 | $4,520 | 0.0501 |
| 647 | 647 | 100 | 547 | 100 | $2,647 | 0.0501 |

regression coefficient for two effect sizes: $r=.20$ and $r=.10$. (All other assumptions from Fig. 13.1 are retained in Table 13.5).

When $r=.20$, the optimal TMM design was the 4875/150 design, that is, $N=4875$ participants provide cheap (self-report) data and $N=150$ of those participants also provide expensive (TLFB) data. When $r=.10$, the optimal TMM design was the 5875/100 design, that is, $N=5875$ participants provide cheap (self-report) data and $N=100$ of those participants also provide expensive (TLFB) data.

However, for the alcohol use study we described, taking advantage of the benefits of the two-method measurement design may not be feasible because of the difficulty in finding 5,875 students for whom course credit could be given for taking part in the study. Thus, rather than holding costs constant and examining the increase in SE benefits, we now hold the SE (and statistical power) constant, and examine the total cost benefits of performing the study with various versions of the two-method measurement design (see Table 13.6).

The figures for the cost results when holding statistical power constant are shown in Table 13.6 (we focus on the smaller effect size, $r=.10$, in this table). Taking this approach, the TMM design shown in the bottom row of the table ($N=647$ participants provide data for the cheap measures, and $N=100$ of these also provide data for the expensive measures) is just over a third the cost of a complete-cases design (with $N_{CC}=375$) having the same statistical power.

## *Calculating Cost Ratio and Estimating Benefits in Studies with Broad Focus*

Now, consider a study with a much broader focus. When the study focus is broad, the cost ratios of cheap and expensive measures will be smaller. As we just saw above with a narrow-focus study, the cost differential between measures can be quite large (e.g., the 20:1 ratio just described would not be uncommon). However, with a broad-focus study, the cost differential for the same measures might be much more modest (as low as 1:1 or even lower). This is because the costs for the other aspects of the study will be much larger for the broad-focus study; these additional costs are added to the costs of the cheap measure when calculating the cost ratios of cheap to expensive measures.

**Table 13.7** SE benefits of the two-method measurement design, hold costs constant (1:1 cost ratio)

| N total | N cheap (SR) | N expensive (TLFB) | N partial (SR only) | N complete (SR and TLFB) | Total costs | SE $r=.20$ | $r=.10$ |
|---|---|---|---|---|---|---|---|
| 375 | 375 | 375 | 0 | 375 | $15,000 | 0.0485 | 0.0501 |
| 400 | 400 | 350 | 50 | 350 | $15,000 | 0.0486 | 0.0485 |
| 450 | 450 | 300 | 150 | 300 | $15,000 | 0.0487 | 0.0486 |
| 500 | 500 | 250 | 250 | 250 | $15,000 | 0.0489 | 0.0488 |
| 550 | 550 | 200 | 350 | 200 | $15,000 | 0.0494 | 0.0491 |
| 600 | 600 | 150 | 450 | 150 | $15,000 | 0.0501 | 0.0494 |
| 650 | 650 | 100 | 550 | 100 | $15,000 | 0.0516 | 0.0500 |

Consider a broad-focus version of the college alcohol study just described. Suppose students were asked to complete a relatively long survey that, in addition to self-report measures tapping many other constructs, included the same self-report measures of recent alcohol use from the previous example. In a recent study much like this, students were paid $20 for 1 h of work. As before, we might then sample students at random and ask them to spend an additional 15–30 min with the more in-depth TLFB procedure to assess their recent alcohol use. In this context, the cost ratio is a much more modest 1:1.

The direct benefits of the two-method measurement design in this context are shown in Table 13.7. With the larger effect size ($r=.20$), the most powerful design in this instance was the complete-cases design with $N=375$. With the smaller effect size ($r=.10$), the optimal design was the 400/350 version of the TMM design (i.e., $N=400$ participants provide self-report data and $N=350$ of those participants also provide TLFB data). To be sure, the direct benefits of the TMM design are minimal in this context.

On the other hand, although the cost ratios with broad-focus studies tend to be smaller, there are hidden, or indirect, benefits of the TMM design in such research situations. Focus for the moment on the rightmost column of Table 13.7. When $r=.10$, the SE for the 650/100 version of the TMM design is virtually the same as the SE for the complete case design (with $N_{cc}=375$). So what is the benefit?

The benefit stems from the very fact that the study has a broad focus. With the complete-cases design ($N_{cc}=375$), ALL hypotheses, even those having little or nothing to do with alcohol use, must be tested with $N=375$. And there will be many such hypotheses in this type of study given its broad focus. However, as shown in the bottom row of Table 13.7, the 650/100 version of the two-method measurement design allows the researcher to test all hypotheses having little or nothing to do with alcohol use with $N=650$.

Statistical power for various effect sizes tested with $N=375$ and $N=650$ is shown in Table 13.8. For some effect sizes ($r=.07-.08$), power is low with either design. But even for these effect sizes, the probability of detecting a significant effect is 56–58 % higher with the TMM design than with the financially equivalent

**Table 13.8** Statistical power various effect sizes with two sample sizes

| | N | | |
|---|---|---|---|
| r | 375 | 650 | power ratio |
| .07 | .273 | .431 | 1.58 |
| .08 | .341 | .532 | 1.56 |
| .09 | .415 | .632 | 1.52 |
| .10 | .492 | .724 | 1.47 |
| .11 | .569 | .803 | 1.41 |
| .12 | .644 | .866 | 1.34 |
| .13 | .714 | .914 | 1.28 |
| .14 | .777 | .948 | 1.22 |
| .15 | .831 | .970 | 1.17 |
| .16 | .876 | .984 | 1.12 |
| .17 | .912 | .992 | 1.09 |
| .18 | .939 | * | 1.06 |
| .20 | .974 | * | 1.03 |
| .25 | * | * | 1.00 |

\* = power > .995. Power ratio is power $_{N=650}$/power $_{N=350}$

complete-cases design. For other effect sizes ($r=.09-.14$), power to detect an effect with the TMM design is sufficient, and substantially greater than power offered by the complete-cases design costing the same. Finally, for effect sizes greater than $r=.14$, both the TMM design and the financially equivalent complete-cases design perform well with respect to statistical power and the power difference between competing designs is smaller.

## The Full Bias-Correction Model

An important assumption Graham et al. (2006) made regarding the model shown in Fig. 13.1 was that the correlation between the bias factor and the outside variable ("Health" in Fig. 13.1) is zero. We will refer to this outside variable generically as "Y"; thus the assumption is $r_{Bias,Y}=0$. If this assumption is met, then the power benefits of the two-method measurement design will be achieved as described above, and the estimate of the relationship between the substantive factor ("Smoking" in Fig. 13.1) and the outside variable ("Health") will be unbiased. However, to the extent that $r_{Bias,Y}>0$, the estimate of the relationship between the substantive factor and the outside variable will be biased.

When the assumption that $r_{Bias,Y}=0$ is not met, Graham et al. (2006) suggested that other models were possible that would allow this nonzero correlation to be estimated. One obvious model is shown in Fig. 13.4. With this model, one simply

# The Full Bias-Correction Model

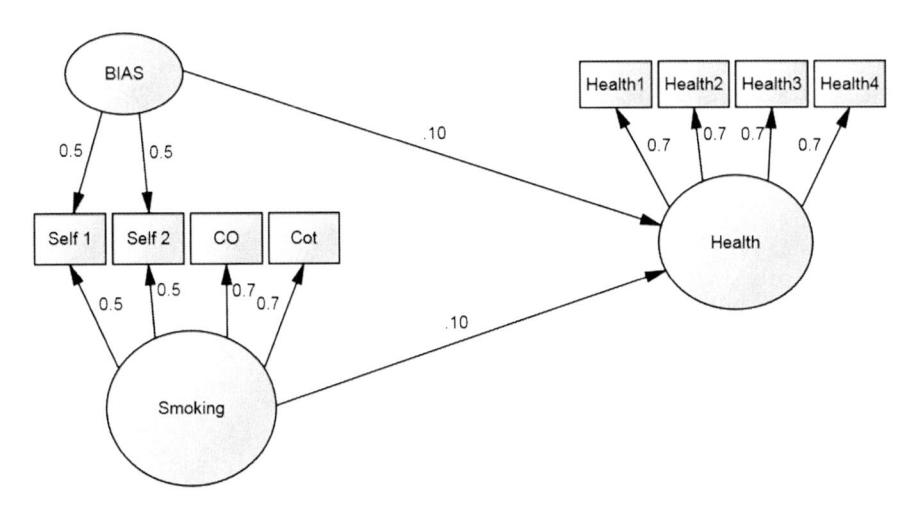

**Fig. 13.4** Full bias-correction model

estimates the relationship between the bias factor and the outside factor. This relationship can be modeled either as a factor regression (as shown in Fig. 13.4) or as a factor correlation.

In our earlier work, we found that the model depicted in Fig. 13.4 did provide unbiased estimates of the key factor associations. However, we also found that the sample size and power benefits of the two-method measurement model disappeared when we estimated this bias-Y relationship.

Recent work, however, shows that this pessimistic conclusion was only partially correct. With the parameter values shown in Fig. 13.4, the two-method measurement design offered no benefits over the financially equivalent complete-cases design (see Configuration 1 in Table 13.9). One key factor in Configuration 1 is the 3:1 cost ratio between measures. According to the simulations in Graham et al. (2006), a 3:1 cost ratio is modest by today's standards. Note that these values are comparable to those shown in the Graham et al. simulations as having the greatest effect when the $r_{\text{Bias,Y}}=0$ assumption holds. In Configuration 15, factor loadings and factor correlations are held constant, but the cost ratio between measures is a more pronounced 10:1. In the Graham et al. (2006) simulations, this configuration of the TMM design produced an $N_{\text{EFF}}$ Increase Factor of 3.47. However, with the full bias-control model, the benefit produced by the TMM design was much more modest ($N_{\text{EFF}}$ Increase Factor = 1.02).

We explored how changing various parameter values might increase the $N_{\text{EFF}}$ Increase Factor. In Table 13.9, Configurations 2–5 show what happens when just one of the factor loadings was varied. For example, in Configuration 2, increasing the expensive measure factor loading on the valid factor from .70 to .89 produced only minimal power benefits. Decreasing the factor loading for the cheap measure

**Table 13.9** Benefits of two-method measurement "full" bias control model

| Config-uration | Factor loadings | | | Factor correlations | | | Cost ratio | $N_{EFF}$ increase factor (NIF) |
|---|---|---|---|---|---|---|---|---|
| | Expensive measure | Cheap measure valid factor | Cheap measure bias factor | Valid-Y | Bias-Y | | | |
| 1 | .70 | .50 | .50 | .10 | .10 | | 3:1 | 1.00 |
| 2 | .89 | .50 | .50 | .10 | .10 | | 3:1 | 1.01 |
| 3 | .70 | .50 | .30 | .10 | .10 | | 3:1 | 1.00 |
| 4 | .70 | .70 | .50 | .10 | .10 | | 3:1 | 1.01 |
| 5 | .70 | .86 | .50 | .10 | .10 | | 3:1 | 1.07 |
| 6 | .70 | .86 | .30 | .10 | .10 | | 3:1 | 1.09 |
| 7 | .89 | .86 | .50 | .10 | .10 | | 3:1 | 1.21 |
| 8 | .89 | .86 | .30 | .10 | .10 | | 3:1 | 1.27 |
| 9 | .89 | .86 | .30 | .10 | −.10 | | 3:1 | 1.27 |
| 10 | .89 | .86 | .30 | −.10 | −.10 | | 3:1 | 1.27 |
| 11 | .89 | .86 | .30 | −.10 | −.05 | | 3:1 | 1.27 |
| 12 | .89 | .86 | .30 | −.10 | 0 | | 3:1 | 1.33 |
| 13 | .89 | .86 | .30 | .27 | −.16 | | 3:1 | 1.47 |
| 14 | .89 | .86 | .30 | .43 | −.26 | | 3:1 | 1.76 |
| 15 | .70 | .50 | .50 | .43 | −.26 | | 5:1 | 1.02 |
| 16 | .86 | .57 | .68 | .10 | .10 | | 10:1 | 1.12 |
| | | | | .36 | .21 | | 3:1 | |

$N_{EFF}$ Increase Factor = 1.00 means no benefit of TMM design compared to the complete-cases design costing the same

on the bias factor from .50 to .30 produced no benefit (Configuration 3). In Configuration 4, increasing the factor loading of the cheap measure on the valid factor from .50 to .70 produced a small benefit ($N_{EFF}$ Increase Factor = 1.01). As shown in Configuration 5, further increasing the cheap measure factor loading to .86 produced a slightly higher benefit ($N_{EFF}$ Increase Factor = 1.07).

As shown in Configurations 6 and 7 of Table 13.9, improving two of the factor loadings produced additional power benefits over the financially equivalent complete-cases design. Improving all three factor loadings (Configuration 8) provided benefit of $N_{EFF}$ Increase Factor = 1.27. As shown in Configurations 9–11, changing the value of $r_{Bias,Y}$ had no impact on the $N_{EFF}$ Increase Factor. On the other hand, increasing $r_{Valid,Y}$ did have an effect, as shown in Configurations 12 and 13. With the values shown for Configuration 13, the $N_{EFF}$ Impact Factor = 1.47 was the largest benefit observed for the 3:1 cost ratio. Configuration 14 shows the further benefit of increasing the cost ratio to 5:1 ($N_{EFF}$ Increase Factor = 1.76).

The conclusion we draw here is that the benefits from the full bias-control model can be substantial. But perhaps those benefits emerge with a somewhat smaller set of parameter values. As with the partial bias-control model, where $r_{Bias,Y} = 0$ is tenable, the cost ratio is a major factor in determining the power benefits produced by the TMM design. Also, increases in the valid factor loading for the cheap measures yielded $N_{EFF}$ Increase Factor benefits. When the cheap measures had high factor loadings for the valid factor, combined with low factor loadings on the bias factor, $N_{EFF}$ Increase Factor benefits were especially pronounced. In contrast with the partial bias-control model, the full bias-control model yielded greater benefits with larger effect sizes.

## *A Note on Estimation Bias*

An issue that arises with the full bias-control model is estimation bias. When the model generating the data specifies $r_{Valid,Bias} = 0$, the parameter estimates for $r_{Valid}$ with the complete-cases model are unbiased. However, with the missing data models, a small amount of bias is introduced in the $r_{Valid}$ estimate. However, in our experience, the degree of bias tends to be small and can be considered to be tolerably small (see Chaps. 1 and 10).

## Assumptions

Below we describe two assumptions about research scenarios in which the TMM design might be applied.

## *Assumption 1: The Expensive Measure is More Valid than the Cheap Measure*

When does this assumption hold? Virtually all of the expensive measures we have discussed above have biases; in other words, they are all impacted by sources of variance that are different from the construct under study (e.g., see Palmer et al. 2002). For example, all things considered, saliva cotinine is a very good (objective) measure of cigarette smoking. But because it is a metabolite of nicotine, cotinine levels will also be high if the person has consumed smokeless tobacco but has not smoked cigarettes. Expired CO is also a good (objective) indicator of cigarette smoking. However, because it detects any burned substance, the CO value will be high if the person has smoked marijuana or has been in close contact with others who smoke cigarettes, or even if the person lives in a highly industrialized part of a city or in close proximity to a freeway. Similarly, uniaxial accelerometers are sensitive to many factors that are largely irrelevant to the amount of PA the subject has engaged in. Subjects who have walked or run on the hardest surfaces (e.g., concrete) will appear to have done more PA than will those who have walked or run on the softest surfaces (e.g., grass). Also, uniaxial accelerometers only capture up and down movements; because the mechanics of running change as people run faster, these devices are less well suited for capturing the fastest running. In the extreme, uniaxial accelerometers cannot distinguish between fast walking and the fastest running.

Although these kinds of biases exist, they often have relatively little impact on the utility of these measures. Other kinds of bias, on the other hand, are more of a problem for measures that are purported to be objective indicators of some construct. The word "objective" implies that the scores from the measure are not subjective (i.e., they are not under the subject's control). But some measures that are often accepted as objective indicators are, at least to an extent, under the subject's control. A good example of this is the uniaxial accelerometer described above. The biases related to the device's inability to capture nonvertical movement are largely out of the subject's control; however, there is another bias we describe as noncompliance bias that is entirely dependent on the subject's level of adherence to study protocol. The individual subject is often given the accelerometer device and instructed to wear it every waking minute (except when in contact with water). But whether or not the person actually does wear the device as instructed is completely up to the subject.

This kind of bias poses a special problem for at least two reasons. First, especially with younger subjects, failing to wear the device could be very common. Second, there could be systematic reasons that individuals fail to wear the devices. For example, some children may choose not to wear the device when they are being most active, perhaps out of fear that the device could be damaged or lost. Or the child may find the device a bother during the most demanding physical activities (e.g., playing full-court basketball). This reason for noncompliance would have a rather substantial effect on the correlation between self-reported PA and the accelerometer data. This would be particularly bad if the person took off the device for a relatively short period of highest activity, but then wore it again for the remainder of the (relatively sedentary) day, such that the accelerometer data would appear to have come from a valid day of wearing.

The bias resulting from the first of these two scenarios should be relatively minor if the failure to wear the device were largely a random process, or if the bias could reasonably be modeled as a random process. However, in the second scenario, the noncompliance bias is clearly nonrandom. Even this might also be less of a problem if there were some way of knowing which days the device was not worn (e.g., from diary data). But these measures, themselves, are susceptible to self-report biases and are less than a fully satisfying solution for the problems associated with the accelerometers.

The problem with noncompliance bias is that the supposedly "objective" measure (such as the uniaxial accelerometer) may need to be modeled as also loading on the self-report bias factor. However, the very thing that allows the TMM models to be estimated is that it is reasonable to assume that the expensive measures have loadings of "0" on the bias factor. The upshot when these loadings must be different from "0" is that more parameters must be estimated in the model than are possible. That is, these models are not "identified" (in terms of simple algebra, these models have too few "equations" for the number of "unknowns"). The bottom line is that with biases like noncompliance bias, the TMM models we have described in this chapter (the partial- and full bias-correction models) are no longer tenable.

## *Assumption 2: The Model Will "Work" Once You Have Collected the Data*

### Realities of All Bias-Control Models

One of the realities of bias-control models is that the models tend to be unstable. With careful planning and data collection that is aimed at this kind of analysis, this type of instability should be minimized. If the following conditions are met, this problem should be minimized:

- *Have at least two cheap measures* (and possibly three) of the substantive factor. The key here is that the two or three cheap measures are all associated with the same response bias. When the cheap measures share the same response bias, the bias can be modeled (and controlled for) as shown in Figs. 13.1 and 13.4.
- *Have at least two expensive measures of the substantive factor* (although one expensive measure may work in some instances). It is important to choose an expensive measure that has no known subjective biases; alternatively, at a minimum, the expensive measure should be universally considered superior to the cheap measure.[1]

---

[1] We do have some question about whether the universal acceptance of a measure as being better than, say, self-reports, is sufficient to mean that such measures will work well in TMM models. A good counter example is that the uniaxial accelerometer has long been virtually universally accepted as an appropriate validator for self-reported PA; but as we have argued in this chapter, this practice may not be justified.

- *Ensure that the factor loadings on the substantive factor are substantial.* This can be accomplished if data collection procedures are built around the TMM approach. Substantive factor loadings are much less likely to be substantial if the data were collected before the TMM analysis approach was decided upon. Pilot testing can be very valuable here.
- *Ensure that the factor loadings on the substantive factor for cheap and expensive items are at least similar* (e.g., no more than .20–.30 difference). This is also much more likely if data collection is built around TMM. Pilot testing can be very valuable here as well.
- *Ensure that the zero-order correlation between cheap and expensive measures is at least modest* (e.g., at least $r=.20$). Problems with bias-control models often stem from the fact that the cheap and expensive measures are not highly correlated. Again, pilot testing will provide insight into the extent to which the cheap and expensive measures are correlated.

**When the Bias-Y Correlation Is Substantial**

As described above, one assumption underlying the TMM design is that the bias factor and the outside variable (e.g., "Health" in Fig. 13.1) are uncorrelated. If this assumption is met, then the power benefits of the two-method measurement design are more likely to be achieved, and the estimate of the relationship between the substantive factor (e.g., "Smoking") and the outside variable (e.g., "Health") will be unbiased. However, to the extent that the bias factor and outside variable are correlated, the parameter estimate of substantive interest (i.e., between the substantive factor and the outside variable) will be biased. We have noted above that the full bias-correction model (see Fig. 13.4) may be used successfully in this context, but the true power benefits will depend more heavily on factor loadings, factor correlations, and especially on the true cost ratio.

# Individual Versus Group Level Focus of the Research

The TMM models described in this chapter apply when the researcher is interested in group-level statistics. That is, these models apply to the sample as a whole and not to individual participants. One good example of this point relates using the TMM approach to the study of blood pressure assessment. The TMM approach has been shown to work exceptionally well in this context (e.g., see Zawadzki et al. in press), in the sense that the TMM models were highly successful in modeling the kinds of bias commonly observed in assessments of BP taken in doctors' offices ("white-coat hypertension" and "masked hypertension"). However, it is not possible at present to use the bias-control models to determine which individual patients exhibited white coat or masked hypertension with the typical clinic BP assessments.

## Alternative Model: The Auxiliary Variable Model

The power and cost benefits of the TMM models described in this chapter derive from the fact that all participants in a study sample provide data for the cheap measure, and that only a small random sample of participants also provide data for the expensive measure. When the TMM models described in this chapter cannot be estimated in a particular research context, for example, when only a single cheap measure is available, it is still possible to estimate an auxiliary variable model that will achieve some of the benefits shown with the full TMM models. As shown in Chap. 11, auxiliary variable models work best when the correlation is high between the auxiliary variable and the variable that is sometimes missing.

It will generally be true that auxiliary variable models will provide $N_{EFF}$ benefits that are modest in comparison to the benefits that are possible with the full TMM model. For example, look again at the data forming the basis for Table 13.1. Suppose there was only a single cheap measure and only a single expensive measure. Under those circumstances, the full TMM model could not be estimated. In those data, the correlation between the cheap and expensive measures was $r=.78$. Using the auxiliary variable utility described in Chap. 11, it is easy to see that under these circumstances, the optimal auxiliary variable model yields $N_{EFF}=367$ (compared to the optimal $N_{EFF}=542$ shown in Table 13.1).

However, it will sometimes happen that correlations higher than $r=.78$ are observed. Researchers studying body composition, for example, may find that the auxiliary variable model is particularly useful. Because the cheapest measure of body composition typically used (BMI) is just a single measure, the TMM model is not readily applied to this type of data. However, with body composition measures it is also not unusual for the correlation between the cheap measure (BMI) and the expensive measure (DEXA) is greater than $r=.78$. We did find one study (Bowden et al. 2005), who found only $r=.55$ between BMI and DEXA in a sample of sedentary college students. On the other hand, Lintsi et al.(2004) found and average $r=.825$ between BMI and DEXA. If all the other correlations were the same as observed in Table 13.1, the auxiliary variable model would yield $N_{EFF}=400$. Lindsay et al. (2001) observed an average correlation of $r=.88$ between BMI and DEXA in a child and adolescent sample. If all the other correlations were the same as observed in Table 13.1, the auxiliary variable model would yield $N_{EFF}=466$ in this instance. Finally, the highest correlation observed between BMI and DEXA by Lindsay et al. (2001) was $r=.94$ (in their sample of 5–9-year-old males). If all the other correlations were the same as observed in Table 13.1, the auxiliary variable model would yield $N_{EFF}=620$! Clearly, there will be times when the auxiliary variable model will be a valuable alternative to a complete-cases model.

# References

Avesani, C. M., Draibe, S. A., Kamimura, M. A., Cendoroglo, M., Pedrosa, A., Castro, M. L., & Cuppari, L. (2004). Assessment of body composition by dual energy X-ray absorptiometry, skinfold thickness and creatinine kinetics in chronic kidney disease patients. *Nephrology Dialysis Transplantation, 19*, 2289–2295.

Berman, J. S., & Kenny, D. A. (1976). Correlational bias in observer ratings. Journal of Personality and Social Psychology, 34, 263–273.

Biglan, A., Gallison, C., Ary, D., & Thompson, R. (1985). Expired air carbon monoxide and saliva thiocyanate: Relationships to self-reports of marijuana and cigarette smoking. *Addictive Behaviors, 10*, 137–144.

Bowden, R. G., Lanning, B. A., Doyle, E. I., Johnston, H. M., Nassar, E. I., Slonaker, B., Scanes, G. (2005). Comparison of body composition measures to dual-energy X-ray absorptiometry. *Journal of Exercise Physiology online, 8*, 1–9.

Eid, M. (2000). A multitrait-multimethod model with minimal assumptions. *Psychometrika, 65*, 241–261.

Etter, J. F., Duc, T. V., and Perneger, T. V. (2000). Saliva cotinine levels in smokers and non-smokers. *American Journal of Epidemiology, 151*, 251–258.

Fisher, J. O., Johnson, R. K., Lindquist, C., Birch, L. L., & Goran, M. I. (2000). Influence of body composition on the accuracy of reported energy intake in children. *Obesity Research, 8*, 597–603.

Gerin, W., Ogedegbe, G., Schwartz, J., Chaplin, W. F., Goyal, T., Clemow, L., et al. (2006). Assessment of the white-coat effect. *Journal of Hypertension, 24*, 67–74.

Glindemann, K. E., Ehrhart, I. J., Drake, E. A., & Geller, E. S. (2007). Reducing excessive alcohol consumption at university fraternity parties: A cost-effective incentive/reward intervention. *Addictive Behaviors, 32*(1), 39–48.

Graham, J. W., & Collins, N. L. (1991). Controlling correlational bias via confirmatory factor analysis of MTMM data. Multivariate Behavioral Research, 26, 607–629.

Graham, J. W., Taylor, B. J., Olchowski, A. E., & Cumsille, P. E. (2006). Planned missing data designs in psychological research. *Psychological Methods, 11*, 323–343.

Hoyt, W. T. (2000). Rater bias in psychological research: When is it a problem and what can we do about it? Psychological Methods, 5, 64–86.

Kenny, D. A., & Kashy, D. A. (1992). Analysis of the multitrait-multimethod matrix by confirmatory factor analysis. *Psychological Bulletin, 112*, 165–172.

Lindsay, R. S., Hanson, R. L., Roumain, J., Ravussin, E., Knowler, W. C., and Tataranni, P. A. (2001). Body mass index as a measure of adiposity in children and adolescents: relationship to adiposity by dual energy X-ray absorptiometry and to cardiovascular risk factors. Journal of Clinical Endocrinology and Metabolism, 86, 4061–4067.

Lintsi, M., Kaarma, H., and Kull, I. (2004). Comparison of hand-to-hand bioimpedance and anthropometry equations versus dual-energy X-ray absorptiometry for the assessment of body fat percentage in 17–18-year-old conscripts. *Clinical Physiology and Functional Imaging, 24*, 85–90.

Lohman, T. G. (1996). Dual energy x-ray absorptiometry. In A. F. Roche, S. B. Heymsfield, & T. G. Lohman (Eds.), *Human body composition* (pp. 63–78). Champaign, IL: Human Kinetics Books.

Luepker, R.V., Pechacek, T.F., Murray, D.M., Johnson, C.A., Hurd, P., & Jacobs, D.R. (1981). Saliva thiocyanate: A chemical indicator of smoking in adolescents. *American Journal of Public Health, 71*, 1320–1324.

O'Brien, E., Mee, F., Atkins, N., and O'Malley, K. (1991). Accuracy of the SpaceLabs 90207 determined by the British Hypertension Society protocol. *Journal of Hypertension, 9*, 573–574.

Palmer, R. F., Graham, J. W., Taylor, B. J., & Tatterson, J. W. (2002). Construct validity in health behavior research: Interpreting latent variable models involving self-report and objective measures. Journal of Behavioral Medicine, 25, 525–550.

Roubenoff, R., Kehayias, J. J., Dawson-Hughes, B., & Heymsfield, S. B. (1993). Use of dual-energy x-ray absorptiometry in body composition studies: Not yet a "gold standard." *American Journal of Clinical Nutrition, 58*, 589–591.

Sallis, J. F., and Saelens, B. E. (2000). Assessment of physical activity by self-report: status, limitations, future directions. *Research Quarterly for Exercise and Sport, 71*, 1–14.

Sobell, L. C., & Sobell, M. B. (1990). Self-report issues in alcohol abuse: State of the art and future directions. *Behavioral Assessment, 12*, 77–90.

Sobell, L. C., & Sobell, M. B. (1992). Time line follow-back: A technique for assessing self-reported alcohol consumption. In R. Z. Litten & J. P. Allen (Eds.), *Measuring alcohol consumption: Psychosocial and biochemical methods*, pp. 41–72. Totowa, NJ: Humana Press.

Verdecchia, P., Schillaci, G., Reboldi, G., Franklin, S. S., and Porcellati, C. (2001). Different prognostic impact of 24-hour mean blood pressure and pulse pressure on stroke and coronary artery disease in essential hypertension. *Circulation, 103*, 2579–2584.

West, S. G., Hecker, K. D., Mustad, V. A., Nicholson, S., Schoemer, S. L., Wagner, P., Hinderliter, A. L., Ulbrecht, J., Ruey, P., and Kris-Etherton, P. M. (2005). Acute effects of monounsaturated fatty acids with and without omega-3 fatty acids on vascular reactivity in individuals with type 2 diabetes. *Diabetologia, 48*, 113–122.

West, S. G., Wagner, P., Schoemer, S. L., Hecker, K. D., Hurston, K. L., Likos Krick, A., Boseska, L., Ulbrecht, J., and Hinderliter, A. L. (2004). Biological correlates to day-to-day variation in flow-mediated dilation in individuals with Type 2 diabetes: a study of test-retest reliability. *Diabetologia, 47*, 1625–1631.

Zawadzki, M. J., Graham, J. W., and Gerin, W. (in press). Increasing the Validity and Efficiency of Blood Pressure Estimates Using Ambulatory and Clinic Measurements and Modern Missing Data Methods. *American Journal of Hypertension.*

Printed by Publishers' Graphics LLC
AMZ20130210.19.19.108